Receive your CME certificate immediately...

log on to www.theclinics.com/home/cme to take and score your test online.

CONTINUING MEDICAL EDUCATION SUPPLEMENT

PEDIATRIC CLINICS OF NORTH AMERICA

Sponsored by
The University of Virginia School of Medicine
Charlottesville, Virginia

Karen S. Rheuban, MD
ASSOCIATE DEAN FOR CONTINUING MEDICAL EDUCATION
MEDICAL DIRECTOR, OFFICE OF TELEMEDICINE
PROFESSOR OF PEDIATRICS
UNIVERSITY OF VIRGINIA HEALTH S`
CHARLOTTESVILLE, VIRGINIA

Based on the issue
**Common Respiratory Symptoms and Ill_____ ____u Evidence-Based
Approach (Vol 56:1)**

This activity has been planned and implemented in accordance with the Essential Areas and Policies of the Accreditation Council for Continuing Medical Education (ACCME) through the joint sponsorship of the University of Virginia School of Medicine and Elsevier. The University of Virginia School of Medicine is accredited by the ACCME to provide continuing medical education for physicians.

The University of Virginia School of Medicine designates this educational activity for a maximum of 15 AMA PRA Category 1 Credits™ for each issue, 90 credits per year. Physicians should only claim credit commensurate with the extent of their participation in the activity.

The American Medical Association has determined that physicians not licensed in the US who participate in this CME activity are eligible for 15 AMA PRA Category 1 Credits™.

Test expires 12 months following publication date.

Publication Date: February 2009   Test expires: March 31, 2010

TEST NO. PCL56:1   •   FEBRUARY, 2009

W. B. SAUNDERS COMPANY
An imprint of Elsevier, Inc.

Elsevier Inc.
1600 John F. Kennedy Blvd., Suite 1800
Philadelphia, PA 19103-2899

http://www.us.elsevierhealth.com

CONTINUING MEDICAL EDUCATION
SUPPLEMENT TO PEDIATRIC CLINICS OF NORTH AMERICA
ISSN 1557-8135 **FEBRUARY 2009**

CHANGE OF ADDRESS
We cannot score tests submitted after the 12-month deadline has expired. Please notify us immediately of any change in address to ensure that your test booklet reaches you in a timely manner. Send address changes, along with a copy of the mailing label from your test booklet, to:

> W. B. Saunders Company
> Periodicals Fulfillment
> 6277 Sea Harbor Drive
> Orlando, FL 32887–4800

Customer Service: 1-800-654-2452 (US). From outside of the US, call 1-407-345-1000.
E-mail: JournalsCustomerService-usa@elsevier.com

TEST NO. PCL56:1 • FEBRUARY, 2009

CONTINUING MEDICAL EDUCATION SUPPLEMENT

GOAL

The goal of *Pediatric Clinics of North America* is to keep practicing pediatricians and pediatric residents up to date with current clinical practice in pediatrics by providing timely articles reviewing the state of the art in patient care.

OBJECTIVES

After reading the issue, the participants will be able to:
- understand the evidence for diagnosis and treatment of upper and lower respiratory tract disease in children
- learn the differential diagnosis of chest pain in children
- understand the causes of acute and chronic cough in pediatric patients

ACCREDITATION

Pediatric Clinics of North America is planned and implemented in accordance with the Essential Areas and Policies of the Accreditation Council for Continuing Medical Education (ACCME) through the joint sponsorship of the University of Virginia School of Medicine and Elsevier. The University of Virginia School of Medicine is accredited by the ACCME to provide continuing medical education for physicians.

The University of Virginia School of Medicine designates this educational activity for a maximum of 15 *AMA PRA Category 1 Credits*[TM] for each issue, 90 credits per year. Physicians should only claim credit commensurate with the extent of their participation in the activity.

The American Medical Association has determined that physicians not licensed in the US who participate in this CME activity are eligible for 15 *AMA PRA Category 1 Credits*[TM].

Category 1 credit can be earned by reading the text material, taking the CME examination online at http://www.theclinics.com/home/cme, and completing the evaluation. After taking the test, you will be required to review any and all incorrect answers. Following completion of the test and evaluation, your credit will be awarded and you may print your certificate.

FACULTY DISCLOSURES/CONFLICT OF INTEREST

The University of Virginia School of Medicine, as an ACCME accredited provider, endorses and strives to comply with the Accreditation Council for Continuing Medical Education (ACCME) Standards of Commercial Support, Commonwealth of Virginia statutes, University of Virginia policies and procedures, and associated federal and private regulations and guidelines on the need for disclosure and monitoring of proprietary and financial interests that may affect the scientific integrity and balance of content delivered in continuing medical education activities under our auspices.

The University of Virginia School of Medicine requires that all CME activities accredited through this institution be developed independently and be scientifically rigorous, balanced and objective in the presentation/discussion of its content, theories and practices.

All authors/editors participating in an accredited CME activity are expected to disclose to the readers relevant financial relationships with commercial entities occurring within the past 12 months (such as grants or research support, employee, consultant, stock holder, member of speakers bureau, etc.). The University of Virginia School of Medicine will employ appropriate mechanisms to resolve potential conflicts of interest to maintain the standards of fair and balanced education to the reader. Questions about specific strategies can be directed to the Office of Continuing Medical Education, University of Virginia School of Medicine, Charlottesville, Virginia.

Disclosure of Discussion of non-FDA approved uses for pharmaceutical products and/or medical devices:
The University of Virginia School of Medicine, as an ACCME provider, requires that all faculty presenters identify and disclose any "off label" uses for pharmaceutical and medical device products. The University of Virginia School of Medicine recommends that each physician fully review all the available data on new products or procedures prior to instituting them with patients.

Please note the disclosure information in the front of the *Clinics* issue.

TEST NO. PCL56:1 • FEBRUARY, 2009

INSTRUCTIONS FOR COMPLETING THE EXAMINATION FOR CREDIT

The test booklet has been mailed to you for your convenience; however, all examinations must be taken online in order to receive credit.

Please register online at www.theclinics.com/home/cme using the account number provided on the mailing label of this test booklet. Instructions for completing the test are provided on the website. With the online service, readers will benefit from the convenience of instant scoring and credit.

Test questions will be available online for 12 months.

Technical support is available Monday through Friday during the hours of 7:30 am to 6:00 pm EST:

Customer Service Department
6277 Sea Harbor Drive
Orlando, FL 32887 USA
(800) 654-2452 (Toll Free US & Canada)
(407) 345-4299 (Outside US & Canada)

FAX: (407) 363-9661
E-mail: JournalsCustomerService-usa@elsevier.com

If you do not have access to a computer, please call Customer Service to obtain an answer sheet and envelope. Please return your answer sheet via mail in the envelope provided; *faxed answer sheets will not be accepted.* Remember to complete both the test and the subsequent program evaluation. Please allow 4 to 6 weeks for processing and scoring answer sheets submitted in this manner.

TEST NO. PCL56:1 • FEBRUARY, 2009

1. All but which of the following is TRUE regarding the pathophysiology of cough?

    A. laryngeal cough is a reflex cough that protects against aspiration
    B. tracheobronchial cough is always reflexive
    C. tracheobronchial cough can be mechanically stimulated
    D. tracheobronchial cough can be stimulated by chemoreceptors

2. The overall management of cough includes which of the following?

    A. evaluation of etiology
    B. defining exacerbation factors
    C. defining the effect on the patient and family
    D. all of the above

3. Chronic cough is defined as cough persisting more than:

    A. 1 week
    B. 2 weeks
    C. 4 weeks
    D. none of the above

4. A "pertussis like cough" can also be caused by which of the following agents?

    A. mycoplasma
    B. parainfluenza virus
    C. respiratory syncytial virus
    D. all of the above

TEST NO. PCL56:1 • FEBRUARY, 2009

5. Which of the following accurately reflects the role of over the counter remedies for chronic cough in children?

   A. little evidence that they are effective in management of chronic cough
   B. side effects may be significant
   C. unintentional ingestions pose additional risks
   D. all of the above

6. Demographics of chest pain in children seen in the emergency department include all but which of the following?

   A. most children report chest pain to be of a moderate to severe degree regardless of etiology
   B. most are fearful of a cardiac etiology
   C. chest pain is the presenting complaint in 3% of all pediatric visits to the doctor
   D. chest pain is the second most common cause for referral to a pediatric cardiologist

7. Cardiac causes of chest pain include all but which of the following?

   A. atrial septal defect
   B. aortic stenosis
   C. hypertrophic cardiomyopathy
   D. Kawasaki disease

8. Chest pain with fever may represent which of the following?

    A. myocarditis
    B. pericarditis
    C. pneumonia
    D. all of the above

9. Although a thorough history and physical examination is often sufficient to exclude heart disease, which of the following requires more detailed assessment and/or referral?

    A. family history of Marfan syndrome
    B. crushing chest pain
    C. palpitations
    D. all of the above

10. Gastrointestinal causes of chest pain include which of the following?

    A. reflux
    B. gastritis
    C. foreign body
    D. all of the above

11. Chest pain that is reproduced by palpation most likely represents:

    A. musculoskeletal chest pain
    B. arrhythmia
    C. reactive airways disease
    D. none of the above

12. Pulmonary causes of chest pain include:

    A. pneumonia
    B. pulmonary embolus
    C. pneumothorax
    D. all of the above

13. Symptoms associated with pectus excavatum include all but which of the following?

    A. impaired cardiac output with exercise
    B. syncope
    C. chest pain
    D. dyspnea

14. Chest pain in Marfan syndrome may represent all but which of the following?

    A. costochondritis
    B. pneumothorax
    C. aortic dissection
    D. aortic aneurysm

15. In acute initial rhinosinusitis, evidence demonstrates no significant effects in prevention of disease or duration of symptoms following treatment with:

    A. echinacea
    B. vitamin C
    C. zinc
    D. all of the above

16. In persistent rhinosinusitis, all but which of the following shortened the course of illness?

    A. vitamin C
    B. intranasal steroids
    C. antibiotics
    D. none of the above

17. Clinical signs that predict streptococcal infection in 50% of children include:

    A. fever greater than 38°C
    B. exudative pharyngitis
    C. tender adenopathy and absence of cough
    D. all of the above

18. What percentage of cases of streptococcal pharyngitis resolve by 1 week even without therapy?

    A. 25%
    B. 50%
    C. 85%
    D. 100%

19. All but which of the following are complications of untreated strep pharyngitis?

    A. peritonsillar abcess
    B. rheumatic fever
    C. epiglottis
    D. otitis media

20. Although any of the following respiratory viruses can present with a host of clinical phenotypes, which of the following represent common associated symptoms?

    A. parainfluenza – croup
    B. respiratory syncytial virus – bronchiolitis
    C. rhinovirus – asthma exacerbation
    D. all of the above

21. Which of the following recommendations about the use of bronchodilators in bronchiolitis is TRUE?

    A. inhaled bronchodilators are generally not helpful in patients with acute infection and bronchial thickening with secretions
    B. inhaled bronchodilators may be useful in patients with underlying reactive airways disease who develop obstruction due to inflammation and bronchospasm
    C. use of bronchodilators must be weighed against the potential adverse effects in the face of limited therapeutic efficacy
    D. all of the above

22. The differential diagnosis of stridor in a young infant/child includes which of the following in addition to viral larygotracheobronchitis?

    A. epiglottitis
    B. foreign body
    C. retropharyngeal abcess
    D. all of the above

23. Agents shown to be beneficial in acute croup include:

    A. oral corticosteroids
    B. nebulized corticosteroids
    C. epinephrine by nebulization
    D. all of the above

24. Treatment for moderate to severe tracheobronchomalacia includes all but which of the following?

    A. continuous positive airway pressure (CPAP)
    B. surgical or stent therapy
    C. salbutamol
    D. bi-level positive airway pressure (Bi-PAP)

25. The British Thoracic Society guidelines for hospital admission for pneumonia in pediatric patients include which of the following?

    A. oxygen saturation less than 92%
    B. respiratory rate >50 in children, >70 in infants
    C. apnea or grunting
    D. all of the above

26. Treatment of choice for community acquired pneumonia in preschool children is:

    A. amoxicillin or coamoxyclavulinic acid for 5–7 days
    B. co-trimoxazole therapy
    C. erythromycin
    D. none of the above

TEST NO. PCL56:1 • FEBRUARY, 2009

27. Common bacterial organisms causing pneumonia in neonates include:

   A. group B streptococcus
   B. *E. coli*
   C. listeria
   D. all of the above

28. Which of the following is TRUE regarding vaccine prevention of pneumonia in children?

   A. *S. Pneumoniae* vaccine is effective
   B. *H. Influenza* vaccine is effective
   C. most populations with the highest mortality from pneumonia do not have access to vaccines
   D. all of the above

29. Which of the following regarding tuberculosis in children is NOT true?

   A. increasing incidence worldwide reported
   B. diagnosis is based on clinical findings and smear and culture
   C. CT should regularly be performed to assess for mediastinal adenopathy
   D. in young children, gastric aspirates may be useful when sputum cannot be obtained

30. Proper treatment of tuberculosis includes which of the following?

   A. at least 6 months therapy, beginning with 3–4 drugs for 2 months, continuing with INH and rifampin
   B. 12 months therapy with rifampin alone
   C. administration of medication should be supervised
   D. A and C

TEST NO. PCL56:1 • FEBRUARY, 2009

PROGRAM EVALUATION

1. Rate this *Clinics* issue for its coverage of the topic (identifies major controversies, alternative approaches, etc.)

   A. excellent
   B. satisfactory
   C. unsatisfactory

2. Rate this *Clinics* issue for its balance, scientific integrity, and freedom from commercial bias.

   A. excellent
   B. satisfactory
   C. unsatisfactory

3. Rate the appropriateness of the level sophistication of this *Clinics* issue for the intended audience.

   A. excellent
   B. satisfactory
   C. unsatisfactory

4. How relevant were the topics presented in this *Clinics* issue to the patients in your practice?

   A. very relevant
   B. slightly relevant
   C. not at all relevant

5. Do you plan to make changes in your practice as a result of reading this issue?

   A. yes, definitely
   B. possibly
   C. no

6. Rate the test for its coverage of the topics in this issue.

    A. excellent
    B. satisfactory
    C. unsatisfactory

7. Rate the appropriateness of the level of complexity of the test for the intended audience.

    A. excellent
    B. satisfactory
    C. unsatisfactory

8. Rate the format and functionality of the online test. Were the instructions clear and was the process intuitive?

    A. excellent
    B. satisfactory
    C. unsatisfactory

What did you like most about this *Clinics* issue?

What can we do to improve the *Clinics*?

Please list the topics that you would like presented in future issues.

Approximately how many hours did your spend reading this issue?

Common Respiratory Symptoms and Illnesses: A Graded Evidence-Based Approach

Guest Editor

ANNE B. CHANG, MBBS, MPHTM, FRACP, PhD

PEDIATRIC CLINICS
OF NORTH AMERICA

www.pediatric.theclinics.com

February 2009 • Volume 56 • Number 1

SAUNDERS an imprint of ELSEVIER, Inc.

W.B. SAUNDERS COMPANY
A Division of Elsevier Inc.

1600 John F. Kennedy Boulevard • Suite 1800 • Philadelphia, Pennsylvania 19103-2899

http://www.theclinics.com

THE PEDIATRIC CLINICS OF NORTH AMERICA Volume 56, Number 1
February 2009 ISSN 0031-3955, ISBN-13: 978-1-4160-5795-6, ISBN-10: 1-4160-5795-1

Editor: Carla Holloway
Developmental Editor: Theresa Collier

The Pediatric Clinics of North America (ISSN 0031-3955) is published bimonthly by Elsevier Inc., 360 Park Avenue South, New York, NY 10010-1710. Months of publication are February, April, June, August, October, and December. Business and Editorial Offices: 1600 John F. Kennedy Blvd., Suite 1800, Philadelphia, PA 19103-2899. Customer Service Office: 11830 Westline Industrial Drive, St. Louis, MO 63146. Periodicals postage paid at New York, NY and additional mailing offices. Subscription prices are $162.00 per year (US individuals), $350.00 per year (US institutions), $220.00 per year (Canadian individuals), $466.00 per year (Canadian institutions), $262.00 per year (international individuals), $466.00 per year (international institutions), $81.00 per year (US students and residents), and $138.00 per year (international and Canadian residents and students). To receive students/resident rare, orders must be accompanied by name of affiliated institution, date of term, and the signature of program/residency coordinator on institution letterhead. Orders will be billed at individual rate until proof of status is received. Foreign air speed delivery is included in all Clinics subscription prices. All prices are subject to change without notice. **POSTMASTER:** Send address changes to *The Pediatric Clinics of North America*, Elsevier Journals Customer Service, 11830 Westline Industrial Drive, St. Louis, MO 63146. **Customer Service: 1-800-654-2452 (US and Canada). From outside of the US and Canada: 1-314-453-7041. Fax: 1-314-453-5170. For print support, e-mail: JournalsCustomerService-usa@elsevier.com. For online support, e-mail: JournalsOnlineSupport-usa@elsevier.com.**

Reprints. For copies of 100 or more, of articles in this publication, please contact the Commercial Reprints Department, Elsevier Inc., 360 Park Avenue South, New York, NY 10010-1710. Tel.: 212-633-3812; Fax: 212-462-1935; E-mail: reprints@elsevier.com.

The Pediatric Clinics of North America is also published in Spanish by McGraw-Hill Inter-americana Editores S.A., Mexico City, Mexico; in Portuguese by Riechmann and Affonso Editores, Rua Comandante Coelho 1085, CEP 21250, Rio de Janeiro, Brazil; and in Greek by Althayia SA, Athens, Greece.

The Pediatric Clinics of North America is covered in *MEDLINE/PubMed (Index Medicus), Excerpta Medica, Current Contents, Current Contents/Clinical Medicine, Science Citation Index, ASCA, ISI/BIOMED,* and *BIOSIS.*

Printed in the United States of America.

GOAL STATEMENT

The goal of the *Pediatric Clinics of North America* is to keep practicing physicians and residents up to date with current clinical practice in pediatrics by providing timely articles reviewing the state-of-the-art in patient care.

ACCREDITATION

The *Pediatric Clinics of North America* is planned and implemented in accordance with the Essential Areas and Policies of the Accreditation Council for Continuing Medical Education (ACCME) through the joint sponsorship of the University of Virginia School of Medicine and Elsevier. The University of Virginia School of Medicine is accredited by the ACCME to provide continuing medical education for physicians.

The University of Virginia School of Medicine designates this educational activity for a maximum of 15 *AMA PRA Category 1 Credits*™. Physicians should only claim credit commensurate with the extent of their participation in the activity.

The American Medical Association has determined that physicians not licensed in the US who participate in this CME activity are eligible for 15 *AMA PRA Category 1 Credits*™.

Credit can be earned by reading the text material, taking the CME examination online at http://www.theclinics.com/home/cme, and completing the evaluation. After taking the test, you will be required to review any and all incorrect answers. Following completion of the test and evaluation, your credit will be awarded and you may print your certificate.

FACULTY DISCLOSURE/CONFLICT OF INTEREST

The University of Virginia School of Medicine, as an ACCME accredited provider, endorses and strives to comply with the Accreditation Council for Continuing Medical Education (ACCME) Standards of Commercial Support, Commonwealth of Virginia statutes, University of Virginia policies and procedures, and associated federal and private regulations and guidelines on the need for disclosure and monitoring of proprietary and financial interests that may affect the scientific integrity and balance of content delivered in continuing medical education activities under our auspices.

The University of Virginia School of Medicine requires that all CME activities accredited through this institution be developed independently and be scientifically rigorous, balanced and objective in the presentation/discussion of its content, theories and practices.

All authors/editors participating in an accredited CME activity are expected to disclose to the readers relevant financial relationships with commercial entities occurring within the past 12 months (such as grants or research support, employee, consultant, stock holder, member of speakers bureau, etc.). The University of Virginia School of Medicine will employ appropriate mechanisms to resolve potential conflicts of interest to maintain the standards of fair and balanced education to the reader. Questions about specific strategies can be directed to the Office of Continuing Medical Education, University of Virginia School of Medicine, Charlottesville, Virginia.

The faculty and staff of the University of Virginia Office of Continuing Medical Education have no financial affiliations to disclose.

The authors/editors listed below have identified no financial or professional relationships for themselves or their spouse/partner:
Mutasim N. Abu-Hasan, MD; ChunTing Au, MPhil, RPSGT; Andrew Bush, MBBS(Hons), MA, MD, FRCP, FRCPCH; Vargilia P. Carnielli, MD; Anne B. Chang, MBBS, MPHTM, FRACP, PhD (Guest Editor); Diletta de Benedictis, MD; Fernando M. de Benedictis, MD; Mark L. Everard, MB, ChB, FRCP, DM; Janaki Gokhale, MD; Carla Holloway (Acquisitions Editor); J. Declan Kennedy, MD, FRCP, FRACP; A. James Martin, MRCP, FRACP; Ian Brent Masters, MBBS, FRACP, PhD; Craig Mellis, MBBS, MPH, MD, FRACP; Peter S. Morris, MBBS, PhD, FRACP; Sarath C. Ranganathan, MBChB, PhD; Gregory J. Redding, MD; Karen Rheuban, MD (Test Author); Steven M. Selbst, MD; Samatha Sonnappa, MBBS, MD; and Miles Weinberger, MD.

The authors/editors listed below identified the following professional or financial affiliations for themselves or their spouse/partner:
Ian M. Balfour-Lynn, MBBS, MD, FRCP, FRCPCH, FRCS(Ed), DHMSA jointly runs a company receiving sponsorship from Carburos Mettallicos.
Albert Martin Li, MD has received a grant from Johnson & Johnson.
Paul D. Robinson, MBChB, MRCPCH, FRACP has received a grant from Pharmaxis.
Peter Van Asperen, MBBS, MD, FRACP is an independent contractor for MSD, Pharmaxis, and UCB, and serves on the Advisory Board for MSD.

Disclosure of Discussion of Non-FDA Approved Uses for Pharmaceutical and/or Medical Devices:
The University of Virginia School of Medicine, as an ACCME provider, requires that all authors identify and disclose any "off label" uses for pharmaceutical and medical device products. The University of Virginia School of Medicine recommends that each physician fully review all the available data on new products or procedures prior to clinical use.

TO ENROLL

To enroll in the *Pediatric Clinics of North America* Continuing Medical Education program, call customer service at 1-800-654-2452 or visit us online at www.theclinics.com/home/cme. The CME program is available to subscribers for an additional fee of $195.00.

Contributors

GUEST EDITOR

ANNE B. CHANG, MBBS, MPHTM, FRACP, PhD
Professor and Pediatric Respiratory and Sleep Physician, Menzies School of Health Research, Charles Darwin University; and Queensland Children's Respiratory Centre, Royal Children's Hospital, Brisbane, Queensland, Australia

AUTHORS

MUTASIM ABU-HASAN, MD
Clinical Associate Professor of Pediatrics, Pediatric Allergy and Pulmonary Division, Pediatrics Department, University of Iowa Children's Hospital, University of Iowa College of Medicine, Iowa City, Iowa

CHUN TING AU, MPhil, RPSGT
Department of Pediatrics, Prince of Wales Hospital, The Chinese University of Hong Kong, Shatin, Hong Kong

IAN M. BALFOUR-LYNN, MBBS, MD, FRCP, FRCPCH, FRCS(Ed), DHMSA
Consultant in Pediatric Respiratory Medicine, Department of Pediatric Respiratory Medicine, Royal Brompton Hospital, London, United Kingdom

ANDREW BUSH, MBBS (Hons), MA, MD, FRCP, FRCPCH
Professor of Pediatric Respirology, Imperial School of Medicine at National Heart and Lung Institute; and Honorary Consultant Pediatric Chest Physician, Royal Brompton Hospital, London, United Kingdom

VIRGILIO P. CARNIELLI, MD
Director, Division of Neonatology, Department of Neonatal Medicine, Salesi Children's University Hospital, Ancona, Italy

ANNE B. CHANG, MBBS, MPHTM, FRACP, PhD
Professor and Pediatric Respiratory and Sleep Physician, Menzies School of Health Research, Charles Darwin University; and Queensland Children's Respiratory Centre, Royal Children's Hospital, Brisbane, Queensland, Australia

DILETTA DE BENEDICTIS, MD
Department of Pediatrics, Post-Graduate School of Pediatrics, S. Maria della Misericordia Hospital, University of Perugia, Perugia, Italy

FERNANDO M. DE BENEDICTIS, MD
Director, Division of Pediatric Medicine, Department of Pediatrics, Salesi Children's University Hospital, Ancona, Italy

MARK L. EVERARD, MB, ChB, FRCP, DM
Consultant and Honorary Reader in Pediatric Respiratory Medicine, Department of Respiratory Medicine, Sheffield Children's Hospital, Sheffield, United Kingdom

JANAKI GOKHALE, MD
Pediatric Resident, Jefferson Medical College, Philadelphia, Pennsylvania; A.I. DuPont Hospital for Children, Wilmington, Delaware

J. DECLAN KENNEDY, MD, FRCP, FRACP
Associate Professor, Discipline of Pediatrics, Department of Pulmonary Medicine, Child, Youth, and Women's Health Service, University of Adelaide, Women's and Children's Hospital, North Adelaide, South Australia, Australia

ALBERT MARTIN LI, MD
Department of Pediatrics, Prince of Wales Hospital, The Chinese University of Hong Kong, Shatin, Hong Kong

A. JAMES MARTIN, MRCP, FRACP
Director, Discipline of Pediatrics, Department of Pulmonary Medicine, Child, Youth, and Women's Health Service, University of Adelaide, Women's and Children's Hospital, North Adelaide, South Australia, Australia

IAN BRENT MASTERS, MBBS, FRACP, PhD
Director, Queensland Children's Respiratory Centre, Royal Children's Hospital, Brisbane, Queensland, Australia

CRAIG MELLIS, MBBS, MPH, MD, FRACP
Professor and Associate Dean, Central Clinical School, University of Sydney, Royal Prince Alfred Hospital, Sydney, New South Wales, Australia

PETER S. MORRIS, MBBS, PhD, FRACP
Associate Professor and Deputy Leader, Child Health Division, Menzies School of Health Research; Institute of Advanced Studies, Charles Darwin University; and Northern Territory Clinical School, Flinders University, Darwin, Australia

SARATH C. RANGANATHAN, MBChB, PhD
Department of Respiratory Medicine, Royal Children's Hospital Melbourne, Parkville; Infection, Immunity, and Environment Theme, Murdoch Children's Research Institute; and Department of Pediatrics, University of Melbourne, Melbourne, Australia

GREGORY J. REDDING, MD
Professor, Department of Pediatrics, University of Washington School of Medicine; and Chief, Pulmonary Division, Seattle Children's Hospital, Seattle, Washington

PAUL D. ROBINSON, MBChB, MRCPCH, FRACP
Department of Respiratory Medicine, The Children's Hospital at Westmead; and The Children's Hospital at Westmead Clinical School, Discipline of Pediatrics and Child Health, Faculty of Medicine, University of Sydney, Westmead, Sydney, Australia

STEVEN M. SELBST, MD
Professor of Pediatrics, Vice-Chair for Education, and Pediatric Residency Program Director, Pediatric Residency Program, Jefferson Medical College, Philadelphia, Pennsylvania; A.I. DuPont Hospital for Children, Wilmington, Delaware

SAMATHA SONNAPPA, MBBS, MD
Department of Respiratory Medicine, Great Ormond Street Hospital; and Portex Anesthesia, Intensive Therapy and Respiratory Medicine Unit, Institute of Child Health, London, United Kingdom

PETER VAN ASPEREN, MBBS, MD, FRACP
Department of Respiratory Medicine, The Children's Hospital at Westmead; and The Children's Hospital at Westmead Clinical School, Discipline of Pediatrics and Child Health, Faculty of Medicine, University of Sydney, Westmead, Sydney, Australia

MILES WEINBERGER, MD
Director, Pediatric Allergy and Pulmonary Division; and Professor, Pediatrics Department, University of Iowa Children's Hospital, University of Iowa College of Medicine, Iowa City, Iowa

Contents

The principle weakness when reviewing therapeutic interventions for acute bronchiolitis is the lack of a clear diagnostic test or definition. Current evidence suggests that oxygen is the only useful pharmacologic agent for correcting hypoxia.

Ian M. Balfour-Lynn

Domiciliary oxygen is used increasingly in pediatric practice, and the largest patient group to receive it is ex-premature babies with chronic neonatal lung disease. Because of a scarcity of good evidence to inform clinicians, there is a lack of consensus over many issues, even those as fundamental as the optimum target oxygen saturation. Nevertheless, many children benefit from receiving supplemental oxygen at home, particularly because it helps to keep them out of the hospital.

THE CLINICS ARE NOW AVAILABLE ONLINE!

Access your subscription at:
www.theclinics.com

Preface

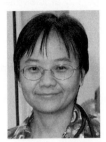

Anne B. Chang, MBBS, MPHTM, FRACP, PhD
Guest Editor

"Hi Doc. John keeps getting respiratory infections. What should I do?"
"Jane has been coughing for 5 weeks and we have had little sleep. Can you give her something to stop this cough?"

Such scenarios are regularly seen by most clinicians whose practice includes children. Indeed, children who have respiratory symptoms and signs or illness are among the most common presentations to medical practitioners. In this issue of *Pediatric Clinics of North America*, an evidence-based approach to common scenarios in pediatric respiratory care is emphasized, because significant advances in clinical care have occurred when long held dogma were questioned and evidence applied.[1] William Silverman eloquently articulated this in his book *Where's the Evidence?*[1] He further challenges clinicians to reflect on where the line between "knowing" (the acquisition of new medical information) and "doing" (the application of that new knowledge) is drawn.

In this issue, authors with significant clinical and research expertise from the United States, Europe, Asia, and Australia have utilized the GRADE[2] system for each recommended approach. As these articles were written well before the *British Medical Journal* GRADE series were published, the short GRADE system was utilized.[2] The steps in each article are designed to answer the questions: "What is the evidence-based approach?" and "What is the strength of the evidence of the approach?" The first five articles focus on common respiratory symptoms that are encountered by clinicians, such as respiratory noises and cough. The remaining articles are disease specific, designed as an evidence-based approach to guide the clinician when a child who has an illness such as pneumonia presents.

A significant limiting factor in almost all of the articles in this issue is the lack of randomized controlled trials for the suggested approach taken. Indeed, even for the very common symptoms of cough[3] or wheeze[4] in the young child, there is a glaring lack of high level evidence, let alone for the less common but significant symptoms of chest pain and shortness of breath. We have a long way to go to achieving complete evidence-based medicine in the respiratory care of children. However, this issue

Pediatr Clin N Am 56 (2009) xv–xvi
doi:10.1016/j.pcl.2008.11.001
0031-3955/08/$ – see front matter © 2009 Elsevier Inc. All rights reserved.

provides a succinct approach that highlights the evidence, or lack of, to managing respiratory symptoms and conditions, which general practitioners and pediatricians are likely to encounter in a child. I hope readers will find the articles useful in their clinical practice and stimulate some to conduct clinical research to improve the management of common respiratory conditions in childhood. I thank the authors for their valuable contributions to this issue.

Anne B. Chang, MBBS, MPHTM, FRACP, PhD
Child Health Division
Menzies School of Health Research
Charles Darwin University
Brisbane
Australia

Queensland Children's Respiratory Centre
Royal Children's Hospital
Herston Road
Herston, Brisbane
Queensland 4006
Brisbane
Australia

E-mail address:
annechang@ausdoctors.net

REFERENCES

1. Silverman WA. Where's the evidence? Debates in modern medicine. New York: Oxford University Press; 1999.
2. GRADE Working Group. Grading quality of evidence and strength of recommendations. BMJ 2004;328:1490–7.
3. Chang AB, Glomb WB. Guidelines for evaluating chronic cough in pediatrics: ACCP Evidence-Based Clinical Practice Guidelines. Chest 2006;129:S260–83.
4. Brand PL, Baraldi E, Bisgaard H, et al. Definition, assessment and treatment of wheezing disorders in preschool children: an evidence-based approach. Eur Respir J 2008;32:1096–110.

Respiratory Noises: How Useful are They Clinically?

Craig Mellis, MBBS, MPH, MD, FRACP

KEYWORDS

• Noisy breathing • Validity and reliability
• Wheeze • Rattle • Stridor

As the parents of infants and young children will attest, "noisy breathing" is extremely common in this age group. Whereas a multitude of different noises have been described in the literature, the most frequently used terms are "wheeze," "rattle," "stridor," "snore," and "nasal snuffle/snort." Conventional wisdom, based on empiric evidence and basic physiology, is that these noises emanate from specific anatomic sites within the respiratory system (**Table 1**). Thus, correctly identifying these noises is of major clinical relevance, in terms of localizing both the site of obstruction, and the most likely underlying cause.

There is a vast array of underlying conditions, both congenital and acquired, that can produce these noises. For example, in a major textbook on pediatric respiratory disease there are more than 35 listed causes of wheeze, and a similar number for stridor.[1] However, for practical purposes, most noises will be attributable to a relatively small number of common, underlying conditions. **Table 2** lists the most common acute and persistent causes of these noises.

Although the clinical utility of these respiratory noises is often assumed, unfortunately, distinguishing these noises from each other can be very difficult. Many children will have multiple noises, as the obstruction to airway is often extensive (eg, inflammation involving both upper and lower airways), the noise may vary from minute to minute, and some noises will not clearly fit one of these simple descriptors. This difficulty in categorizing the noise is worse when the noise is intermittent, described by the child's parent, and not confirmed by the clinician. Further, even when heard by the clinician agreement between clinicians on the terminology of these noises is far from perfect.

Because these noises can be considered as either a symptom (when reported on history by a parent) or a sign (when confirmed on physical examination by a clinician) it is crucial that we have high-quality research evidence regarding both the validity (accuracy or closeness to the truth, when compared with a "gold standard") and

Central Clinical School, Room 406, Blackburn Building D06, University of Sydney, Royal Prince Alfred Hospital, Sydney, NSW 2006, Australia
E-mail address: c.mellis@usyd.edu.au

Pediatr Clin N Am 56 (2009) 1–17
doi:10.1016/j.pcl.2008.10.003
0031-3955/08/$ – see front matter © 2009 Elsevier Inc. All rights reserved.

Table 1	
Common noises and the site of origin	
Noise	**Site of Origin**
Wheeze	Intrathoracic airways
Rattle	Either or both intra- and extrathoracic airways
Stridor	Extrathoracic airways
Snore	Oro-naso-pharyngeal airway
Snuffle/snort	Nasal passages/naso-pharynx
Grunt	Alveoli/lung parenchyma

the reliability (repeatability) of these symptoms and signs.[2] Reliability includes both intraobserver reliability (ie, whether the clinician will agree with himself/herself when observing the same sign on two separate occasions), and between-observer reliability (ie, whether two clinicians, or parent and clinician, will agree when both observe the same physical sign).

The purpose of this article is to appraise the published research evidence concerning respiratory noises in infants and young children, with particular emphasis on the validity and reliability of these noises, and their subsequent clinical relevance and diagnostic significance. Numerous textbooks and narrative reviews have comprehensive descriptions of the clinical features of the conditions that can cause noisy breathing, and these will not be elaborated on here. Rather, this review will focus on evidence relating to validity and reliability of these noises (symptoms and signs), and whether we can improve the utility of these reported and observed noises by the use of technology, such as video recordings or computerized acoustic analysis.

It must be pointed out that despite noisy breathing being an extremely common clinical problem, there is a paucity of high-quality clinical research evidence concerning these key questions. The available evidence is from observational studies, and using the Grade approach[3] is automatically assigned as "low" level evidence. There are also inconsistencies and the data are sparse. Moreover, it is clear that much of the evidence has come predominantly from several research groups, particularly in the United Kingdom. Consequently, further research could have an important impact on the conclusions drawn from the current evidence presented here.

Table 2		
Common clinical causes of noisy breathing		
Noise	**Acute**	**Persistent**
Wheeze	Intermittent asthma/Viral-induced wheeze	Infants: Transient early wheeze (TEW)
		Older children: Persistent asthma
Rattle	Acute viral bronchitis	Chronic sputum retention (neuromuscular disorders)
Stridor	Acute laryngotracheobronchitis (or viral "croup")	Laryngomalacia (or "infantile larynx")
Snore	Acute tonsillitis/pharyngitis	Chronically enlarged tonsils and adenoids
Snuffle	Acute viral head cold ("coryza")	Allergic rhinitis

DEFINITIONS
Wheeze

Wheeze is a high-pitched, continuous musical noise, often associated with prolonged expiration. While predominantly heard in the expiratory phase, wheeze can occur throughout the respiratory cycle. Basic respiratory physiology tells us that wheeze emanates from the intrathoracic airways, and can be produced by pathology either in the large, central airways, or the small, peripheral airways. The intensity of the wheeze is a poor indicator of the severity of the obstruction. Indeed, if the obstruction is extremely severe the wheeze may become inaudible.

Wheeze as a result of large airways obstruction

When a structural lesion obstructs airflow in the large airways (intrathoracic trachea and major bronchi), the resultant noise is a result of turbulent airflow at the point of narrowing (**Fig. 1**). Thus, the wheeze may be quite localized on auscultation, and is classically termed "monophonic."[4] Although asthma is the commonest cause of wheeze, there are numerous other potential causes, many of which are serious and require specific, urgent interventions. These include inhaled foreign body, endobronchial tuberculosis, and bronchial adenoma. Extrinsic compression of a large, central airway will produce a similar type of wheeze. Causes include rare, but important conditions, such as enlarged mediastinal lymph nodes, benign or malignant mediastinal tumors, and achalasia.

Wheeze as a result of small airways obstruction

In the presence of extensive small airway narrowing, the resultant high pleural pressure swings can cause compression (inward collapse) of the large airways during expiration, producing generalized expiratory wheezing (**Fig. 2**). The very young are particularly prone to this because their large airways are relatively soft ("floppy") and more prone to collapse. Because the specific site of the large airway obstruction noise is variable, the noise is termed "polyphonic."[4] This is common in infants with acute viral bronchiolitis, where the audible wheeze is usually accompanied by extensive inspiratory crackles on auscultation. Abnormal "floppiness" of the walls of large, central airways can produce an identical noise during normal respiration, and is characteristically seen in the various forms of tracheomalacia and/or bronchomalacia.

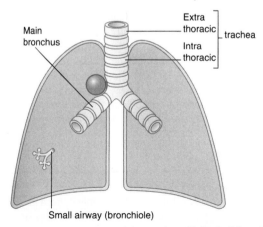

Fig. 1. Wheeze attributable to large airways obstruction. (*Adapted from* Henry R. Wheezing disorders other than asthma. In: Roberton DM, South M, editors. Practical paediatrics. 6th edition. Edinburgh: Churchill Livingstone; 2007. p. 493; with permission.)

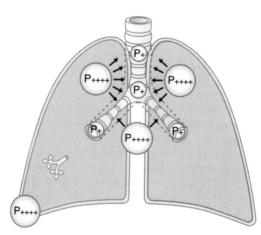

Fig. 2. Wheeze attributable to small airways obstruction. (*From* Henry R. Wheezing disorders other than asthma. In: Roberton DM, South M, editors. Practical paediatrics. 6th edition. Edinburgh: Churchill Livingstone; 2007. p. 493; with permission.)

While the now well-characterized "transient early wheeze" (TEW) is assumed to be a result of congenitally abnormal small-caliber airways,[5] some studies have questioned this assumption.[6] Typically, infants with TEW wheeze persistently through the first year, do not have inspiration crackles, are not troubled by either cough or shortness of breath, and cease wheezing by age 18 to 24 months.

Assessing wheeze

In evaluating a young child with parent-reported wheeze, the first step is to determine exactly what the parents mean by that term. In particular, whether wheeze is being used in a generic sense to describe any noise, particularly a "rattly" chest. Quality of Evidence (GRADE):[3] Moderate. Data are from observational studies, which is the appropriate study design. However, studies are predominantly small cohorts and cross-sectional studies, with some conflicting data.

In young children who, on examination, have a combination of generalized, polyphonic wheeze, asthma (or viral-induced wheeze), is likely. Additional clinical information should be sought to rule this in or out, such as overinflation of the chest, prolonged expiration, or a trial of bronchodilator therapy (see article on asthma elsewhere in this issue).

In a young child, with either localized wheeze or monophonic wheeze, particularly if accompanied by asymmetric breath sounds (that is, uneven air entry), a focal lesion must be ruled out. This could include an endobronchial obstruction (eg, foreign body) or a mass lesion compressing a major bronchus. Thus, further investigations (eg, chest radiograph) and probable bronchoscopy are indicated. Quality of Evidence (GRADE): Moderate to high. Appropriately, data are from observational studies, predominantly cohorts and case series.

Assessing infants with wheeze

In infants (younger than 12 months), a polyphonic wheeze on auscultation, particularly if accompanied by generalized inspiratory crackles, indicates probable acute viral bronchiolitis. Interventions should be considered only if there is significant breathlessness resulting in difficulty feeding. Apart from supplementary oxygen, adequate fluid intake, and careful nursing care, no other intervention is of proven benefit. Quality of evidence for no benefit: High for inhaled beta-agonists, adrenaline, and systemic corticosteroids.

In infants with recurrent or persistent polyphonic wheezing, not associated with significant cough, inspiratory crackles, or significant increase in the work of breathing, the most likely diagnosis is TEW. Quality of evidence: High. Multiple birth cohorts, consistent findings.

However, if the wheeze is associated with any of the above features, then asthma is likely, and a trial of treatment appropriate (see article on asthma in this issue). In this age group, the possibility of a rare congenital malformation of the airways also needs to be considered.

Rattle

The current belief is that a rattle is a result of excessive secretions in the large airways, which are presumably moving with normal respiration.[7] Rattles may be heard in either, or both, inspiration and expiration. A research group in Yorkshire, United Kingdom, coined the term "ruttle" to describe this coarse respiratory noise.[7] However, because the term "rattle" is far more widely recognized, "ruttle" is best avoided, as there is already considerable confusion concerning the numerous terms used to describe noisy breathing. A rapid improvement in rattles (measured objectively with acoustic analysis) after inhalation of anticholinergics suggests these rattling noises are attributable to coughing or clearance of sputum, rather than alterations in bronchomotor tone.[8] Parents will often comment that as well as being able to hear the rattle, they can feel the rattle (as a vibration), when placing their hands over the child's chest wall. Unfortunately, parents commonly mislabel the rattle as a "wheeze," resulting in overdiagnosis of asthma (and unnecessary antiasthma treatment).

Assessing rattle

In an infant or young child with a rattle observed on examination, the most likely cause is acute viral bronchitis. Further inquiry should be made concerning any associated cough or rattle. Quality of evidence: Moderate. One small randomized trial of inhaled anticholinergics reduced rattle.

If the child has an underlying chronic neurologic or neuromuscular condition, the most likely explanation is inability to cough and/or swallow normal secretions, and appropriate investigation to rule out pulmonary aspirations is indicated. Specific interventions are rarely indicated. Quality of evidence: Low. Paucity of data.

Stridor

In contrast to wheeze, stridor is predominantly inspiratory, and indicates obstruction to airflow in the extrathoracic airways down to the level of the thoracic inlet. However, wheeze and stridor can occur in both phases of respiration, particularly when the obstruction is severe. Because stridor is a sign of upper airway obstruction, it should never be ignored. At this point in the respiratory tract there is only a single air passage. Thus, if there is severe obstruction, respiratory arrest can occur, as there is no alternate route for air entry.

The upper airway is a complex anatomic region, which is best divided into supraglottic, glottic, and subglottic areas. The supraglottic area includes the epiglottis, aryepiglottic folds, and false vocal cords. Because this area is composed of soft tissue and muscle, it is prone to inward collapse, resulting in obstruction. This typically occurs in infants with laryngomalacia ("infantile larynx").[9] Laryngomalacia is by far the most common cause of stridor in infants, and is a result of collapse of the supraglottic structure during inspiration. The noise varies in intensity depending on the respiratory effort, typically louder with crying and feeding, softer when quietly sleeping. Although classically causing inspiratory stridor, it is often associated with other noises such as "stertor" (or "clucking" noise), but a normal cry (voice), and normal cough.

Although acute epiglottitis (caused by *Haemophilius influenzae* type B) is now rare because of widespread vaccination, the noise produced by this condition is typically a soft vibrating "snoring" sound, rather than a harsh inspiratory stridor. Further, there is usually no associated cough, and certainly no loud barking "croupy" cough.

The glottic area includes the true vocal cords. Typically, pathology at this level causes a soft, hoarse cry (voice) as well as inspiratory stridor. Examples include vocal cord paresis, laryngeal web, and laryngeal warts.

The subglottic area includes the extrathoracic trachea, down to the level of the thoracic inlet. Although supported by cartilage, this can collapse inwards in the presence of large pleura pressure swings. Acute stridor at this anatomic level in infants and young children is usually caused by viral "croup" (laryngotracheobronchitis).[10] Typically, the stridor is loud and harsh, together with a loud brassy, honking cough, and signs of a viral respiratory tract infection.

Assessing stridor

In infants with persistent stridor, but no significant increase in the work of breathing, no cough, normal cry, no apnea or cyanotic episodes, and thriving, then laryngomalacia is the most likely cause. No further investigation is warranted apart from follow-up review. Quality of evidence: High. Large observational studies with consistent findings.

If stridor is persistent and associated with any of the above features, then consider significant upper airway pathology, and probable larangoscopy and bronchoscopy. Quality of evidence: Moderate. Mostly from small cohorts and case series.

If stridor is acute, and associated with symptoms and signs of a viral respiratory tract infection plus a brassy (croupy) cough, then viral croup (larynotracheobronchitis) is most likely. If the stridor is present at rest, the obstruction should be considered moderately severe and systemic corticosteroids or inhaled corticosteroids are indicated. Quality of evidence: High. Systematic reviews.

If the acute stridor occurs in the absence of a viral respiratory tract infection, then the possibility of a large ingested foreign body should be considered, particularly if there is any difficulty in swallowing. Quality of evidence: Moderate. Small cohorts and case series.

Snore

Although snoring is generally more obvious in inspiration, the noise is frequently audible throughout the respiratory cycle. The noise arises from an increase in the resistance to airflow through the upper airways, predominantly in the region of the nasopharynx and oropharynx. During rapid eye movement (REM) sleep there is relaxation of the oropharyngeal musculature, thus further compromising the narrow air passages, resulting in the vibratory noise we all recognize as "snoring." Predictably, in young children the usual cause is enlarged tonsils and/or adenoids.

The major issue clinically, is whether the snoring is of any relevance to the child's health. Distinguishing primary snoring from pathologic obstructive sleep apnea-hypopnea (OSAH) is difficult clinically.[11] If there are associated symptoms suggesting OSAH, a formal sleep study may be indicated. Symptoms that suggest genuine OSAH include observed apnea, excessive daytime sleepiness, and behavior or learning problems.[12] This noise will not be discussed in detail here, as it is covered in another article in this issue.

Snuffles and Snorts

The terms "snuffles" and "snorts" are used to describe respiratory noises emanating from the nasal passages. Snuffle has also been used to describe any discharge from the nasal passages, and is sometimes used to describe a minor viral upper respiratory tract infection ("head cold"). The term was originally used in relation to congenital syphilis. These nasal noises are frequently audible in both inspiration and expiration, and often associated with visible secretions from the nares.

Assessing snuffles and snorts

In young infants with persistent nasal obstruction, nasal patency needs to be assessed to rule out choanal atresia. Bilateral nasal obstruction in older children suggests either perennial allergic rhinitis or, rarely, nasal polyps (usually in association with cystic fibrosis). If persistent, purulent nasal secretions consider chronic bacterial rhinosinusitis. Latter is suggestive of underlying presence of suppurative airways disease (eg, cystic fibrosis, immune deficiency syndromes, and ciliary dysfunction).

Grunt

An expiratory grunt is classically seen in the presence of extensive alveolar pathology and is considered a sign of serious disease. Grunting is particularly seen in hyaline membrane disease (neonates) and lobar pneumonia (infants and children). However, in both these situations, other clinical features of the underlying problem (especially respiratory distress) are far more impressive, and of far greater diagnostic relevance, than the noise per se. The expiratory grunt is a natural form of continuous positive airway pressure (CPAP), aimed at improving oxygenation, and is mechanistically similar to "pursed lips breathing" in adults with chronic dyspnea.

PREVALENCE OF NOISY BREATHING

Although wheeze is well studied, there are few observational studies of infants addressing the question of "how common are *all* forms of noisy breathing?" To answer this question Thornton and colleagues[13] studied a birth cohort of almost 300 randomly chosen, normal-term infants in Cambridge, England. This cohort was followed longitudinally from birth to 6 months. Mothers were interviewed at home about any concerns they had regarding their infant's health. In addition, mothers were questioned in detail about 28 specific symptoms to determine the incidence, severity, and duration of these specific symptoms.

Respiratory symptoms were by far the dominant concern. The commonest concern expressed by these mothers was "noisy breathing," followed by common cold symptoms, running nose, cough, and breathing difficulties. More than 80% of the mothers reported 1 or more of the 28 specific symptoms in the previous 24 hours. "Noisy breathing" was reported in 30% and was second only to "cold peripheries" (39%). Further, of those mothers reporting noisy breathing, 20% classified this as "moderate or severe," and almost half stated that the noisy breathing was "always present." Clearly, the prevalence of respiratory symptoms, particularly noisy breathing, is very high in apparently healthy, term infants.

A further observational study from the United Kingdom investigated both the frequency of noisy breathing and the terminology used by parents to describe noisy breathing in infants younger than 18 months of age.[7] Part of this study included a community survey, using a postal questionnaire about noisy breathing, to 200 parents of infants. Of these 200, only 62 responded and, of these, 39 reported noisy breathing. Clearly, with this low response rate, the 63% prevalence is an overestimate of the true prevalence, and further high-quality research on this question is needed.

On the other hand, rates of wheeze in infants have been the subject of numerous birth cohorts, the most notable being that from Tucson, Arizona.[5] The latter study introduced the now commonly used term "transient early wheeze" (TEW) to describe otherwise healthy infants who wheeze in infancy but cease wheezing by age 3 years. Most studies of TEW indicate that theses infants have abnormal lung function from birth (ie, smaller than normal-caliber airways). Large birth cohort studies from a number of countries including the United Kingdom,[14,15] Sweden,[16] France,[17] and Brazil[18] have been studied to ascertain the rate of parent-reported wheeze (or whistling from the chest). Although rates vary slightly, most indicate that approximately 30% to 40% of parents report infant wheeze; however, few studies have validated these parental reports.

One of the few studies that compared parent reported respiratory illness in infants with clinical diagnosis was from New Mexico.[19] An active illness surveillance system was established over the first year of life in a large birth cohort (n = 1200). This included a daily symptom diary kept by parents plus a telephone interview every 2 weeks. If a respiratory illness was reported, infants were visited at home by a nurse practitioner and specimens for virology collected. Each child contributed an average of 429 observation days. Most respiratory illnesses diagnosed by the nurse practitioner as "lower" respiratory (LRI) were accompanied by a parent report of either "wheeze" or "wet cough." LRI with wheeze was less frequent than LRI with wet cough (6% versus 33%). Thus, in infancy coughing illnesses are far more frequent than wheezing illnesses. However, as many of the infants with "LRI and wet cough" had a "rattly, bubbly chest," parents are likely to have reported the noise as "wheeze" (if they had not been seen, and confirmed as "non-wheeze," by a clinician). These results highlight the likely overdiagnosis of parent-reported wheeze in infants.

Reported rates of wheeze in older children has also been extensively studied. By far the best data currently available are from the International Study of Asthma and Allergies in Childhood (ISAAC) study.[20] This is a worldwide, systematic study using identical methodology to measure the rates of reported wheeze in both younger (6- to 7-year-olds) and older children (13- to 14-year-olds). For the younger children, rates of "recent wheeze" were as reported by parents (ie, "Has your child had wheezing or whistling in the chest in the past 12 months?"), and for the older children, self-reported rates of "recent wheeze" (ie, "Have you had wheezing or whistling in the chest in the past 12 months?"). To assess time trends, these studies have now been repeated. The results are available from the most recent cross-sectional questionnaire survey of almost 200,000 6- to 7-year-olds in 37 countries and over 300,000 13- to 14-year-olds in 56 countries. For 6- to 7-year-olds, parent-reported rates of "recent wheeze" varied from a low of 2.8% (Indonesia) to a high of 37.6% (Costa Rica). High rates were also reported in New Zealand (22.2%), United Kingdom (20.9%), Australia (20%), and North America (Canada, 18.2%). For 13- to 14-year-olds, self-reported rates of recent wheeze were in a similar range, with a low of 3.4% (Albania) and a high of 31.2% (Isle of Man). High rates were again reported for Costa Rica (27.3%), New Zealand (26.7%), United Kingdom (24.7%), and North America (United States, 22.3%).

However, a major question with all these questionnaire studies is exactly what do parents and/or children understand by the term "wheeze"? In particular, whether many of those with reported wheeze have other respiratory noises (such as rattle, stridor, or snore) which is being misinterpreted as a wheeze.

WHAT DO PARENTS UNDERSTAND BY WHEEZE?

This question was addressed in a hospital-based observational study of older children.[21] A total of 139 children (aged 4 months to 15 years, median 2.5 years) were assessed in the emergency department (ED) to measure the agreement between clinician and parent report on the noise. There was a less than 50% agreement between a clinician's finding wheeze and parents' report of wheeze. That is, in children presenting to

ED with wheeze (or asthma), where the doctor finds wheeze, 39% of the parents use words other than wheeze (particularly cough and/or difficult breathing). Also, when the doctor does not find wheeze (especially with upper airway noises), 14% of parents use the term wheeze to describe this noise. Clearly, parents and clinicians differ widely in the use of the term wheeze in children with acute symptoms in an ED setting.

In the same study, 160 parents attending the outpatient chest clinic, because of wheeze, were asked, "What do you understand by wheeze, and how do you recognize wheeze in your child?" Terms used by parents to describe the noise included hissing, squeaking, whistle, and rasp. Surprisingly, almost a quarter of these parents did not equate wheeze with a noise. Forty percent of parents stated they used nonauditory cues when asked, "How do they know when your child is wheezy?" It is clear that for a substantial proportion of parents, wheeze has a very different meaning to that used by clinicians.

The implication of these findings on the accuracy of numerous pediatric epidemiology studies that routinely report the rates of "Has your child wheezed in the past 12 months?" or "Has your child ever wheezed?" as "asthma symptoms" are obvious.

VALIDATION OF RESPIRATORY QUESTIONNAIRE TO MEASURE WHEEZE

A study from Brazil attempted to validate a questionnaire on wheeze in infancy.[22] In this study of young children presenting to the ED with an acute respiratory illness, parents answered a questionnaire on wheezing (adapted from the International Study of Wheezing in Infants).[22] A total of 209 infants aged 12 to 15 months were assessed. Fifty-six of these were reported to be currently wheezing and this was confirmed in 43. A further 153 parents reported "no current wheeze" and this absence of wheeze was confirmed clinically in 146.

Assuming the ED clinician is the "gold standard," the sensitivity and specificity of parent-reported wheeze was 0.86 and 0.92 respectively (that is, a positive likelihood ratio of >10). This is considerably more accurate than that seen in most other similar studies in infants and toddlers. This suggests that using a questionnaire can be more accurate than simply asking the parent to nominate a single term to describe the noise.

COMPARING THE SEVERITY OF PARENT-REPORTED WHEEZE WITH CLINICIAN-CONFIRMED WHEEZE

One observational study measured the lung function of children with "confirmed" (by clinicians) with "unconfirmed" (parent-reported) wheeze.[23] This study was part of a large UK birth cohort (n = 1000) and describes a subgroup of 454 children followed to the age of 3 years. A total of 186 (41%) of these children had "parent-reported wheeze," and in 130 (29%) the wheeze was "confirmed" by a clinician. Specific airway resistance (sRaw) was measured at the age of 3 by plethysmography. The major finding was that sRaw was significantly higher (reflecting greater airflow limitation) in those children with "clinician confirmed" wheeze, compared with children who had "never wheezed," and those with "parent-reported" wheeze. In short, children with clinically confirmed wheeze in the first 3 years of life have more abnormal lung function, suggesting a more clinically relevant degree of airway pathology, than those with parent-reported wheezing (and those who have never wheezed).

UTILITY OF VIDEOS AS A "GOLD STANDARD"

An observational study from the United Kingdom investigated the terminology used by parents to describe noisy breathing in infants younger than 18 months of age.[7] The parents of approximately 100 infants with noisy breathing were interviewed. These infants were from three separate populations: hospital inpatients (n = 44), hospital outpatients (n = 19), and a community sample (n = 29). Almost half the parents used the term "wheeze" (or whistle/musical sound) to describe noisy breathing initially, while the term "rattle" (or "ruttle"/ bubbly chest) was used almost as frequently. The terms "stridor" (5%), "snuffly" (5%), and "snore" (3%) were far less commonly used.

To evaluate the accuracy of these terms, the parents of 72 of these infants were shown a series of videos specifically displaying footage of infants with typical wheeze, rattle, or stridor. After viewing these videos, parents were then asked to choose the term that best matched their child's noisy breathing. Approximately a third of the parents changed from their initial term "wheeze," to "rattle." If we assume the video is the "gold standard," these numbers translate to a sensitivity of 0.63 and a specificity of 0.68 for parents' use of the term "wheeze." That is, a false positive rate of 32%, and false negative rate of 37%. For parent-reported "rattle," the corresponding figures are 0.45 and 0.81 (sensitivity and specificity respectively), or a false positive rate of 20% and false negative rate of 55%! An additional finding from this study was that giving parents a list of terms to describe their infants' noise was unhelpful. Although these parents reported that an adult imitating the noise was of limited value, they found the video clips of infants with specific, single noises to be the most useful method of assessing their infants' respiratory noises.

Clearly, the terminology used by parents is very prone to misclassification. Thus, it is essential that clinicians and epidemiologists attempt to clarify what parents really mean by these commonly used terms, such as wheeze and rattle. Evidence suggests the term "wheeze" is overused by parents, while the term "rattle" is underused. Adding to the difficulty, it is apparent that some infants will have, simultaneously, both a "wheeze" and a "rattle." Moreover, infants will switch over time from a predominant "wheeze" (eg, early in the course of viral bronchitis with wheeze) to a predominant "rattle" (eg, resolving stage of viral bronchitis). The major clinical implication of these data is that clinicians should not equate "wheeze" (particularly wheeze reported by parents, and unconfirmed by a clinician) with asthma. When assessing children with parent-reported wheeze, clinicians need to question further as to what the parents are really describing as a wheeze.

In a further attempt to evaluate the accuracy of parents' descriptions of noisy breathing, Cane and McKenzie[24] assessed the utility of video clips of children demonstrating noisy breathing. These videos included both typical wheeze and other noises, such as stridor, snore, and stertor (ie, "a clucking hen" noise). The parents of 190 children younger than 8 years were shown these videos. Parents were a mix of those with and without a child with asthma (or other respiratory complaints). Videos were shown to parents who were then asked what word they would use to describe these noises. In addition, parents were asked where they believed these noises were coming from, ie, chest, throat, or nose. The first major finding was the difficulty the authors had with clinicians agreeing on what the actual video noises were demonstrating. Agreement among clinicians was poor — in only 10 of the 15 videos was there unanimous agreement on the term used to describe the noise. This was despite the videos demonstrating a distinct, typical single sound, which is obviously far removed from real life, clinical situations.

As with the previous study using videos, 30% of the parents (whether they had a wheezy child or not) used terms other than "wheeze" to describe the video of wheezing. A further 30% of these parents falsely labeled other sounds (stridor, snore, or stertor) as "wheeze." Although parents' reports of symptoms were in poor agreement with clinicians, the ability of parents to identify the origin (or location) of the noise was in relatively good agreement with the clinicians. This study supports other studies indicating that video clips are a method of improving the accuracy of parental terms used to describe noisy breathing, especially "wheeze."

Video questionnaires have been used to validate measures of wheeze in older children. The ISAAC written and video questionnaires were compared in 317,000 adolescents (aged 13 to 14 years old) in 40 countries.[25] As expected, responses to the video gave lower prevalences of wheeze symptoms. Chance corrected agreement (Kappa) was also generally low. Initial pilot studies, using hypertonic saline bronchial challenges in 393 school children (age 13 to 15 years) to validate the ISAAC questionnaire found low sensitivity (47%), but high specificity (92%) when compared with a positive response to the question regarding "current wheeze."[26] Similar results were found for a 6-minute exercise challenge (sensitivity = 46%; specificity = 88%). Similar findings have been published more recently from Germany as part of the ISAAC Phase II study.[27] Although the high specificity is encouraging (to rule asthma "in"), a bronchial challenge test is not generally considered an adequate "gold standard" for the diagnosis of wheeze or asthma.

NATURAL HISTORY/PROGNOSIS OF NOISY BREATHING

An important question is whether early respiratory noises predict subsequent wheeze. The study by Turner and colleagues[28] described the natural history of the full range of these early respiratory noises. This observational study was part of a large Scottish birth cohort of approximately 2000 infants. A respiratory questionnaire (modified ISAAC questionnaire) was administered at the age of 2 and 5 years. The key findings were the following: children with a "whistle" at age 2 were more likely to wheeze (73%), and were more likely to be receiving asthma treatment (40%) at age 5 years, compared with children with a "rattle" at 2 years (34% and 11% respectively), or who "purred" (39% and 18% respectively). Further, children with a "whistle" at 2 years are more likely to have a mother with asthma (38%). Children with a "rattle" or a "purr" at 2 years are more likely to have been exposed to tobacco smoke at home, compared with those with either a "whistle," or no noise at 2 years. This is in keeping with the belief that a rattle is attributable to hypersecretion of mucus and/or recurrent or persistent bronchitis, possibly related to exposure to environmental tobacco smoke.

While "rattle" and "purr" (at 2 years) resolved in the majority by age 5 years, of real concern is that approximately half of these children (with a rattle or a purr) were diagnosed as having asthma. On the other hand, whistle (or wheeze) at 2 years persisted in a substantial proportion at 5 years, and proved to be a strong predictor of ongoing wheeze and subsequent need for asthma treatment. These authors also made the important observation that "most parents seem to think that wheeze is any respiratory noise, of which a whistle is one sub-set [of wheeze]."[28]

The natural history of wheeze in infancy has been studied extensively, particularly by Martinez and colleagues.[5] This birth cohort from Tucson, Arizona, has been studied again in adolescence[29] and early adulthood.[30] The key findings are that three phenotypes of wheeze are identifiable in early childhood, namely, transient early wheeze (TEW), persistent wheeze (PW), and late-onset wheeze (LOW). As discussed above, infants with TEW have abnormal lung function before the onset of their wheeze. However, a more recent assessment of this cohort at age 22 years[30] found the TEW group (with reduced airway function at birth) continued to have reduced airflow, and therefore may be at increased risk of subsequent chronic obstructive pulmonary disease. Those with PW (ie, wheezed both in the first 3 years and beyond) appear to have definite atopic asthma. Those with LOW have no wheeze in the first 3 years, but wheezed after the age of 3 years. Children with LOW have been termed non-atopic wheezers (or viral-induced wheeze), and appear to have a very mild form of asthma.[29] The distribution of these phenotypes in early childhood is as follows: approximately 50% of the Tucson cohort had never wheezed; 20% had TEW; 15% had LOW; and 15% PW. These figures indicate that most infants who wheeze in the first year of life do *not* have asthma.

DO PARENTS AND CHILDREN AGREE ON SYMPTOMS OF WHEEZE?

In an attempt to validate parent-reported exercise wheeze in older children (age 6 to 18 years), 97 children were assessed in summer camps in California.[31] Both criterion validity and construct validity were assessed by comparing reported symptoms on exercise with measured lung function following an exercise provocation test. Parents completed a telephone survey of their child's symptoms with exercise. As expected, parents generally report fewer exercise-related symptoms of wheeze than their children. Although there was some correlation between the variables on lung function testing with those reported by parents, these were generally weak. These results confirm other studies indicating that school-age children are more accurate reporters of wheeze than their parents. These data have important implications for the clinical care of asthma in school-age children.

ACOUSTIC ANALYSIS

Adult studies have highlighted problems with both accuracy (validity) and reliability (or repeatability) of respiratory signs using a stethoscope.[32–34] Given the increased difficulty of examining young, uncooperative children, the assumption is that errors will be substantially greater in pediatric practice. In an attempt to improve the utility of respiratory noises, computerized acoustic analysis has been evaluated. Most studies have been in adults and the published data in children are limited.

A small study (n = 15) of infants suggested a potential role for acoustic analysis.[32] In particular, the ability of acoustic analysis to clearly distinguish wheeze from rattle. Elphick and colleagues[32] found the acoustic properties of wheeze and rattle were quite distinct. Wheeze was characterized by a sinusoidal waveform, with several distinct peaks in the power spectrum display (**Fig. 3**). Rattle ("ruttle") was characterized by an irregular nonsinusoidal waveform, with diffuse peaks in the power spectrum display (**Fig. 4**). The rattle also had a more intense sound at a frequency of less than 600 Hz. Although the results in this study were encouraging, the 15 infants were carefully chosen to ensure they had only one distinct sound (7 with wheeze, 8 with a rattle).

Unfortunately, in a more recent study of young children by the same authors,[33] acoustic analysis proved to be disappointing. This study assessed the validity and reliability of acoustic analysis of respiratory noises in infants younger than 18 months. A total of 102 infants (mean age 5 months) who were in hospital with noisy breathing were evaluated. Each child was tested independently with both a stethoscope (by two experienced clinicians) and with acoustic analysis (also interpreted independently by two observers). There was effective blinding of those performing each of these measurements, and all measurements were taken either concurrently or immediately sequentially. All measures were taken in the right upper zone during tidal breathing. Most of these infants had acute viral bronchiolitis (58%) or an acute respiratory infection (eg, pneumonia, atelectasis, and cystic fibrosis). The investigators used predefined definitions for wheeze, rattle, and crackle on stethoscope, and predefined patterns for these three sounds on acoustic analysis.

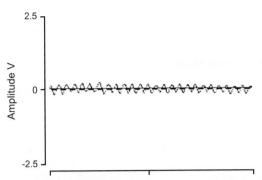

Fig. 3. Wheeze with characteristic sinusoidal pattern. (*From* Elphick HE, Ritson S, Rodgers H, et al. When a "wheeze" is not a wheeze: acoustic analysis of breath sounds in infants. Eur Respir J 2000;16:594; with permission.)

Both acoustic and stethoscope data were available for 100 infants. Agreement between stethoscope examination and acoustic analysis, using the Kappa (k) statistic (agreement over and above chance agreement)[35] was poor for both wheeze (k = 0.07) and rattles (k = 0.11), and fair only (k = 0.36) for crackles. Further, the ability to distinguish between the two audible noises (wheeze and rattles) using both stethoscope and acoustic analysis was poor. These validity results are similar, or worse, than those previously reported in adults. This is understandable, given the majority of the infants had acute bronchiolitis, which characteristically causes multiple noises on auscultation. Measures of reliability were also poor. There was poor agreement between the two experienced observers using a stethoscope for wheeze (k = 0.18), although for rattles and crackles, agreement was moderate (k = 0.53 and k = 0.46, respectively). Two observers also assessed the acoustic analysis results. Between-observer agreement using acoustic analysis was poor for both wheeze and rattles (k = 0.24 and 0.22, respectively), but moderate for crackles (k = 0.44).

In summary, in a study using vigorous methodology for evaluating a diagnostic test, the results for both validity and reliability of both the stethoscope and acoustic analysis were poor. Although it is possible that future development of acoustic analysis techniques could result in improved validity and reliability, at present it appears acoustic analysis has little to offer over the stethoscope in real life clinical situations in infants

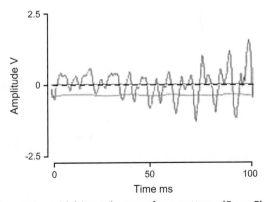

Fig. 4. Ruttles with nonsinusoidal irregular waveform pattern. (*From* Elphick HE, Ritson S, Rodgers H, et al. When a "wheeze" is not a wheeze: acoustic analysis of breath sounds in infants. Eur Respir J 2000;16:594; with permission.)

with noisy breathing. Moreover, there is poor agreement among clinicians when listening to infants and young children with common respiratory noises.

UTILITY OF TRACHEAL SOUND RECORDINGS

Several groups have used tracheal sound recordings in children, particularly to explore this method as a more sensitive indicator of wheeze in bronchial provocation testing of very young children. Godfrey and colleagues[36,37] used nebulized AMP challenge in 80 preschool children and found detection of wheeze acoustically to be a more sensitive way of detecting airway obstruction than the stethoscope (PC wheeze), thus enabling the challenge to be ceased earlier (and safer). Pediatric studies have also analyzed lung sounds and breathing patterns in infants with acute viral bronchiolitis to assess response to bronchodilators.[38] This group noted complex waveforms that differed from the sinusoidal waveforms described as typical of wheeze, indicating that multiple noises are characteristic of this clinical situation.[38]

Several studies have found tracheal sounds to be more sensitive than the stethoscope for detecting wheeze[39-41] in children with exercise-induced asthma. These findings support those of Godfrey and colleagues,[36] namely, that amplification of wheeze enables the clinician to detect this earlier than with a stethoscope. Further, continuous tracheal sound recording appears to be of more substantial value in objectively measuring cough, especially night cough.[40]

USE OF VIDEO QUESTIONNAIRES TO IDENTIFY STRIDOR

Video questionnaire has been used to identify upper airway abnormalities.[42] A group of 43 preschoolers (range 3 to 58 months, median 17 months) with noisy breathing were studied via fiberoptic bronchoscopy. Thirty (70%) had wheeze as their main symptom, 19 were clinician confirmed, whereas the other 11 had only parent-reported wheeze. Parents were shown previously validated video clips of wheeze, stridor, and other airway noises. Ten of the 30 parents who initially reported wheeze identified the noise as upper airway noise or stridor on the video. Of these 10 children, 7 had abnormal upper or central airway pathology on bronchoscopy. Conversely, none of the children whose parents correctly identified wheeze (on the video questionnaire) had an abnormality on bronchoscopy.

Thus, a validated video questionnaire can improve the ability of parents to identify upper airway abnormalities in children with parent-reported wheeze.

Unfortunately, clinicians do have problems distinguishing stridor from wheeze. The entity "exercise-induced inspiratory stridor" (or vocal cord dysfunction [VCD]) is an excellent illustration of the difficulty clinicians have distinguishing wheeze from stridor. Despite the noise being predominantly inspiratory in most patients, this condition is almost invariably incorrectly diagnosed as exercise-induced asthma (EIA). This is despite the noise being predominately inspiratory, coming on during, rather than after, exercise, rapid recovery, and lack of effect of short-acting beta-agonists. In a large case series (n = 95) of predominantly young women with VCD, almost half also had genuine asthma. However in those with VCD and no asthma, asthma had been misdiagnosed for an average of 5 years.

SUMMARY

A number of conclusions can be drawn from the research evidence on noisy breathing (**Box 1**). It is clear that there are major problems with both the accurate (valid) and

> **Box 1**
> **Summary points**
>
> - Noisy breathing is a common symptom in infants.
> - Parent-reported wheeze does not mean the infant or child has a wheeze.
> - Many infants and children with parent-reported wheeze have a "rattle" rather than wheeze.
> - A "rattle" should not be considered an "asthma symptom."
> - Clinicians do not always agree on the terminology of these common noises.
> - A major potential error is misclassifying stridor as a wheeze, and missing significant upper airway obstruction.
> - Published epidemiology rates of asthma in young children are based on "parent-reported" wheeze, and are clearly erroneous.
> - The use of videos of typical noises can improve the accuracy of parents' descriptions of noises.
> - Current technology (such as acoustic analysis) to improve the utility of these noises is disappointing.
> - More high-quality research is needed to establish the clinical utility of these noises.

reliable (reproducible) identification of "respiratory noises." This is particularly so when the noise is "parent reported," and not confirmed by a clinician.

Clearly, clinicians must exercise great care when diagnosing specific types of noisy breathing to ensure it is not incorrectly labeled. An error in recognition will result in the clinician assuming a specific anatomic level of airway obstruction, a misleading differential diagnosis, inappropriate investigation, and treatment. Clinicians need to consider the whole constellation of symptoms and signs, and not totally focus on the specific "type" of noise. In particular, any associated symptoms or signs, such as breathlessness, cough, voice changes, and signs of a viral respiratory infection. This is especially so with misclassification of a "rattle" as a wheeze, resulting in unnecessary and useless asthma treatment. This is of real concern with inhaled corticosteroids, because the lack of response can result in an escalation of the dose, resulting in side effects. A more sinister error is misclassifying stridor as wheeze, and running the risk of missing potentially severe, life-threatening upper airway obstruction.

Given the high error rate with "parent-reported wheeze" there is a need to reexamine the extensive literature on the epidemiology of wheeze in infants and young children, since this is derived from parent-reported wheeze (ie, unconfirmed by a clinician). Clearly a large percentage of these children have a "rattle" rather than a wheeze, and it is inappropriate to call parent-reported wheeze an "asthma symptom."[20] This inflation of the rate of childhood asthma symptoms is particularly prominent in infants and preschool young children. Finally, it is obvious we need more high-quality research evidence to derive better evidence on the clinical utility of these noises, and their natural history (see **Box 1**).

REFERENCES

1. Brown M, Wayne J. Clinical assessment and diagnostic approach to common problems. In: Taussig L, Landau LI, editors. Pediatric respiratory medicine. Missouri: Mosby; 1999. p. 136–52.
2. McGee S. Understanding the evidence: diagnostic accuracy of physical findings. Evidence-based physical diagnosis. Philadelphia: W.B Saunders Company; 2001. p. 3–23.

3. GRADE Working Party. Grading quality of evidence and strength of recommendations. BMJ 2004;328:1–8.

4. Fakhoury K, Seilheimer D, Hoppin A. Approach to wheezing in children. 2008. Available at: http://www.uptodate.com. Accessed April 17, 2008.

5. Martinez F, Wright A, Taussig L, et al. Asthma and wheezing in the first six years of life. The Group Health Medical Associated. N Engl J Med 1995;332(3):133–8.

6. Turner S, Palmer L, Rye P, et al. The relationship between infant airway function, childhood airway responsiveness, and asthma. Am J Respir Crit Care Med 2004; 169(8):921–7.

7. Elphick H, Sherlock P, Foxall G, et al. Survey of respiratory sounds in infants. Arch Dis Child 2001;84:35–9.

8. Elphick H, Ritson S, MI E. Differential respónse of wheezes and ruttles to anticholinergics. Arch Dis Child 2002;86:280–1.

9. Olney D, Greinwald JJ, Smith R, et al. Laryngomalacia and its treatment. Laryngoscope 1999;109(11):1770–5.

10. Quintero D, Fakhoury K. Assessment of stridor in children. 2008. Available at: http://www.uptodate.com. Accessed April 17, 2008.

11. Gozal D, Burnside M. Increased upper airway collapsibility in children with obstructive sleep apnea during wakefulness. Am J Respir Crit Care Med 2004; 169:163–7.

12. Sterni L. Evaluation of snoring or suspected obstructive sleep-hypopnea in children. 2008. Available at: http://www.uptodate.com. Accessed April 17, 2008.

13. Thornton A, Morley C, Hewson P, et al. Symptoms in 298 infants under 6 months old, seen at home. Arch Dis Child 1990;65:280–5.

14. Lewis S, Richards D, Bynner J, et al. Prospective study of risk factors for early and persistent wheezing in childhood. Eur Respir J 1995;8(3): 349–56.

15. Butland B, Strachan D. Asthma onset and relapse in adult life: the British 1958 birth cohort study. Ann Allergy Asthma Immunol 2007;98(4):337–43.

16. Kull I, Bergstrom A, Lilja G, et al. Fish consumption during the first year of life and development of allergic diseases during childhood. Allergy 2006;61(8):1009–15.

17. Clarisse B, Demattei C, Nikasinovic L, et al. Bronchial obstructive phenotypes in the first year of life among Paris birth cohort infants. Pediatr Allergy Immunol 2008; [epub ahead of print].

18. Menezes A, Hallal P, Muino A, et al. Risk factors for wheezing in early adolescence: a prospective birth cohort study in Brazil. Ann Allergy Asthma Immunol 2007;98(5):427–31.

19. Samet J, Cushing A, Lambert W, et al. Comparability of parent reports of respiratory illness with clinical diagnosis in infants. Am Rev Respir Dis 1993;148:441–6.

20. Asher M, Montefort S, Bjorksten B, et al. Worldwide time trends in the prevalence of symptoms of asthma, allergic rhinoconjuctivits, and eczema in childhood: ISAAC phases one and three repeat multicountry cross-sectional surveys. Lancet 2006;368:733–43.

21. Cane R, Ranganathan S, McKenzie S. What do parents of wheezy children understand by "wheeze"? Arch Dis Child 2000;82:327–32.

22. Chong Neto H, Rosario N, Dela Bianca AC, et al. Validation of a questionnaire for epidemiologic studies of wheezing in infants. Pediatr Allergy Immunol 2007;18:86–7.

23. Lowe L, Murray C, Martin L, et al. Reported versus confirmed wheeze and lung function in early life. Arch Dis Child 2004;89:540–3.

24. Cane R, McKenzie S. Parents' interpretations of children's respiratory symptoms on video. Arch Dis Child 2001;84:31–4.

25. Crane J, Mallol J, Beasley R, et al. Agreement between written and video questions for comparing asthma symptoms in ISAAC. Eur Respir J 2003;21(3):455–61.
26. Riedler J, Reade T, Dalton M, et al. Hypertonic saline challenge in an epidemiological survey of asthma in children. Am J Respir Crit Care Med 1994;150(6 Pt 1):1632–9.
27. Buechele G, Rzekhak P, Weinmayr G, et al. Assessing bronchial responsiveness to hypertonic saline using the Stepwise Protocol of Phase Two of the International Study of Asthma and Allergies in Childhood (ISAAC II). Pediatr Pulmonol 2007; 42:131–40.
28. Turner S, Leone C, Harbour P, et al. Early rattles, purrs and whistles as predictors of later wheeze. 2008. Available at: http://adc.bmjjournals.com. Accessed April 17, 2008.
29. Morgan W, Stern D, Sherrill D, et al. Outcome of asthma and wheezing in the first 6 years of life. Am J Respir Crit Care Med 2005;172(10):1253–8.
30. Stern D, Morgan W, Wright A, et al. Poor airway function in early infancy and lung function by age 22 years: a non-selective longitudinal cohort study. Lancet 2007; 370(9589):717–9.
31. Lara M, Duan N, Sherbourne C, et al. Differences between child and parents of symptoms among Latino children with asthma. 1998;106(2). Available at: http://www.pediatrics.org. Accessed April 17, 2008.
32. Elphick H, Ritson S, Rodgers H, et al. When a "wheeze" is not a wheeze: acoustic analysis of breath sounds in infants. Eur Respir J 2000;16:593–7.
33. Elphick H, Lancaster G, Solis A, et al. Validity and reliability of acoustic analysis of respiratory sounds in infants. Arch Dis Child 2004;89:1059–63.
34. Dalmay F, Antonini M, Marquest R, et al. Acoustic properties of the normal chest. Eur Respir J 1995;8:1761–9.
35. Altman D. Some common problems in medical research—inter-rater agreement. Practical statistics for medical research. London: Chapman & Hall; 1991. p. 404–8.
36. Godfrey S, Uwyyed K, Springer C, et al. Is clinical wheezing reliable as the endpoint for bronchial challenges in preschool children? Pediatr Pulmonol 2004;37:193–200.
37. Godfrey S, Shlomo C, Avital A, et al. Timing and nature of wheezing at the endpoint of a bronichial challenge in preschool children. Pediatr Pulmonol 2005;39:262–7.
38. Tal A, Sanchez I, Pasterkamp H. Respirosonography in infants with acute bronchiolitis. Am J Dis Child 1991;145(12):1405–10.
39. Rietveld S, Dooijes E. Characteristics and diagnostic significance of wheezes during exercise-induced airway obstruction in children with asthma. Chest 1996;110(3):624–31.
40. Rietveld S, Lous H, Rijssenbeek-Nouwens L. Diagnostics of spontaneous cough in childhood asthma. Results of continuous tracheal sound recording in the homes of children. Chest 1998;113(1):50–4.
41. Rietveld S, Oud M, Rijssenbeek-Nouwens L, et al. Characteristics and diagnostic significance of spontaneous wheezing in children. J Asthma 1999;36(4):351–8.
42. Saglani S, McKenzie S, Bush A, et al. A video questionnaire identifies upper airway abnormalities in preschool children with reported wheeze. Arch Dis Child 2005;90:961–4.

Cough

Anne B. Chang, MBBS, MPHTM, FRACP, PhD

KEYWORDS

- Cough • Evidence-based medicine • Children
- Systematic review • Clinical evaluation • Protocol

The prevalence of chronic cough (5%–10%)[1,2] is likely dependent on the setting, age of the cohort studied, instrument used, and definition of chronic cough.[3] Cough as a symptom is almost ubiquitous for the entire respiratory system, ranging from uncomplicated minor respiratory tract infections (RTI) to major illnesses, such as cystic fibrosis. Rarely, it may be a symptom of extrapulmonary disease, such as cardiac abnormalities. Most acute cough in children is related to RTIs. Not surprisingly, cough is often trivialized. Cough, however, especially when chronic, significantly impacts on parents' quality-of-life scores.[4,5]

THE BURDEN AND BRIEF PATHOPHYSIOLOGY OF COUGH

The burden of cough is also reflected in the billions of dollars spent annually on over-the-counter (OTC) cough medications,[6] and the number of consultations sought for cough. In an Australian study, the number of medical consultations for coughing illness in the last 12 months was high: more than 80% of children had greater than or equal to five doctor visits, and 53% had greater than 10.[5] Parents of children with chronic cough did not have symptoms of anxiety or depression but were stressed.[5] This is in contrast to adults with chronic cough, which is associated with the presence of depression and anxiety.[7,8] Clinicians need to be cognizant of the stress parents have when dealing with children with chronic cough. The reasons for parental fears and concerns included cause of the cough, fear of choking, and long-term respiratory damage.[1,5,9]

Physiologically, cough has three phases: (1) inspiratory, (2) compressive, and (3) expiratory.[10] The inspiratory phase consists of inhaling a variable amount of air, which serves to lengthen the expiratory muscles, optimizing the length-tension relationship. The compressive phase consists of a very brief (200 millisecond) closure of the glottis to maintain lung volume as intrathoracic pressure builds (up to 300 mm Hg in adults) because of isometric contraction of the expiratory muscles against a closed glottis. The expiratory phase starts with opening of the glottis, releasing a brief (30–50

A.B. Chang is funded by the Royal Children's Hospital Foundation and the National Health and Medical Research Council, Australia.

Menzies School of Health Research, Charles Darwin University, Queensland Children's Respiratory Centre, Royal Children's Hospital, Herston Road, Brisbane, Queensland 4029, Australia
E-mail address: annechang@ausdoctors.net

Pediatr Clin N Am 56 (2009) 19–31
doi:10.1016/j.pcl.2008.10.002
0031-3955/08/$ – see front matter © 2009 Elsevier Inc. All rights reserved.

pediatric.theclinics.com

millisecond) supramaximal expiratory flow[11] (up to 12 L/s in adults, also termed the "cough spike") followed by lower (3–4 L/s) expiratory flows lasting a further 200 to 500 millisecond.[10] Dynamic compression of the airways occurs during the expiratory phase and the high-velocity expulsion of gas (air) sweeps airway debris along. Airway debris and secretions are also swept proximally by ciliary activity. Cough also enhances mucociliary clearance in both healthy individuals and those with lung disease.[12]

Cough can be voluntarily initiated or suppressed, except when it is part of the laryngeal expiratory reflex when the larynx is mechanically stimulated by foreign materials. Physiologists describe two basic types of cough: laryngeal cough (a true reflex, also known as "expiratory reflex") and tracheobronchial cough. Laryngeal cough protects the airways from airway aspiration. Tracheobronchial cough is initiated distal to the larynx and can be volitional. It is primarily stimulated by chemoreceptors in the lower airways and can also be mechanically stimulated.[3] The primary function of tracheobronchial cough is airway clearance and maintenance of the mucociliary apparatus. It has been argued that differentiating the types of cough and what constitutes as a cough is important.[13] Clinicians remain certain, however, what cough is in the clinical setting.

The knowledge of cough neurophysiology has significantly advanced in recent years, although much of the work is based on animal models and may have limited applicability to humans because significant interspecies differences exist.[14] Readers are referred to recent reviews[14–17] for in-depth aspects of cough-related neurophysiology. As a gross oversimplification, the cough pathway can be compartmentalized to the afferent arms (from cough stimulus to the respiratory center) and efferent arms (from respiratory center to respiratory muscles, larynx, and pelvic muscles) of the cough pathway; they are likely to be influenced by a bidirectional feedback loop, but this has not yet been clearly established. Receptors involved in cough are terminations of vagal afferents in airway mucosa and submucosa.[14,18,19] These afferent receptors have different sensitivity to different stimuli and are unequally distributed in the airways; generally, the larynx and proximal large airways are more mechanosensitive and less chemosensitive than peripheral large airways. The existence of distinct cough receptors, widely assumed to be present and first proposed by Widdicombe,[20] was only recently proved.[15,18] Generation of action potentials (depolarization of the terminal membrane) from these receptors is subclassified into ionotropic receptors (they cause generator potentials by acting on ligand-gated ion channels) and metabotropic receptors (they act indirectly on ligand-gated ion channels by G-protein coupled receptors).[17,21]

These cough and airway receptors mediated through the vagus nerve, jugular, and nodose ganglions extend to the nucleus tractus solitaris, which is the first central nervous system synaptic contact of these afferent fibers.[22] Second-order neurons from the nucleus tractus solitaris have polysynaptic connections with the central cough generator, which is also the respiratory pattern generator.[16,22] Nucleus tractus solitaris is postulated to be the site of greatest modulatory influence and plasticity. The mechanisms underpinning chronic cough have been likened to that of chronic pain,[3] and increased neurogenic markers have been described in children with increased cough receptor sensitivity.[23] The intrathoracic pressure and effects of it generated by cough may also perpetuate the chronic cough cycle as suggested by a recent animal study that showed pressure effects enhance cough sensitivity.[24]

An effective cough is dependent on generation of high linear velocities and interaction between flowing gas and mucus in the airways.[10] This is dependent on the integrity of the mechanisms described previously. Other physical characteristics also influence cough efficiency: adequate airway caliber (efficiency decreased in presence of flow-limitation[25] [eg, severe tracheomalacia]); mucous physical properties (sputum tenacity, adhesiveness, water content, and so forth);[10] and respiratory muscle strength.[10] The importance of the integrity of the cough reflex is reflected when it is impaired. Aspiration lung disease occurs in those with a dysfunctional laryngeal reflex (eg, central neurologic problems and multiple organ dysfunction).[26] When the muscular apparatus for an effective cough is impaired (eg, muscular dystrophy), recurrent mucus retention and atelectasis occurs.

MANAGEMENT OF THE SYMPTOM OF COUGH

The overall management of cough entails an evaluation for the following: (1) etiology, which includes assessing if further tests or treatment are required; (2) defining exacerbation factors (eg, exposure to environmental tobacco smoke); and (3) defining the effect on the child and parents.

Defining the Etiology of the Cough

The most likely etiology depends on the setting, selection criteria of children studied, follow-up rate, depth of clinical history, examination, and investigations performed. In defining the etiology, it is helpful to define cough types in accordance to different constructs. Pediatric cough can be classified in several constructs based on (1) timeframe (acute, chronic); (2) likelihood of an identifiable underlying primary etiology (specific and nonspecific cough); and (3) characteristic (moist versus dry). For clinical practicality timeframe is commonly used, divided into acute (<2 weeks), subacute (2–4 weeks), and chronic (>4 weeks) cough. There are no studies that have clearly defined when cough should be defined as chronic (variably defined from >4–8 weeks).[27–29] Cough related to an upper RTI resolves within 10 days in 50% of children and by 25 days in 90%;[30] arguably, childhood chronic cough should be defined as persistent daily cough of greater than 4 weeks. Chronic cough is further subdivided into specific cough (cough associated with other symptoms and signs that are suggestive of an associated or underlying problem) and nonspecific cough (dry cough in the absence of any identifiable respiratory disease or known etiology). These classifications, however, are not mutually exclusive.

Acute cough and expected cough

Although acute RTIs are the most common cause of acute cough in children, all children should be assessed for symptoms and signs of more serious cause, such as inhaled foreign body. In 8% to 12% of children with upper RTIs complications develop.[30] These conditions are discussed elsewhere in this issue.

Expected cough is the presence of cough in situations where cough is the norm, such as during an acute respiratory infection. In most children, acute cough is self-limiting and treatment, if any, should be directed at the cause rather than the symptom of cough. OTC medications for cough confer no benefit in the symptomatic control of cough or on the sleep pattern of children or parents and may cause harm. Steam inhalation, vitamin C, zinc, and Echinacea for upper RTI have little benefit, if any, for symptomatic relief of cough. Systematic reviews have also shown that oral or inhaled β_2-agonists also confer no benefit in children with acute cough and no evidence of airflow obstruction. Antimicrobials are nonbeneficial in acute cough associated with colds. In contrast, honey (0.5–2 teaspoons depending on age) has been shown to be useful in reducing nocturnal cough and improving sleep quality of parents and children with an acute upper RTI-associated cough (**Table 1**).[31]

Table 1
Recommendations for possible interventions for nonspecific cough in children

Therapy	Recommendation	Grade[a]	Type and Strength of Evidence	Time to Response[b]
Antihistamines				
Nonsedating	Not generally recommended unless symptoms of rhinitis coexist	Moderate	SR with RCTs[57,58]	1 wk
Sedating	Sedating antihistamines should not be used, strong			Not relevant
Antimicrobials	For wet cough only, strong	High	SR with RCTs[40]	1–2 wk
Asthma-type therapy				
Cromones	Not recommended, weak	Very low	SR with single open trial[59]	2 wk
Anticholinergics	Not recommended, weak	Very low	SR, no studies in children RCTs[60]	No data
Inhaled CS	Not generally recommended unless symptoms of asthma present, strong	Moderate	SR with RCTs[50,51]	2–4 wk
Oral CS	Not recommended, weak	Low	No data	
β_2-agonist (oral or inhaled)	Not generally recommended unless symptoms of asthma present, weak	Moderate	SR with RCTs[61] RCT[50]	Not relevant
Theophylline	Not recommended, weak	Very low	SR, no studies[62]	1–2 wk
Leukotriene receptor antagonist	Not recommended unless symptoms of asthma present, weak	Very low	SR, observational study[63]	2–3 wk

	Recommendation[a]	Grading[a]	Evidence	Length[b]
GERD therapy				
Motility agents	Not recommended as empiric therapy, weak	Very low	SR with single trial[64]	Not relevant
Acid suppression	Not recommended as empiric therapy, weak	Very low	SR with no RCTs in children[64]	
Food-thickening or antireflux formula	Consider if other symptoms of reflux present (infants only), weak	Moderate	SR with RCTs[64]	1 wk
Fundoplication			Systematic review[64]	
Herbal antitussive therapy	Not recommended, weak	Very low	No data	
Nasal therapy				
Nasal steroids	Not generally recommended unless symptoms of rhinitis coexist, weak	Low	RCT[65] Beneficial when combined with antibiotics for sinusitis[66]	1–2 wk
Other nasal sprays	Not recommended, strong	Very low	No data	
Over-the-counter cough medications	Not recommended, strong	High	SR with RCTs[57,67–69]	Not relevant
Other therapies				
Steam, vapor, rubs	Consider rubs but not vapor or steam, weak	Low	No data	
Honey	Recommended if no contraindications for using of honey, strong	Moderate	Single RCT on acute cough[31]	1 d
Physiotherapy	Not recommended unless cough related to suppurative lung disease, weak	Very low	No data in cough that is unrelated to suppurative-like lung diseases	

Abbreviations: CS, corticosteroids; GERD, gastro-esophageal reflux disease; RCT, randomized controlled trials; SR, systematic review.

[a] Grading of evidence and recommendations.[70]
[b] Length in time for cough to resolve or substantially improve as reported by trialists.

Subacute and chronic cough

Chronic cough differs from acute cough in its management and etiologic factors. The timeframe chosen for chronic cough is similar in the Australian[27] and American[28] guidelines, but differs from the British guidelines.[29] The difference likely reflects the lack of evidence. It is unknown whether the primary stimulus for chronic cough in many children is identical to that for acute cough. Further, it is unknown why the cough associated with common acute viral upper RTIs resolves in most, yet persists in some. Presumably, however, both the specific microbe (eg, cough is more likely to be prolonged after a potent respiratory infection, such as pertussis) or host factors (eg, genetic predisposition to bronchitis) play a role. Unfortunately, there are no studies that have clearly defined when cough should be defined as chronic. Studies have shown that cough related to upper RTIs resolves within 1 to 3 weeks in greater than 90% of children.[30,32] It is logical to define chronic cough as daily cough lasting greater than 4 weeks; published definitions of chronic cough in children have varied from 3 to 12 weeks.[33] In contrast, the current definition of chronic cough in adults is 8 weeks. The pediatric definition is based on the natural history of acute upper RTIs in children[30,32] and the knowledge that pediatric respiratory illness has important differences than that in adults.[33] For example, such conditions as a missed foreign body, which is more common in children (especially in those aged ≤5 years), can lead to permanent lung damage.[34]

Classically recognizable cough

Certain cough characteristics, such as "croupy or brassy cough," are classically taught to point to specific etiologies in children. Data on the sensitivity and specificity of each classic recognizable cough type are limited; the data for brassy cough (for tracheomalacia diagnosed at bronchoscopy) were 0.57 and 0.81, respectively.[35] Kappa value for interobserver agreement for brassy cough was good at 0.79 (95% confidence interval [CI], 0.73–0.86).[35] Although a pertussis-like cough in children is generally caused by *Bordetella pertussis* infection, it may also be caused by adenovirus, parainfluenza viruses, respiratory syncytial virus, and mycoplasma.[36] By contrast, the quality of cough has been shown to be of little use in adults.[37] Chronic productive purulent cough is always pathologic. In obtaining a history in a child with chronic cough, questions specific for classically recognizable cough, such as an exposure to illness history (eg, pertussis and tuberculosis), should be obtained.

Wet-moist-productive cough versus dry cough

Even when airway secretions are present, young children rarely expectorate sputum; hence, "wet-moist" cough is the preferable term rather than "productive" cough.[38,39] The distinction of dry and wet-moist cough has been shown to be both valid and reliable. In a study of 106 children, cough quality (wet or dry) assessed by clinicians had good agreement with parents' assessment (K = 0.75; 95% CI, 0.58–0.93), and had good sensitivity (0.75) and specificity (0.79), when compared with bronchoscopy findings.[35] The use of wet versus dry cough for predicting etiology of cough or response to treatment has not been shown in children, except in protracted bronchitis.[40]

Specific and nonspecific chronic cough

Clinical signs and symptoms that are suggestive of an underlying pulmonary or systemic disorder are termed "specific cough pointers" (**Box 1**).[27] When any of these pointers are present, the cough is referred to as "specific cough." If specific cough pointers are present, further investigations and management of the primary pulmonary pathology is usually warranted. If not, a counsel, watch, wait, and review approach is suggested. This approach is suggested for nonspecific cough (dry cough in the

---

Box 1
Pointers for presence of specific cough

Auscultatory findings (wheeze, crepitations or crackles, differential breath sounds)

Cough characteristics (eg, cough with choking, cough quality, cough starting from birth)

Cardiac abnormalities (including murmurs)

Chest pain

Chest wall deformity

Daily moist or productive cough

Digital clubbing

Dyspnea (exertional or at rest)

Exposure to pertussis, tuberculosis, and so forth

Failure to thrive

Feeding difficulties or dysphagia (including choking or vomiting)

Hemoptysis

Immune deficiency

Medications or drugs (angiotensin-converting enzyme inhibitor)

Neurodevelopmental abnormality

Recurrent pneumonia

---

absence of specific cough pointers). Such cough is more likely to undergo natural resolution.[41] A dry cough may be the early phase of a wet cough,[42] however, and children should be reviewed and attention to exacerbation factors and parental concerns (see later) are warranted.

In selected children with nonspecific cough, diagnoses with simple treatment options, (eg, asthma and complications of upper RTIs, such as sinusitis and bronchitis) may be considered. The evidence for the association between asthma[3,43] and upper airway disorders and cough is not as straightforward in children, however, as it is in adults.[33,44] The use of isolated cough as a marker of asthma is controversial with more recent evidence (clinical and community epidemiologic studies) showing that in most children, isolated cough does not represent asthma.[3,45]

Investigations

As a minimum, all children with chronic cough should have a spirometry (if age appropriate) and chest radiograph performed.[27,28] The validity of this has been shown.[41] When a chest radiograph taken for chronic cough is abnormal, the odds ratio of an specific etiology was 3.16 (95% CI, 1.32–7.62).[41] Other tests to identify the etiology of nonspecific cough have limited applicability in pediatrics. Identification of airway hyperresponsiveness, diagnostic for asthma in adults, is of limited use in children because of interpretation difficulties, and reliable tests can only be performed in older children in whom cough is less common. The three most common causes of chronic cough in adults (gastroesophageal reflux disease, asthma, and upper airways syndrome)[46] are not as common in children.[47] Increased cough sensitivity is found in most conditions causing chronic cough but its use is limited to research.[28]

Except when classical asthma is the etiology, children with specific cough usually require additional tests (chest high-resolution CT scan, bronchoscopy, video fluoroscopy, echocardiograph, sleep polysomnography, nuclear medicine scans, immunologic assessment, and so forth). The role of these tests for evaluation of lung disease is beyond the scope of this article because it encompasses the entire spectrum of pediatric respiratory illness.

MEDICATIONS

Treatment for subacute and chronic cough should be etiologically based, and that for specific cough is beyond the scope of this article. Cough is subjected to the period-effect (ie, spontaneous resolution of cough); the benefit of placebo treatment for cough has been reported to be as high as 85% and non–placebo-controlled intervention studies have to be interpreted with caution.[3] Evidence (or lack of) on treatment trials for nonspecific cough are summarized in **Table 1**. Systematic reviews have concluded that OTC cough remedies have little benefit in the symptomatic control of childhood cough. Significant morbidity and mortality[48] from OTC cough remedies can occur and OTC drugs are common unintentional ingestions in children aged less than 5 years.[49] Cochrane reviews on symptomatic treatment of cough have shown that diphenhydramine is not beneficial for pertussis-related cough; cromones and anticholinergics have little, if any, role in nonspecific chronic childhood cough; and 10 days of antimicrobials reduces persistent cough in children with chronic nasal discharge but benefits are modest (number needed to treat was 8). Antimicrobials may be indicated for subacute and chronic moist cough; two randomized controlled trials (RCTs) showed predominance of *Moraxella catarrhalis*. Meta-analysis on antimicrobials for acute bronchitis in older children (aged >8 years) and adults showed a small benefit of 0.58 days but with significantly more adverse events. Systematic review of uncomplicated sinusitis in children showed that the clinical improvement rate was 88% with antimicrobial and 60% on no antimicrobial. There are only two published RCTs on inhaled corticosteroids for nonspecific cough in children and both groups cautioned against prolonged use.[50,51] In the North American guidelines for pediatric gastroesophageal reflux, the conclusion on cough and gastroesophageal reflux disease section was "there is insufficient evidence and experience in children for a uniform approach to diagnosis and treatment."[52]

If medications are trialed for nonspecific cough, the child should be reviewed and time to response considered. For example, in asthma-related cough, earlier non-RCT studies in adults and children that used medications for asthma for the era (ie, nonsteroidal anti-inflammatory drugs, theophylline, terbutaline, major tranquillizers) reported that cough completely resolved by 2 to 7 days.[3] Time to response is defined as the expected length of time cough resolution occurred in studies where the cough treated was related to the etiology defined.

Defining Exacerbation Factors

When reviewing any child with cough irrespective of the etiology, exacerbation factors should be explored, although no RCTs have examined the effect of cessation of environmental pollutants on cough. There is little doubt that children with environmental tobacco smoke exposure have increased risk of having chronic[53,54] and recurrent cough.[55] The American Academy of Pediatrics policy on tobacco includes recommendations for tobacco cessation.[56] Other exacerbation factors include exposure to pollutants and secondary gains from having a cough.

Defining Effect on Child and Parent

Parents presenting to doctors for their children's cough have significant concerns that causes parental stress.[5] The most significant concerns and worries expressed by

---

Box 2
When a child with chronic cough presents

1. A complete medical examination with particular attention to the cardiorespiratory systems and a focus on

    a. The clinical pattern

       Characteristic cough (eg, pertussis, tracheomalacic cough, see **Box 1**)

   Wet or dry cough? Protracted bronchitis?

       Presence of specific cough pointers to differentiate specific from nonspecific cough, (**Table 2**) (GRADE, moderate; Level of evidence, cohort studies)[41,47]

    b. Presence of exacerbation factors (eg, environmental tobacco smoke, curtailment of physical activity)

    c. Effect of the cough on the child and parents, and explore their concerns (see previously) (GRADE, moderate; Level of evidence, cohort studies)

2. All should undergo

   Chest radiograph

   Spirometry (if aged >3 years) (GRADE, moderate; Level of evidence, cohort studies)

3. They should be further investigated and likely require referral if

   Specific cough pointers are present (other than asthma) (see **Table 2**)

   Cough has not resolved with treatment trials (GRADE, moderate; Level of evidence, cohort studies)

4. A "wait, reassess, and review" approach is recommended for children with nonspecific cough because medications are generally not efficacious for nonspecific cough (see **Table 1**). If medications are trialed, a reassessment is recommended in 2 to 3 weeks, which is the time to response for most medications.[27,28] (GRADE, moderate; Level of evidence, cohort studies and RCTs)

---

parents are feelings of frustration, upset, sleepless nights, awakened at night, helplessness, stress, and feeling sorry for the child. Items that bothered the parents most were the cause of cough, cough relating to a serious illness, child not sleeping well, and cough causing damage.[5] Previous studies have described parental fears

---

Table 2
Characteristic or classical types of cough

Cough Type	Suggested Underlying Process
Barking or brassy cough	Croup, tracheomalacia, habit cough
Honking	Psychogenic
Paroxysmal (± inspiratory "whoop")	Pertussis and parapertussis
Staccato	Chlamydia in infants
Cough productive of casts	Plastic bronchitis or asthma
Chronic wet cough in mornings only	Suppurative lung disease

Data from Chang AB, Glomb WB. Guidelines for evaluating chronic cough in pediatrics: ACCP evidence-based clinical practice guidelines. Chest 2006;129:260S–83S; and Chang AB. Causes, assessment and measurement in children. In: Chung KF, Widdicombe JG, Boushey HA, editors. Cough: causes, mechanisms and therapy. London: Blackwell Science; 2003. p. 57–73.

of their child dying from choking, asthma attack, or cot death, and permanent chest damage, disturbed sleep, and relief of discomfort.[1,9] These concerns are often not appreciated by health professionals and exploration of parental expectations and fears is valuable when managing a child with a chronic cough.

Providing parents with information on the expected time length of resolution of RTIs may reduce anxiety in parents and the need for medication use. Parental and professional expectations and doctors' perception of patients' expectations influences consulting rates and prescription of medications in RTIs. Educational input is best done with consultation about the child's specific condition because written information without consultation has only modest benefit in changing perceptions and behavior. It is also known that information available from the Internet provides incorrect advice on the home management of cough in children.

SUMMARY

Box 2 lists the steps to take when a child with chronic cough presents to the clinician.

REFERENCES

1. Faniran AO, Peat JK, Woolcock AJ. Persistent cough: is it asthma? Arch Dis Child 1998;79:411–4.
2. Faniran AO, Peat JK, Woolcock AJ. Measuring persistent cough in children in epidemiological studies: development of a questionnaire and assessment of prevalence in two countries. Chest 1999;115:434–9.
3. Chang AB. State of the art: cough, cough receptors, and asthma in children. Pediatr Pulmonol 1999;28:59–70.
4. Newcombe PA, Sheffield JK, Juniper EF, et al. Development of a parent-proxy cough-specific QOL questionnaire: clinical impact vs psychometric evaluations. Chest 2008;133:386–95.
5. Marchant JM, Newcombe PA, Juniper EF, et al. What is the burden of chronic cough for families? Chest 2008;134:303–9.
6. Irwin RS. Introduction to the diagnosis and management of cough: ACCP evidence-based clinical practice guidelines. Chest 2006;129:25S–7S.
7. Dicpinigaitis PV, Tso R, Banauch G. Prevalence of depressive symptoms among patients with chronic cough. Chest 2006;130:1839–43.
8. Ludviksdottir D, Bjornsson E, Janson C, et al. Habitual coughing and its associations with asthma, anxiety, and gastroesophageal reflux. Chest 1996;109: 1262–8.
9. Cornford CS, Morgan M, Ridsdale L. Why do mothers consult when their children cough? Fam Pract 1993;10:193–6.
10. McCool FD. Global physiology and pathophysiology of cough. Chest, in press.
11. Bennett WD, Zeman KL. Effect of enhanced supramaximal flows on cough clearance. J Appl Phys 1994;77:1577–83.
12. Oldenburg FA, Dolovich MB, Montgomery JM, et al. Effects of postural drainage, exercise and cough on mucus clearance in chronic bronchitis. Am Rev Respir Dis 1979;120:739–45.
13. Widdicombe J, Fontana G. Cough: what's in a name? Eur Respir J 2006;28:10–5.
14. Canning BJ. Anatomy and neurophysiology of the cough reflex. Chest 2006; 129(Suppl 1):33S–47S.
15. Canning BJ, Mazzone SB, Meeker SN, et al. Identification of the tracheal and laryngeal afferent neurones mediating cough in anaesthetized guinea-pigs. J Physiol 2004;557:543–58.

16. Shannon R, Baekey DM, Morris KF, et al. Production of reflex cough by brainstem respiratory networks. Pulm Pharmacol Ther 2004;17:369–76.
17. Canning BJ. Anatomy and neurophysiology of the cough reflex: ACCP evidence-based clinical practice guidelines. Chest 2006;129:33S–47S.
18. Mazzone SB. Sensory regulation of the cough reflex. Pulm Pharmacol Ther 2004; 17:361–8.
19. Undem BJ, Carr MJ, Kollarik M. Physiology and plasticity of putative cough fibres in the Guinea pig. Pulm Pharmacol Ther 2002;15:193–8.
20. Widdicombe J. The race to explore the pathway to cough: who won the silver medal? Am J Respir Crit Care Med 2001;164:729–30.
21. Lee MG, Kollarik M, Chuaychoo B, et al. Ionotropic and metabotropic receptor mediated airway sensory nerve activation. Pulm Pharmacol Ther 2004;17: 355–60.
22. Bonham AC, Sekizawa S, Joad JP. Plasticity of central mechanisms for cough. Pulm Pharmacol Ther 2004;17:453–7.
23. Chang AB, Gibson PG, Ardill J, et al. Calcitonin gene-related peptide relates to cough sensitivity in children with chronic cough. Eur Respir J 2007;30:66–72.
24. Hara J, Fujimura M, Ueda A, et al. Effect of pressure stress applied to the airway on cough reflex sensitivity in guinea pigs. Am J Respir Crit Care Med 2008;177: 585–92.
25. Smaldone GC, Messina MS. Flow limitation, cough, and patterns of aerosol deposition in humans. J Appl Physiol 1985;59:515–20.
26. Weir K, McMahon S, Barry L, et al. Oropharyngeal aspiration and pneumonia in children. Pediatr Pulmonol 2007;42:1024–31.
27. Chang AB, Landau LI, van Asperen PP, et al. The Thoracic Society of Australia and New Zealand. Position statement. Cough in children: definitions and clinical evaluation. Med J Aust 2006;184:398–403.
28. Chang AB, Glomb WB. Guidelines for evaluating chronic cough in pediatrics: ACCP evidence-based clinical practice guidelines. Chest 2006;129:260S–83S.
29. Shields MD, Bush A, Everard ML, et al. British thoracic society guidelines recommendations for the assessment and management of cough in children. Thorax 2008;63:iii1–iii15.
30. Hay AD, Wilson A, Fahey T, et al. The duration of acute cough in pre-school children presenting to primary care: a prospective cohort study. Fam Pract 2003;20: 696–705.
31. Paul IM, Beiler J, McMonagle A, et al. Effect of honey, dextromethorphan, and no treatment on nocturnal cough and sleep quality for coughing children and their parents. Arch Pediatr Adolesc Med 2007;161:1140–6.
32. Hay AD, Wilson AD. The natural history of acute cough in children aged 0 to 4 years in primary care: a systematic review. Br J Gen Pract 2002;52:401–9.
33. Chang AB. Cough: are children really different to adults? Cough 2005;1:7.
34. Karakoc F, Karadag B, Akbenlioglu C, et al. Foreign body aspiration: what is the outcome? Pediatr Pulmonol 2002;34:30–6.
35. Chang AB, Eastburn MM, Gaffney J, et al. Cough quality in children: a comparison of subjective vs. bronchoscopic findings. Respir Res 2005;6:3.
36. Wirsing von Konig CH, Rott H, Bogaerts H, et al. A serologic study of organisms possibly associated with pertussis-like coughing. Pediatr Infect Dis J 1998;17: 645–9.
37. Mello CJ, Irwin RS, Curley FJ. Predictive values of the character, timing, and complications of chronic cough in diagnosing its cause. Arch Intern Med 1996;156: 997–1003.

38. Chang AB, Masel JP, Boyce NC, et al. Non-CF bronchiectasis-clinical and HRCT evaluation. Pediatr Pulmonol 2003;35:477–83.
39. De Jongste JC, Shields MD. Chronic cough in children. Thorax 2003;58: 998–1003.
40. Marchant JM, Morris P, Gaffney J, et al. Antibiotics for prolonged moist cough in children. Cochrane Database Syst Rev 2005:4.
41. Marchant JM, Masters IB, Taylor SM, et al. Utility of signs and symptoms of chronic cough in predicting specific cause in children. Thorax 2006;61:694–8.
42. Chang AB, Faoagali J, Cox NC, et al. A bronchoscopic scoring system for airway secretions-airway cellularity and microbiological validation. Pediatr Pulmonol 2006;41:887–92.
43. Chang AB, Redding GJ, Everard ML. Chronic wet cough: protracted bronchitis, chronic suppurative lung disease and bronchiectasis. Pediatr Pulmonol 2008;43: 519–31.
44. Kemp AS. Does post-nasal drip cause cough in childhood? Paediatr Respir Rev 2006;7:31–5.
45. McKenzie S. Cough: but is it asthma? Arch Dis Child 1994;70:1–2.
46. Irwin RS, Baumann MH, Bolser DC, et al. Diagnosis and management of cough executive summary: ACCP evidence-based clinical practice guidelines. Chest 2006;129:1S–23S.
47. Marchant JM, Masters IB, Taylor SM, et al. Evaluation and outcome of young children with chronic cough. Chest 2006;129:1132–41.
48. Gunn VL, Taha SH, Liebelt EL, et al. Toxicity of over-the-counter cough and cold medications. Pediatrics 2001;108:E52.
49. Chien C, Marriott JL, Ashby K, et al. Unintentional ingestion of over the counter medications in children less than 5 years old. J Paediatr Child Health 2003;39: 264–9.
50. Chang AB, Phelan PD, Carlin J, et al. Randomised controlled trial of inhaled salbutamol and beclomethasone for recurrent cough. Arch Dis Child 1998;79:6–11.
51. Davies MJ, Fuller P, Picciotto A, et al. Persistent nocturnal cough: randomised controlled trial of high dose inhaled corticosteroid. Arch Dis Child 1999;81:38–44.
52. Rudolph CD, Mazur LJ, Liptak GS, et al. Guidelines for evaluation and treatment of gastroesophageal reflux in infants and children: recommendations of the North American Society for Pediatric Gastroenterology and Nutrition. J Pediatr Gastroenterol Nutr 2001;2(Suppl 32):S1–31.
53. Holscher B, Heinrich J, Jacob B, et al. Gas cooking, respiratory health and white blood cell counts in children. Int J Hyg Environ Health 2000;203:29–37.
54. Jaakkola JJ, Jaakkola MS. Effects of environmental tobacco smoke on the respiratory health of children. Scand J Work Environ Health 2002;2(Suppl 28):71–83.
55. Hermann C, Westergaard T, Pedersen BV, et al. A comparison of risk factors for wheeze and recurrent cough in preschool children. Am J Epidemiol 2005;162: 345–50.
56. American Academy of Pediatrics. Tobacco's toll: implications for the pediatrician. Pediatrics 2001;107:794–8.
57. Schroeder K, Fahey T. Should we advise parents to administer over the counter cough medicines for acute cough? Systematic review of randomised controlled trials. Arch Dis Child 2002;86:170–5.
58. Chang AB, Peake J, McElrea M. Anti-histamines for prolonged non-specific cough in children. Cochrane Database Syst Rev 2008:2.
59. Chang AB, Marchant JM, Morris P. Cromones for prolonged non-specific cough in children. Cochrane Database Syst Rev 2004:1.

60. Chang AB, McKean M, Morris P. Inhaled anti-cholinergics for prolonged non-specific cough in children. Cochrane Database Syst Rev 2003:4.
61. Smucny JJ, Flynn CA, Becker LA, et al. Are beta2-agonists effective treatment for acute bronchitis or acute cough in patients without underlying pulmonary disease? A systematic review. J Fam Pract 2001;50:945–51.
62. Chang AB, Halstead RA, Petsky HL. Methylxanthines for prolonged non-specific cough in children. Cochrane Database Syst Rev 2005:3.
63. Chang AB, Winter D, Acworth JA. Leukotriene receptor antagonist for prolonged non-specific cough in children. Cochrane Database Syst Rev 2006:2.
64. Chang AB, Lasserson T, Gaffney J, et al. Gastro-oesophageal reflux treatment for prolonged non-specific cough in children and adults. Cochrane Database Syst Rev 2005:2.
65. Gawchik S, Goldstein S, Prenner B, et al. Relief of cough and nasal symptoms associated with allergic rhinitis by mometasone furoate nasal spray. Ann Allergy Asthma Immunol 2003;90:416–21.
66. Barlan IB, Erkan E, Bakir M, et al. Intranasal budesonide spray as an adjunct to oral antibiotic therapy for acute sinusitis in children. Ann Allergy Asthma Immunol 1997;78:598–601.
67. Schroeder K, Fahey T. Over-the-counter medications for acute cough in children and adults in ambulatory settings. Cochrane Database Syst Rev 2004:2.
68. Paul IM, Yoder KE, Crowell KR, et al. Effect of dextromethorphan, diphenhydramine, and placebo on nocturnal cough and sleep quality for coughing children and their parents. Pediatrics 2004;114:e85–90.
69. Chang AB. Causes, assessment and measurement in children. In: Chung KF, Widdicombe JG, Boushey HA, editors. Cough: causes, mechanisms and therapy. London: Blackwell Science; 2003. p. 57–73.
70. GRADE Working Group. Grading quality of evidence and strength of recommendations. BMJ 2004;328:1490–7.

Perceptions and Pathophysiology of Dyspnea and Exercise Intolerance

Miles Weinberger, MD*, Mutasim Abu-Hasan, MD

KEYWORDS

- Dyspnea • Exercise • Exercise testing • Respiratory distress
- Ventilation

WHAT IS DYSPNEA?

Dsypnea is derived from the Latin *dyspnoea*, from Greek *dyspnoia* from dyspnoos, and is often described by patients as shortness of breath. It involves the perception of difficulty or painful breathing. It is a common symptom of numerous medical disorders, but psychologic factors can also contribute to the sensation of dyspnea. Dyspnea on exertion, or exertional dyspnea, indicates dyspnea that occurs or worsens during physical activity. This article discusses the physiology, etiologies, evaluative procedures, and treatment of dyspnea.

PATHOPHYSIOLOGY OF DYSPNEA

Dyspnea is a complex psycho-physiologic sensation that occurs in a variety of cardiopulmonary diseases (**Fig. 1**). Increased work of breathing occurs when there is an increase in mechanical loading of the respiratory system, both resistive and elastic.[1,2] The sensation of dyspnea requires intact afferent and efferent pathways for the full perception of the neuromechanical dissociation between the respiratory effort attempted and the work actually accomplished.[3] The sensation is triggered or accentuated by a variety of receptors located in the chest wall, respiratory muscles, lung parenchyma, carotid body, and brain stem.[4] The sensation of dyspnea is stronger in patients with higher scores for anxiety and has been reported in patients with anxiety disorders with no cardiopulmonary disease.[5–9] These observations demonstrate the importance of cerebral cognition in this complex symptom.

Pediatric Allergy and Pulmonary Division, Pediatrics Department, University of Iowa Children's Hospital, University of Iowa College of Medicine, 200 Hawkins Drive, Iowa City IA 52242, USA
* Corresponding author.
E-mail address: miles-weinberger@uiowa.edu (M. Weinberger).

Pediatr Clin N Am 56 (2009) 33–48
doi:10.1016/j.pcl.2008.10.015
0031-3955/08/$ – see front matter
pediatric.theclinics.com

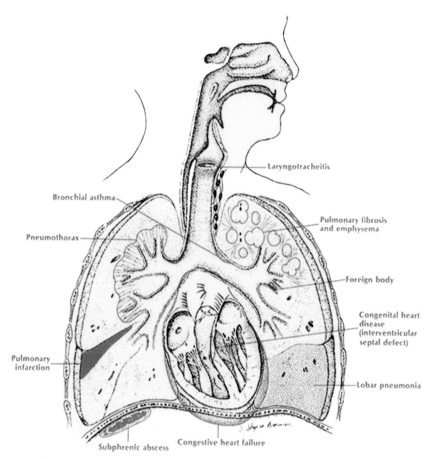

Fig.1. Cardiopulmonary sites that can cause dyspnea. (*From* Collins RD. Differential diagnosis in primary care. 4th edition. Philadelphia: Lippincott Williams & Wilkins; 2008. p. 141; with permission.)

CLINICAL MANIFESTATIONS OF DYSPNEA

People describe dyspnea in different ways. They certainly don't use the word dyspnea. Instead, people will say things such as, "I get tired easily," "I have trouble catching my breath," "I can't take a deep breath," "my throat gets tight," "my chest gets tight," "I can't keep up with the other kids," or simply "I get short of breath." Some of the differences appear to be cultural.[10] Complaints of dyspnea may occur spontaneously and unpredictably, in certain environments or during certain activities. They can be episodic or continuous.

Other differences relate to perception.[11] Differences in perception influence the recognition of asthma. Children with asthma symptoms that have not been recognized by their parents have been shown to perceive dyspnea less readily than those whose asthma has been recognized by their parents.[12] Patients with chronic severe obstructive lung disease, such as asthma and chronic obstructive pulmonary disease, experience adaptation to the sensation of dyspnea. Such patients typically rate their feeling of breathlessness low for severe degrees of obstruction when compared with the acutely ill and with patients with mild chronic disease.[13] Of particular importance is the demonstration that individuals who have experienced near-fatal episodes from asthma have a diminished perception of dyspnea.[14]

When taking a history, it is important to have the patient describe their perception of dyspnea in as much detail as possible. The level of function or dysfunction associated with the dyspnea is also important in assessing the clinical manifestations of dyspnea. In addition to the patient's perception, observations should be obtained from parents, teachers, coaches, or others who have the opportunity to observe the patient for signs of increased work of breathing.

Interestingly, there is a dissociation between dyspnea and actual respiratory effort.[3] Examples include observations in adults with pulmonary embolism or pulmonary hypertension who may report breathlessness out of proportion to respiratory effort, including changes in minute ventilation or pulmonary mechanics. Additionally, induced hypercapnia has been associated with dyspnea accompanied by actual reduction in respiratory effort.[3] Thus, the sensation of dyspnea can reflect either actual increased work of breathing, as in airway obstruction, or the perception of breathlessness, as occurs with acute hypoxemia or hypercapnia.

The feeling of dyspnea or breathlessness can also occur from panic and hyperventilation attacks, where the perception of difficulty breathing is not accompanied by any respiratory pathophysiologic abnormality other than the effects of the hyperventilation itself. Because dyspnea, from whatever cause, depends on perception, attempts have been made to standardize perception. The Borg and the Visual Analog Scales have been the most commonly used measures of dyspnea.[15–17]

PHYSICAL FINDINGS ASSOCIATED WITH DYSPNEA

Physical findings of dyspnea can range from none at all to obvious increased work of breathing manifested by retractions, tachypnea, nasal flaring, use of accessory muscles, and cyanosis. If the dyspnea occurs only during exercise, then reproduction of the exercise-induced dyspnea may require a formal exercise test to reproduce the symptom. This provides the opportunity to observe the patient during the dyspnea and measure cardiopulmonary physiology associated with the dyspnea.

Respiratory sounds may include inspiratory stridor, expiratory wheezing, crackles, or just normal air movement. Identifying respiratory sounds associated with the dyspnea can be helpful in identifying the physiologic abnormality. Inspiratory sounds indicate extrathoracic obstruction, while expiratory sounds indicate intrathoracic obstruction. The pitch of the sounds can also provide clues. Low-pitched inspiratory sounds are typically from supraglottic obstruction, while high-pitched inspiratory sounds are more likely to be from laryngeal or subglottic narrowing. Expiratory wheezing can be monophonic, representing obstruction of one intrathoracic airway, while polyphonic expiratory wheezing indicates more diffuse airway involvement. The extent of the obstruction influences the increased work of breathing to overcome the narrowing of the specific component of the airway.

PHYSIOLOGIC ABNORMALITIES ASSOCIATED WITH DYSPNEA

Both cardiac and pulmonary disease can be associated with dyspnea. Pulmonary edema affects lung compliance and gas exchange. Myocarditis affects cardiac output and limits oxygen delivery to tissues. Pulmonary function testing can differentiate between obstructive and restrictive causes of dyspnea. Obstructive causes are characterized by decreases in flow, while restrictive causes are characterized by decreased lung volumes. Gas exchange abnormalities can be assessed by measurement of oxygenation and pCO_2, while measurement of diffusing capacity can be used to determine if there is a loss of the pulmonary capillary bed, as occurs in interstitial lung disease and pulmonary fibrosis. Exercise testing with cardiopulmonary monitoring can measure oxygen use, CO_2 production, cardiac function, and ventilatory abnormalities.

EXERCISE-INDUCED DYSPNEA

Exercise-induced dyspnea can be present when cardiac or pulmonary function is compromised at an earlier stage in the underlying disease than when dyspnea from those problems occurs at rest. Dyspnea during exercise in patients who otherwise have no known lung or heart disease is therefore a symptom that warrants investigation. It might represent a mild abnormality that is manifested only during exercise, in which increased ventilation and cardiac output are required, or it could be caused by a distinct pathophysiologic abnormality that is induced only by exercise.[18] Of the latter, exercise-induced bronchospasm as a manifestation of asthma is the most widely studied. Its prevalence is very high, but because of poor correlation between the degree of airway obstruction and the sensation of dyspnea, exercise-induced bronchospasm is subject to being unrecognized.[19–21] However, exercise-induced asthma is also subject to being over-reported.[22,23]

Following are selected cases representing common and uncommon examples of dyspnea, which demonstrate the diversity of clinical entities that can present with this symptom.

CASE STUDIES OF DYSPNEA
Case 1

A 10-year-old boy with known asthma comes home from school complaining of difficulty breathing. His mother observes that he has suprasternal retractions. He is taken to the local emergency room, where diffuse polyphonic wheezing is heard and oximetry indicates an O_2 saturation of 93%. Albuterol aerosol is given, his retractions decrease, his O_2 is now 92%, but he states that he feels better and that it is now easier to breath. So what was the mechanism for his dyspnea? Central receptors for hypoxemia? Was he also hypercapneic? Or was it the increased airway resistence from bronchospasm?

It is unlikely that the modest degree of hypoxemia would have been sufficient to make him complain of difficulty breathing. The rapid response to albuterol is consistent with decreasing the resistence to air flow, with consequent lessor effort resulting in chest wall receptors no longer sending signals of increased respiratory effort. Hypoxemia can be from ventilation-perfusion mismatching and commonly occurs early in acute asthma. Because albuterol relaxes pulmonary arteriol smooth muscle in addition to bronchial smooth muscle, ventilation-perfusion mismatching may actually worsen from use of a bronchodilator, even though symptomatic relief results from the decrease in airway resistance from the bronchodilatation. Alternatively, a severe increase in airway resistance greater than can be maintained by the patient results in hypoventilation, with a consequent increase in pCO_2. The rapid relief of dyspnea, despite the continued mild degree of hypoxemia, makes that scenario unlikely in this patient. His dyspnea was therefore a manifestation of the increased work of breathing perceived through receptors in the chest wall.

The presence of continued mild hypoxemia is from the ventilation-perfusion mismatching, resulting from the shunting of pulmonary arterial blood from poorly ventilated areas of the lung to better-ventilated areas. If the same degree of hypoxemia was accompanied by continued increased work of breathing manifested by continued retractions and discomfort, then obtaining a pCO_2 would be critical to identify the potential for early signs of respiratory failure.

Treatment requires a short course of oral corticosteroid to reverse the obstruction from inflammation that results in differential ventilation and the consequent ventilation-perfusion mismatching. Inhaled corticosteroids may then be indicated as long-term maintenance medication if this episode is more than a manifestation of intermittent viral respiratory-induced asthma.[24]

Case 2

A 15-year-old girl takes a typical teenage summer-time job in Iowa, called detasseling. (Detasseling is done to cross-breed, or hybridize, two different varieties of corn. Fields of corn that will be detasseled are planted with two varieties of corn. By removing the tassels from all plants of one variety, all the grain growing on those plants will be fertilized by the other variety's tassels.) She developed severe dyspnea with respiratory sounds that were described as wheezing, and was taken to the local emergency room, where an injection of epinephrine relieved her symptoms. The next day, she again attempted detasseling, with the same result. She then abandoned her goal of detasseling but continued for the next 3 weeks to have similar episodes of dyspnea, described by the patient, emergency room care givers, and her primary care pediatrician as "wheezing." These episodes would occur both spontaneously and with exertion, and would not respond to epinephrine as they did on the first 2 days. Trials by her primary care pediatrician of antiasthmatic medications, including inhaled albuterol, oral corticosteroids, and inhaled corticosteroids, failed to either prevent or relieve acute symptoms when they occurred. Symptoms would last up to several hours, considerably limiting activity of this normally very active adolescent.

After 3 weeks of these daily symptoms, she was referred to the authors' pediatric allergy and pulmonary clinic. She was initially asymptomatic. However, a treadmill exercise reproduced her dyspnea and the respiratory sound previously described as wheezing. The sound precipitated during exercise testing was high-pitched and limited to inspiration. Spirometry before and after the onset of dyspnea demonstrated inspiratory airway obstruction (**Fig. 2**).[25] Flexible laryngoscopy during the episode demonstrated paradoxical vocal cord movement (video with audio can be seen and heard as Video 3 at the following site: http://pediatrics.aappublications.org/cgi/content/full/120/4/855).

This demonstrated that her dyspnea was from the vocal cord dysfunction syndrome. While the evaluation included a large positive skin prick test to corn pollen, which explained the initial episodes as being consistent with laryngeal edema from intense exposure to the corn pollen during the detasseling procedure, the subsequent episodes were from the functional disorder of vocal cord dysfunction with paradoxical motion, whereby the vocal cords paradoxically closed on inspiration with relaxation and consequent opening on expiration.[26]

Instructions by a speech pathologist provided this girl with the ability to stop the paradoxical movement when it would start, but it continued to occur during vigorous activity, interfering with her activities as a cheerleader. Suspecting a vagal mechanism for this, a trial of pre-exercise treatment with an anti-cholinergic inhaler, ipratropium, reliably prevented the exercise-induced vocal cord dysfunction.[27] This regimen allowed her to resume her usual athletic activities, including cheerleading.

Case 3

The 15-year-old girl in Case 3 had a 1.5-year history of recurrent, extremely severe dyspnea. Episodes were sufficiently impressive to observers that paramedics were repeatedly called for urgent transportation to a local hospital emergency room. Symptoms would last for variable periods of time and occurred with sporadic frequency,

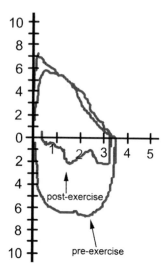

Fig. 2. Spirometry before and after exercise in the girl described in Case 2, showing the marked decrease in the inspiratory portion of the flow-volume loop in association with dyspnea, and an inspiratory wheeze-like sound (technically a high-pitched stridor). (*From* Weinberger M, Abu-Hasan M. Pseudo-asthma: when cough, wheezing, and dyspnea are not asthma. Pediatrics 2007;120(4):860; with permission.)

without apparent inciting factors. She had been treated with various antiasthmatic medications, including inhaled and oral corticosteroids, with no benefit. She had been hospitalized several times, where she received intravenous corticosteroids and vigorous use of inhaled bronchodilators, also without benefit.

The first time this girl was seen at the authors' pediatric allergy and pulmonary clinic, she was free of any symptoms of dyspnea and her physical examination was normal. Initial spirometry was completely normal. To further assess the cause of the dyspnea, a bronchoprovocation with histamine was planned. While preparing the vials of the various concentrations of histamine needed for the progressive inhalational provocation, and before any had been administered, she began having severe respiratory distress, with both inspiratory and expiratory wheezing-like sounds. Her spirometry changed from showing normal inspiratory and expiratory flow to severe obstruction in both phases of respiration (**Fig. 3**). Flexible laryngoscopy during the episode demonstrated virtually complete closure of the vocal cords, leaving only a small aperture for air movement with no abduction, except briefly during speech (video with audio can be seen and heard as Video 4 at the following site: http://pediatrics.aappublica tions.org/cgi/content/full/120/4/855).[25]

Treatment focused on speech pathology, to teach the patient control over her vocal cords when symptoms occurred. Response to treatment was only partially effective. She was able to control some episodes but not others. Lack of continuity for her care hampered progress. She and her single mother subsequently moved to Texas, and she was lost to follow-up.

Case 4

A 9-year-old girl was transferred from a local hospital to the authors' pediatric intensive care unit (PICU) because of progressive dyspnea and hypoxemia. She had a prior history of intermittent asthma, with appropriate responses to conventional measures,

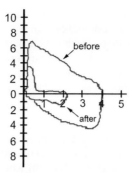

Fig. 3. Spirometry before and after the onset of dyspnea in the girl described in Case 3, showing the marked decrease in the inspiratory and expiratory portion of the flow-volume loop in association with an inspiratory wheeze-like sound (technically a high-pitched stridor on inspiration and a monophonic wheeze on expiration). (*From* Weinberger M, Abu-Hasan M. Pseudo-asthma: when cough, wheezing, and dyspnea are not asthma. Pediatrics 2007;120(4):860; with permission.)

although the authors did not have the medical records for those ambulatory care episodes. On this occasion, progressively greater need for oxygen had been needed to keep O_2 saturations above 90%, despite frequent β_2 agonist (albuterol) aerosol and intravenous corticosteroids. Transfer was arranged when that level of O_2 saturation could not be maintained, even with 100% O_2 by mask. When seen in the PICU, she was severely dyspneic, with rapid respirations and mild intercostal retractions. Despite continuous albuterol aerosol and an intravenous β_2 agonist, her O_2 saturations fell below 70%. She was intubated and ventilated with 100% O_2, but her saturation stayed at 70%. She required only 15-cm H_2O pressure to provide adequate ventilation at an appropriate volume setting for her size. A blood gas demonstrated a pCO_2 of 28 mm Hg at that ventilator setting.

Because there was no evidence of airway obstruction based on the modest pressure requirements for ventilation, it appeared likely that the vigorous use of β_2 agonists was increasing ventilation-perfusion mismatching in a lung disease other than asthma. Stopping all bronchodilator use resulted in oxygen requirements to maintain saturations greater than 90%, rapidly decreasing from 100% to an FiO_2 of 70%. After permitting her to rest overnight on the ventilator with progressively decreasing O_2 requirement, she was extubated the following morning with only 40% O_2 required. The need for oxygen gradually decreased over the ensuing days.

Pulmonary function testing the following day showed no evidence for airway obstruction, but decreased lung volumes and diffusing capacity were observed. This subsequently normalized over several weeks. Recurrences of this restrictive lung disease were observed over subsequent years, but with gradually decreasing frequency. Decreased lung volumes and diffusion capacity for carbon monoxide (DLCO) without airway obstruction was observed with each of these, all of which were self-limited without treatment after a trial of corticosteroids was not found to alter the course. Bronchodilators were avoided and hospitalization was rarely required, and then only with no need for assisted ventilation or intensive care. By the time she started college, these episodes stopped reoccurring.

While the etiology of this apparently interstitial lung disease was never identified, this patient's clinical course shows the potential danger of assuming asthma in all cases of acute respiratory distress in children. Use of β_2 agonists for dyspnea with hypoxemia in the absence of airway obstruction risks substantial worsening of hypoxemia by pulmonary arteriolar dilatation, thereby overcoming the normal protective reflexive pulmonary arteriolar constriction that shunts blood from poorly ventilated to better ventilated areas of the lung. The improvement in ventilation that occurs from the bronchodilatation of a β_2 agonist in asthma generally results in greater overall benefit, whereas the absence a bronchospastic component to the clinical situation results in only worsening of hypoxemia, as occurred in this patient.

Case 5

This 3-year-old boy was admitted to the University of Iowa Children's Hospital because of progressive dyspnea on exertion and recent onset of cyanosis. His mother described him as becoming very short of breath when going up stairs. One month earlier, he had similar symptoms, was hospitalized locally, given antibiotics, and recovered completely within a few days. When seen by the authors, he had rapid respirations with only minimal intercostal retractions. He appeared definitely cyanotic but other than the tachypnea, he did not appear distressed at rest. He was afebrile. An arterial blood gas showed a pO_2 of 50 with a pCO_2 of 32 mm Hg. A chest X-ray showed perihilar and right lower lobe infiltrates (**Fig. 4**).

In investigating the potential etiology, a history of raising doves in the front room of the house was obtained (**Fig. 5**). Examination of the boy's serum identified precipitins to pigeon serum and pigeon droppings (**Fig. 6**). The common precipitin to pigeon droppings and serum in this boy confirm that the lung disease is a manifestation of pigeon breeder's lung disease, an allergic alveolitis.[28] It was the impressive degree of hypoxemia without a major degree of increased work of breathing that suggested an interstitial or alveolar process and not an airway cause for his dyspnea.

Within a few days in the hospital, spontaneous recovery was apparent, with normalization of his blood gases. He was kept in the hospital until his parents could remove

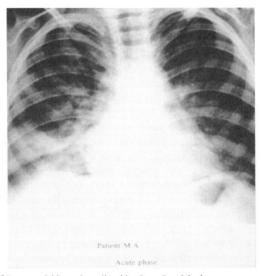

Fig. 4. Chest film of 3-year-old boy described in Case 5, with dyspnea on exertion, tachypnea, cyanosis; he was afebrile, had minimal intercostal retractions, and did not appear to be distressed while at rest. (*From* Wolf SJ, Stillerman A, Weinberger M, et al. Chronic interstitial pneumonitis in a 3-year-old from hypersensitivity to dove antigens. Pediatrics 1987;79(6): 1027; with permission.)

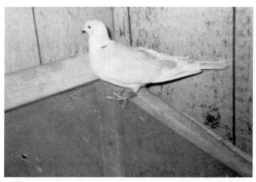

Fig. 5. One of the doves (a pink pigeon) raised in the front room of the home of the child described in Case 5.

the pigeons and clean the front room of the house. He subsequently remained well. In contrast to his complete recovery, repeated exposure over prolonged periods can be associated with irreversible pulmonary fibrosis in someone with allergic alveolitis, also called hypersensitivity pneumonitis.

Case 6

A 16-year-old high school basketball player judged competitive for college scholarships was seen in the Pediatric Allergy & Pulmonary Clinic for exercise-induced dyspnea. Although an excellent and aggressive player, he could not last a quarter without complaining of shortness of breath. The coach would pull him out, and after a few minutes rest he was able to re-enter the game. A previous diagnosis of asthma led to the use of albuterol, without any response.

Physical examination revealed an extremely fit-looking tall adolescent. Baseline pulmonary function was normal. Treadmill running with cardiopulmonary monitoring

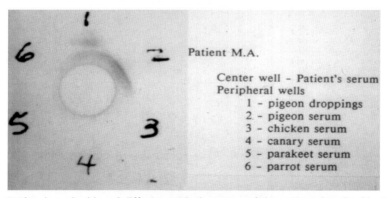

Fig. 6. Ouchterlony double-gel diffusion with the serum of the patient described in Case 5; his serum is in the center well and the indicated antigens are in six surrounding wells on an agar plate. The common precipitin to pigeon droppings and serum in this boy confirm that the lung disease is a manifestation of allergic alveolitis from pigeon breeder's lung disease. (*From* Wolf SJ, Stillerman A, Weinberger M, et al. Chronic interstitial pneumonitis in a 3-year-old from hypersensitivity to dove antigens. Pediatrics 1987;79(6):1027–9; with permission.)

was performed with increasing ramp until his typical symptom of dyspnea was repro-duced (**Fig. 7**).

Although the initial monitoring of cardiac and pulmonary gas exchange was consis-tent with that of a well-conditioned athlete, the onset of his reproduced dyspnea was associated with a sudden increase in the heart rate to 220 beats per minute. Upon cessation of exercise, the heart rate stayed at 220 for up to 10 minutes, when it abruptly dropped to 90. A consult from a cardiac electrophysiologist interpreted the ECG as demonstrating supra-ventricular tachycardia. Electophysiologic studies subsequently identified an alternate conductive pathway to the atrioventricular bundle. A radio-frequency ablation procedure was then performed, after which he was then able to complete quarters in basketball without the previously experienced dyspnea.

The relevance of presenting this patient is the presence of the symptoms, shortness of breath, in the absence of any pulmonary abnormality. At no time did this boy complain of palpitations. In the absence of reproducing his symptoms during appro-priate physiologic monitoring, his treatable problem would not have been identified.

Case 7

A 16-year-old girl was referred to the Pediatric Allergy & Pulmonary Clinic because of exercise-induced dyspnea. She was captain of her basketball team, but continued to

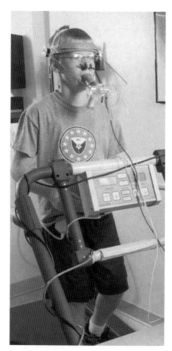

Fig. 7. Treadmill testing with cardiopulmonary monitoring. Oxygen use and carbon dioxide production with breath-by-breath analysis combined with ECG cardiac monitoring permit assessment of physiologic function and physical conditioning. A pressure transducer permits measurement of flow-volume loops during exercise to assess upper or lower airway obstruc-tion during exercise. (*From* Weinberger M, Abu-Hasan M. Pseudo-asthma: when cough, wheezing, and dyspnea are not asthma. Pediatrics 2007;120(4):862; with permission.)

experience exercise-induced symptoms that limited her activity and required her to frequently sit out of the game for a period of time because of dyspnea. These symptoms had been present for at least the two previous years. She had been diagnosed at age 14 with exercise-induced asthma and placed on an inhaled corticosteroid. The dose had been progressively increased because of continued exercise-induced dyspnea. She also used albuterol before exercise. Despite consistent adherence to the prescribed regimen, no benefit was apparent from any of this.

Treadmill exercise testing with cardiopulmonary monitoring was performed while running during a progressively increasing ramp. Based on the heart rate and oxygen use, she demonstrated a high level of cardiovascular function consistent with being a well-conditioned athlete. Her exercise-induced dyspnea was not reproduced until well beyond her anaerobic threshold. Her capillary pH at the end of exercise was 7.18, and a pCO_2 of 42 mm Hg with no apparent cardiac or pulmonary pathophysiology.

The diagnosis of her exercise-induced dyspnea was thus because of reaching normal physiologic limitation. As exercise progressively increases, maximum oxygen use is eventually reached and anaerobic metabolism becomes the eventual source of energy. That produces lactic acid, and the resultant metabolic acidosis is translated by receptors into a demand for greater minute ventilation to create compensatory respiratory alkalosis by decreasing pCO_2. However, increased carbon dioxide is being simultaneously produced and the neurologic demand for increased ventilation encounters the physical limits of ventilation. The continued respiratory drive beyond the capability of the body to meet the demand results in dyspnea, which is interpreted by some as abnormal shortness of breath.

In a study of children and adolescents referred to the authors for exercise-induced dyspnea, most had been previously diagnosed and treated for asthma. The most common cause of exercise-induced dyspnea in these patients, occurring in over half of those tested, was physiologic limitation. It was the perception of these individuals that the dyspnea they were experiencing represented an abnormal physical problem. These patients included the full range of cardiovascular conditioning from highly conditioned competitive athletes to those attempting vigorous exercise with little prior conditioning and consequent below-average cardiovascular conditioning. In the absence of cardiopulmonary monitoring during exercise that reproduced their symptoms, the etiology of the exercise-induced dyspnea would have continued to be inappropriately treated in many of these patients (**Fig. 8**).[22]

Case 8

A 26-year-old pediatric cardiology fellow with a long history of severe chronic asthma entered the authors' care program. She had a documented history of at least one episode of respiratory failure requiring intubation and ventilatory assistance. With appropriate maintenance medication, her asthma had become well controlled until she developed symptoms of a viral respiratory infection associated with disturbing cough. As the cough increased, she became increasingly dyspneic, and came to the University of Iowa Emergency Treatment Center. Because of impressive dyspnea and tachypnea, she was admitted immediately to the medical intensive care unit. A blood gas there showed a pO_2 of 220 on oxygen, a pH of 7.54, and a pCO_2 of 18 mm Hg. The presence of excellent oxygenation with respiratory alkalosis was consistent with hyperventilation, a diagnosis that was as apparent to this medically sophisticated patient as it was to the physicians caring for her.

While the cough was probably a manifestation of her asthma, her experience in the recent past of requiring intubation and assisted ventilation from respiratory failure was

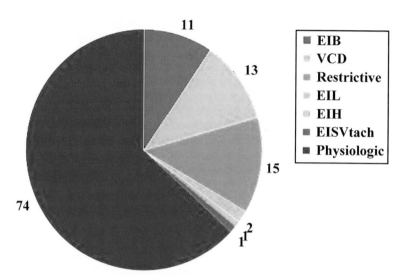

Fig. 8. Diagnoses determined by treadmill exercise testing with physiologic monitoring. *Abbreviations*: EIB, exercise-induced bronchospasm; EIH, exercise-induced hyperventilation; EIL, exercise-induced laryngomalacia; EIVTach, exercise-induced supraventricular tachycardia; Physiologic, normal physiologic limitation without other abnormality; Restrictive, apparent restriction of chest wall movement; VCD, vocal cord dysfunction. (*From* Weinberger M, Abu-Hasan M. Pseudo-asthma: when cough, wheezing, and dyspnea are not asthma. Pediatrics 2007;120(4):862; with permission.)

the likely explanation for the anxiety-induced hyperventilation in this case. The authors present this young adult because this medically sophisticated pediatric cardiology fellow was asked if she could tell the difference between the dyspnea she experienced in this case and dyspnea when she experienced asthma leading to respiratory failure. Her response was that both felt the same. This emphasizes that dyspnea is perceived as dyspnea, whatever the etiology.

The authors have had several children and adolescents with similar histories of life-threatening episodes from acute asthma who subsequently experienced similar symptoms of dyspnea associated with hyperventilation. Unless emergency treatment center physicians are alert to this possibility, inappropriate treatment for asthma will be given that will not relieve the dyspnea and will continue to result in repeated such care requirements. Such patients should be suspected if initial pulse oximetry in a dyspneic asthmatic is in the high 90s while breathing room air. When a blood gas, capillary, or venous is adequate, it can then be determined if the pH is high and the pCO_2 is low, consistent with respiratory alkalosis from hyperventilation. Provision for a means of assessing lung function at home permits the patient to distinguish dyspnea from the airway obstruction of acute asthma from that of anxiety and hyperventilation, thereby preventing unnecessary episodes of urgent medical care.

Case 9

A 16-year-old girl with cystic fibrosis had been admitted to the hospital with an exacerbation of her lung disease. Despite increased cough and decreased spirometric values indicating worsening airway obstruction, she was not initially dyspneic. She was treated with intravenous tobramycin and piperacillin. Three days into treatment, she began to experience increasingly severe dyspnea associated with neither hypoxemia nor hypocapnia. She was transferred to the PICU. Her hemoglobin was found to have dropped to less than 4 mg/dL, in association with severe hemolysis mediated by antibodies to the pipericillin.

This patient illustrates that increased airway obstruction in chronic lung disease, such as cystic fibrosis, is often not associated with dyspnea, despite levels of airway obstruction that would cause dyspnea when occurring acutely in someone with asthma. This patient also demonstrates the potential for dyspnea from the decreased oxygen-carrying capacity of severe anemia, even while blood gases themselves remain normal.

Case 10

A 14-year-old boy with a diagnosis of systemic lupus erythematosis (SLE) made 3 years earlier, with no prior history of respiratory complaints, was admitted to the PICU with a history of progressive fatigue, dyspnea, and chest pain. He had no fever or cough. He was tachypneic and had an O_2 saturation by pulse oximetry of 91%, which increased readily to 99% with supplemental O_2. He appeared to be experiencing increased respiratory effort, but there was minimal inspiratory movement with each breath. He was started on 250 mg of intravenous methylprednisolone every 8 hours.

By the second day of admission, his O_2 saturation normalized although he was still dyspneic. Pulmonary function at that time demonstrated no airway obstruction, but his vital capacity was only 20% of predicted, and his total lung capacity was 34% of predicted. By day five he was no longer dyspneic; his vital capacity and total lung capacity had increased to 31% and 44% of predicted, respectively. His single breath DLCO normalized for alveolar volume (DLCO/Va) was only mildly reduced at 78% of predicted. Continued treatment by the pediatric rheumatologist further improved his vital capacity and total lung capacity to 45% and 57% of predicted, respectively, by 23 days after admission; his DLCO/Va had increased somewhat to 87% of predicted by that time.

While the physiologic mechanism of this uncommon complication of SLE, known as shrinking lung syndrome, is only speculative, it appears to be associated with restricted diaphragmatic movement, which was in fact demonstrated fluoroscopically in this patient.[29] This case illustrates that restrictive changes are well tolerated until a critically low level of ventilation is reached. This patient also demonstrates the value of lung volumes and DLCO in addition to just spirometry in identifying the physiologic abnormality associated with dyspnea. While there is the potential for interstitial lung disease to be associated with collagen-vascular diseases, the modest decrease in the DLCO for this patient did not provide support for that type of physiologic abnormality.

SUMMARY

Dyspnea is a complex psycho-physiologic sensation that has many causes that can be anatomic, physiologic, or psychologic. The entities causing dyspnea include commonly occurring problems, such as asthma, and uncommon but clinically important problems to identify, such as allergic alveolitis and the shrinking lung syndrome of systemic lupus erythematosis. Functional disorders, such as the variations of vocal cord dysfunction and hyperventilation, require identification so those patients can be treated behaviorally and not subjected to inappropriate medication. Exercise-induced dyspnea, while a characteristic of asthma, should not be assumed to be asthma in the absence of other symptoms of asthma and a convincing response to prevention by pretreatment with an albuterol aerosol. Treadmill exercise testing that reproduces symptoms with cardiopulmonary monitoring can identify the physiologic

Table 1
Intervention for dyspnea

Intervention	Recommendation	Grading of Recommendation (Based on Evidence of Benefit)	Quality of Supporting Evidence
Albuterol (salbutamol) aerosol	Only for asthma	Strong	Strong
Corticosteroids, inhaled	Only for chronic asthma	Strong	Strong
Corticosteroids, oral, short course of high dose	For exacerbations of asthma	Strong	Strong
Corticosteroids, oral, short course of high dose	For assessment of response to support the diagnosis of asthma as the cause of dyspnea	Moderate	Moderate
Long acting β_2 agonists	As additive agent to inhaled corticosteroids for chronic asthma	Moderate	Strong
Montelukast	For chronic asthma	Low	Moderate
Epinephrine (adrenalin) injection	For acute laryngeal edema of systemic anaphylactic reaction	High	High
Speech therapy	For recurring spontaneous episodes of vocal cord dysfunction	Moderate	Low
Ipratropium aerosol	For prevention of exercise-induced vocal cord dysfunction	Moderate	Low
Ipratropium aerosol	For severe acute asthma not responding to albuterol	Moderate	Moderate
Environmental adjustment	For allergic asthma	Moderate	Low
Environmental adjustment	For allergic alveolitis	High	Moderate

abnormality, whether exercise-induced bronchospasm, vocal cord abnormalities, or the various other physiologic causes demonstrated to be associated with exercise-induced dyspnea. The following outline (see also **Table 1**) lists the steps health care professionals should follow when a patient presents with dyspnea:

I. A complete medical examination with particular attention to cardiorespiratory systems and a focus on:
  A. Determining its clinical pattern
    1. Present all of the time
    2. Present only during exercise
    3. Present only with specific environmental exposures
  B. Level of respiratory dysfunction (ie, degree of disability)
  C. Observation of level of dysfunction from others
  D. Presence of airway noises
II. Evaluation should include:
  A. Chest X-ray
  B. Baseline oximetry
  C. Blood pH and pCO_2 when oximetry below normal or if dyspnea presents with normal oximetry
  D. Spirometry with considerations for lung volumes and diffusing capacity if patient is able to perform
  E. Cardiorespiratory exercise test to reproduce exercise-induced symptoms if patient is able to do this
III. Referral for further evaluation and management if:
  A. Dyspneic at rest and diagnosis not apparent
  B. Hypoxemic and diagnosis not apparent

REFERENCES

1. Meek PM, Schwartzstein RM, and the ad hoc Committee of the Nursing Assembly of the American Thoracic Society. Dyspnea—mechanisms, assessment, and management: a consensus statement. American Thoracic Society. Am J Respir Crit Care Med 1999;159(1):321–40.
2. O'Donnell DE, Hong HH, Webb KA. Respiratory sensation during chest wall restriction and dead space loading in exercising men. J Appl Phys 2000;88(5):1859–69.
3. Demediuk BH, Manning H, Lilly J, et al. Dissociation between dyspnea and respiratory effort. Am Rev Respir Dis 1992;146(5 pt 1):1222–5.
4. The enigma of breathlessness [editorial]. Lancet 1986;1(8486):891–2.
5. Zealley AK, Aitken RC. Breathlessness and anxiety. Br Med J 1970;2(5705):363.
6. Rietveld S, Everaerd W, van Beest I. Excessive breathlessness through emotional imagery in asthma. Behav Res Ther 2000;38(10):1005–14.
7. Rietveld S, Prins PJ. The relationship between negative emotions and acute subjective and objective symptoms of childhood asthma. Psychol Med 1998;28(2):407–15.
8. Janson C, Bjornsson E, Hetta J, et al. Anxiety and depression in relation to respiratory symptoms and asthma. Am J Respir Crit Care Med 1994;149(4 Pt 1):930–4.
9. Tiller J, Pain M, Biddle N. Anxiety disorder and perception of inspiratory resistive loads. Chest 1987;91(4):547–51.
10. Trochtenberg DS, BeLue R. Descriptors and perception of dyspnea in African-American asthmatics. J Asthma 2007;48(10):811–5.

11. Fosi E, Stendardi L, Binazzi B, et al. Perception of airway obstruction and airway inflammation in asthma: a review. Lung 2006;184(5):251–8.
12. Van Gent R, van Essen-Zandvliet LEM, Rovers MM, et al. Poor perception of dyspnea in 28 children with undiagnosed asthma. Eur Respir J 2007;30(5):887–91.
13. Veen JC, Smits HH, Ravensberg AJ, et al. Impaired perception of dyspnea in patients with severe asthma. Relation to sputum eosinophils. Am J Respir Crit Care Med 1998;158(4):1134–41.
14. Restrepo RD, Peters J. Near-fatal asthma: recognition and management. Curr Opin Pulm Med 2008;14(1):13–23.
15. Borg G. Psychophysical bases of perceived exertion. Med Sci Sports Exerc 1982;14(5):377–81.
16. Gift AG. Validation of a vertical visual analogue scale as a measure of clinical dyspnea. Rehabil Nurs 1989;14(6):323–5.
17. Wilson RC, Jones PW. Differentiation between the intensity of breathlessness and the distress it evokes in normal subjects during exercise. Clin Sci 1991;80(1):65–70.
18. Pratter MR, Curley FJ, Dubois J, et al. Cause and evaluation of chronic dyspnea in a pulmonary disease clinic. Arch Intern Med 1989;149(10):2277–82.
19. Hammerman SI, Becker JM, Rogers J, et al. Asthma screening of high school athletes: identifying the undiagnosed and poorly controlled. Ann Allergy Asthma Immunol 2002;88(47):380–4.
20. Panditi S, Silverman M. Perception of exercise induced asthma by children and their parents. Arch Dis Child 2003;88(9):807–11.
21. Melani AS, Ciarleglio G, Pirelli M, et al. Perception of dyspnea during exercise-induced bronchoconstriction. Respir Med 2003;97(3):221–7.
22. Abu-Hasan M, Tannous B, Weinberger M. Exercise-induced dyspnea in children and adolescents: if not asthma then what? Ann Allergy Asthma Immunol 2005;94(3):366–71.
23. Seear M, Wensley D, West N. How accurate is the diagnosis of exercise induced asthma among Vancouver schoolchildren? Arch Dis Child 2005;90(9):898–902.
24. Abu-Hasan M, Weinberger M. Management of asthma in children: translating patient-oriented evidence into practice. Hosp Physician 2007;43(8):36–49.
25. Weinberger M, Abu-Hasan M. Pseudo-asthma: when cough, wheezing, and dyspnea are not asthma. Pediatrics 2007;120(4):855–64.
26. Christopher KL, Wood RP 2nd, Eckert RC, et al. Vocal-cord dysfunction presenting as asthma. N Engl J Med 1983;308(26):1566–70.
27. Doshi D, Weinberger M. Long-term outcome of vocal cord dysfunction. Ann Allergy Asthma Immunol 2006;96(6):794–9.
28. Wolf SJ, Stillerman A, Weinberger M, et al. Chronic interstitial pneumonitis in a 3-year-old from hypersensitivity to dove antigens. Pediatrics 1987;79(6):1027–9.
29. Ferguson PJ, Weinberger M. Shrinking lung syndrome in a 14 year old boy with systemic lupus erythematosus. Pediatr Pulmonol 2006;41(2):194–7.

Chest Pain and Chest Wall Deformity

Janaki Gokhale, MD[a,b], Steven M. Selbst, MD[a,b],*

KEYWORDS
- Chest pain • Cardiac • Musculoskeletal • Pulmonology
- Pectus deformity • Ischemia

Chest pain is a relatively common complaint among pediatric patients and presents a diagnostic challenge that is associated with significant emotional as well as monetary costs. Patients as well as their families are often concerned about life-threatening causes for the chest pain, although these are rarely identified. There are numerous etiologies for pediatric chest pain and **Box 1** lists the differential diagnosis of chest pain in children.

The clinician's primary goal in evaluating the pain, whether it is in a primary care office, cardiology clinic, or the emergency department (ED) setting, is to identify the serious causes and rule out other organic pathology. Similarly, chest wall deformity can also be of great concern to patients and their families. The goal in evaluation and treatment of patients with chest wall deformity should be to maximize lung growth and function as a child grows and to minimize related psychologic problems.

Table 1 describes the levels of evidence for studies discussed in this paper.

CHEST PAIN

The frequency of pediatric chest pain among different EDs has been shown to be anywhere between 0.3% (Level of evidence [LOE] 2, **Table 1**)[1] and 0.6% of all visits (LOE 2).[2,3] In an earlier study (LOE 2),[4] the occurrence rate of chest pain in the ED, cardiac clinic, and primary care physician's office in one hospital was found to be 0.288%. One of these studies (LOE 2),[1] while finding very few "serious" causes of chest pain, noted that almost 90% of patients considered the pain to be at least "moderate or severe" in intensity; at least half of the patients interviewed by a psychiatrist in another study were worried about the pain being related to their "heart" (LOE 2).[4]

Given the perceived severity of pain and the surrounding anxiety about heart problems and presumably other life-threatening problems, it would be useful to have an evidence-based guide for chest pain that allowed efficient identification of

[a] Jefferson Medical College, Philadelphia, PA 19107, USA
[b] A.I. duPont Hospital for Children, 1600 Rockland Road, Wilmington, DE 19803, USA
* Corresponding author. Department of Pediatrics, A.I. duPont Hospital for Children, 1600 Rockland Road, Wilmington, DE 19803.
E-mail address: sselbst@nemours.org (S.M. Selbst).

Pediatr Clin N Am 56 (2009) 49–65
doi:10.1016/j.pcl.2008.10.001
0031-3955/08/$ – see front matter © 2009 Elsevier Inc. All rights reserved.

Box 1
Differential diagnosis of pediatric chest pain

Cardiac

Coronary artery disease-ischemia/infarction

    Anomalous coronary arteries

    Kawasaki disease (coronary arteritis)

    Diabetes mellitus (long standing)

Arrhythmia

    Supraventricular tachycardia

    Ventricular tachycardia

Structural abnormalities of the heart

    Hypertrophic cardiomyopathy

    Severe pulmonic stenosis

    Aortic valve stenosis

Infection

    Pericarditis

    Myocarditis

Gastrointestinal disorders

    Reflux esophagitis

    Pill induced esophagitis

    Esophageal foreign body

Psychological disorders

    Stress-related pain

Musculoskeletal disorders

    Chest wall strain

    Direct trauma/contusion

    Rib fracture

    Costochondritis

Idiopathic

Pulmonary/Respiratory disorders

    Severe cough

    Asthma

    Pneumonia

    Pneumothorax/pneumomediastinum

    Pulmonary embolism

Miscellaneous disorders

    Sickle cell crisis

    Abdominal aortic aneurysm (Marfan syndrome)

    Pleural effusion (collagen vascular disease)

    Shingles

    Pleurodynia (coxsackievirus)

    Breast tenderness (pregnancy, physiologic)

    Chest mass

Table 1			
Levels of evidence			
Level	Description	No. Papers Cited—Chest Pain	No. papers Cited—Chest Wall Deformity
1	Randomized controlled trials or meta-analysis	0	1
2	Prospective or cohort studies	8	2
3	Case control	2	3
4	Retrospective studies	6	2
5	Case series/case reports, expert opinion/review	3	9

This system of classification was created specifically for the evidence found regarding chest pain and chest wall deformity and has not been previously validated. A common validated method of classification[27] cannot be used accurately in this case because we aim to provide guidance on characterization and diagnosis, as well as management of chest pain. The classification of levels of evidence for each of these goals is different based on this validated method. Therefore, we have provided only a simple guide for the reader to understand the types of studies that are included in this discussion. It is important to note that although a study may be listed as a "LOE 2" it may not necessarily supercede a better-designed case control or evidence stated in a review (LOE 5). Some studies have significant limitations and are discussed in the text where they appear.

life-threatening conditions and correct diagnosis of other etiologies. However, as has been shown by several studies (all LOE 2),[1–4] life-threatening causes of chest pain are rare in the pediatric population. It follows that it would be quite difficult for any randomized, prospective study to have sufficient power to provide evidence necessary to direct diagnostic testing. However, based on the data available, we suggest a commonsense approach that should allow for reasonable use of resources without compromising diagnostic sensitivity (**Table 2**). On review of the few studies that have been devoted to the complaint of pediatric chest pain, one reassuring theme is found: a thorough history and physical examination provide the best clues to determine etiology, and further diagnostic workup is not required in most cases.

Cardiac

As has already been stated, most patients/parents who present with chest pain are concerned about their heart (LOE 2).[4] In fact, chest pain is the second most common cause for referral to a pediatric cardiologist (LOE 5).[5] Although a cardiac problem is generally not found with chest pain (all LOE 2),[1–4] arrhythmias, mitral valve prolapse, and myocarditis/pericarditis are worth discussing. Rarely, one may see aortic dissection or ischemia—the latter with obstructive lesions, cocaine use, coronary artery anomalies, coronary artery occlusion, or myocardial bridging. With more serious, life-threatening causes, there may be a history of Marfan syndrome (see section on Marfan syndrome later in this article) or congenital hyperlipidemia. Chest pain could be the first sign of hypertrophic cardiomyopathy.

Previous studies have shown that a thorough history and physical examination are often enough to identify cardiac causes of chest pain. In one study (LOE 2),[1] of 168 patients who presented to the ED with chest pain, 9 patients were found to have a cardiac-related cause. Symptoms of fever (2/9), dyspnea (3/9), palpitations (5/9), pallor (2/9) and most importantly pathologic heart auscultation (9/9) were found to be statistically significantly related to a cardiac etiology. Interestingly, palpitations were also

Table 2
Worrisome signs and symptoms to prompt further workup in pediatric patients (partial list)

Workup	History/Symptom	Sign
Chest x-ray	Fever	Fever
	Cough	Tachypnea, rales, distress
	Shortness of breath	Ill-appearing/"sick"
	History of trauma	Significant trauma
	Pain wakes from sleep	Extreme tachycardia
	History of drug use (eg, cocaine)	Pathologic auscultation of heart
	Associated with exercise	Absent/decreased breath sounds
	Acute onset of pain	Palpation of subcutaneous air
	Serious medical problems (Marfan, Kawasaki, lupus)	Tall, thin
	Foreign body ingestion (coin, button battery)	Drooling, gagging
Electrocardiogram	Associated with exercise	Pathologic auscultation of heart
	Associated with syncope	Tachycardia (>180 beats per minute)
	History of drug use (eg, cocaine)	Ill-appearing/"sick"
	Consider with fever	Consider with fever

found to be statistically significantly related to a psychogenic cause (5/15 patients), so this may not be a reliable marker for cardiac pain. Pain with exercise has long been considered worrisome for cardiac disease. In this study, chest pain associated with exercise was found in only 6 of 108 patients with chest wall–related pain, but it was not significantly related to cardiac pain either. In the same study, 5 of 69 patients who presented to a pediatric cardiology clinic for chest pain were found to have supraventricular tachycardia. Again, palpitations were significantly correlated (5/5) patients for this category (LOE 2).[1] An earlier prospective study (LOE 2)[2] of children in the ED with chest pain conducted electrocardiograms (EKGs) in 191 of 235 patients with "ill-defined" or "cardiac-related chest pain." Of these, 31 of 235 were found to be abnormal, but only 4 of 235 showed new or "not minor" changes. Three revealed arrhythmias that were noted on physical examination and one showed evidence of pericarditis in a child who had fever and known systemic lupus erythematosis. In this study, these same 235 patients had echocardiograms done, and of these there were four that showed previously unknown mitral valve prolapse. However, these may have been incidental findings not necessarily related to the chest pain. One study (LOE 2)[6] of 106 patients with a chief complaint of "murmur" and "chest pain" (21/106) found EKG and chest radiograph (CXR) to be helpful in evaluation even when no cardiac disease was suspected on history and physical examination. However, a limitation of this study, as noted in the paper, is that the two groups of patients were lumped together and there is not sufficient power to make this conclusion for patients with chest pain alone. Finally, a 1-year prospective study of 336 patients with chest pain from a pediatric ED in Canada (LOE 2)[3] identified only 5 patients with cardiac disease. It seems these were identified purely by clinical suspicion by history and physical examination, or by appropriately directed EKG or (presumably) echocardiogram. Using this approach, the authors point out that misdiagnosis of serious organic etiology is unlikely.

These prospective studies suggest that a careful history and physical examination are generally sufficient to diagnose cardiac-related chest pain. If not, they should at least be sufficient to guide the use of CXRs, EKGs, and echocardiograms. While other diagnoses such as pericarditis and ischemia are not adequately represented in these studies to draw a conclusion, retrospective studies support the prospective studies and commonsense approach outlined in **Table 2**. In a retrospective study of 20 pediatric patients with acute pericarditis, 13 were found to have muffled heart sounds and 7 were found to have a friction rub (LOE 4).[7] The clinical examination "generally showed a sick child" with chest pain, fever, and tachypnea, and all were found to have cardiomegaly on CXR. Regarding ischemia and myocardial infarction, we found two small retrospective studies with nine patients each with myocardial infarction after presenting with chest pain to an ED. In one, the authors describe acute chest pain with a mean duration of 40 hours (LOE 4),[8] and in the second the authors state that each patient had "typical severe retrosternal chest pain radiating to the left arm or jaw" (LOE 4).[9]

Previous case reports and case series have also reported myocardial ischemia in children with a prior history of Kawasaki disease, history of cocaine or amphetamine drug use, familial hypercholesterolemia, hypercoagulability, myocardial tumors, and family history of early coronary heart disease. Based on this evidence (and lack of evidence), we recommend a commonsense approach for suspected ischemia. A history of classic crushing substernal chest pain (not sharp), syncope with chest pain, chest pain associated with exercise, family history for sudden death at a young age, use of drugs like cocaine, or underlying cardiac disease, may imply a need to investigate cardiac etiology for pain. Likewise, findings on physical examination such as decrease in oxygen saturation, or significant changes in heart rate and blood pressure, with acute presentation, abnormal cardiac examination should guide the workup and prompt evaluation with an EKG and CXR. Although chest pain with fever is highly correlated with pneumonia, uncommon cardiac infections such as myocarditis or pericarditis should also be considered in a febrile child with chest pain.

Gastrointestinal

Prospective studies have shown that gastrointestinal (GI) pain can account for to 4% of pediatric chest pain to an ED (LOE 2).[1,2] The exacerbation of pain when eating can be significantly correlated ($P = .0003$) to gastritis, esophagitis, or constipation according to one prospective study of ED patients (LOE 2).[1] One clinical trial showed that many patients who were initially diagnosed with idiopathic chest pain actually had a GI cause for their pain. In that study, 21 of 27 had either esophagitis, gastritis, or esophageal spasm confirmed by esophagogastroduodenoscopy (EGD), esophageal manometry, and Bernstein acid perfusion test (LOE 2).[10] Interestingly, none of the patients had symptoms of heartburn, regurgitation, pain with swallowing, dysphagia, hemorrhage, or "water brash," and instead the pain was described as being over the left side, either central or retrosternal, and lasting less than a minute to several hours. A more recent study showed that patients who presented to a cardiology clinic with chest pain who also had epigastric pain (44 of 132 patients) had positive findings of gastritis on endoscopy (41/44 of these patients). Of these patients, 39 were treated and 38 of these had resolution of symptoms (LOE 2).[11] Based on these findings, we recommend that the suspicion of gastritis or esophagitis must remain on the differential diagnosis of chest pain even without overt symptoms. In the absence of other concerning findings on history and physical examination, it may be reasonable to refer these patients (midsternal "burning" type pain, worse with eating or lying down) to a gastroenterologist or start a trial of H-2 blockers or proton pump inhibitors depending on the clinical setting to see if symptoms of chest pain improve.

Some young children will complain of acute significant chest pain following ingestion of a coin or other foreign body that lodges in the esophagus. Although many such patients are nonverbal, these children may present with obvious discomfort and they may have associated drooling or dysphagia if the coin is trapped in the upper esophagus. Some patients or parents can give a clear history of an ingested foreign body, but in some cases the diagnosis is less obvious. Although there are no studies to provide evidence-based guidance, it seems reasonable to obtain a CXR to look for an esophageal foreign body in a young child with acute onset of midsternal pain, especially if the child is drooling.

Psychiatric

Chest pain related to a psychogenic cause has an incidence of anywhere between 5% (LOE 2)[5] and 9% (LOE 2)[1,2] in children who present to the ED. The pain is generally thought to be precipitated by hyperventilation, stressful life event, depression, or anxiety with no other organic etiology. One study used a specific questionnaire to identify signs of stress and depression, but these questions were not statistically significantly associated with a psychogenic diagnosis (LOE 2),[3] although recurrence of pain was (LOE 2).[3] Another study found psychogenic chest pain to be 2.5 times more likely in adolescents (P = .02) and three times more likely with a family history of chest pain (P = .001) (LOE 2).[2] The association of psychogenic chest pain with children of older age was confirmed by a second study (P = .01) (LOE 2).[1] Finally, one study found that compared with slightly older children referred to a cardiology clinic for benign heart murmur, children with noncardiac chest pain were significantly more likely to have anxiety symptoms (LOE 3).[12]

Currently, although significant demographic associations do seem to exist in previous studies, there are no specific questions that can be used in a practical setting to reliably identify patients with this type of pain. However, the clinician should inquire about possible stressors and significant life events that may correlate with the onset of chest pain. If a stressful life event or history of anxiety is obvious, in patients with no other significant findings on history and physical examination, it may be reasonable to conclude the chest pain is related to stress. In others, where a stressful event is not immediately obvious, it is reasonable to probe further into causes for emotional stress before labeling chest pain as idiopathic.

Musculoskeletal

Musculoskeletal chest pain appears to be a relatively common cause for pediatric chest pain in both the ED and cardiology clinic settings. Studies from the ED put the incidence of costochondritis between 9.0% and 22.5% of patients, trauma-related chest pain to be about 5%, and other musculoskeletal pain such as muscle strain in 5% to 15% of patients (all LOE 2).[2,4,13] Musculoskeletal chest pain is generally considered when pain is reproducible to palpation or suggested by a history of muscle strain or minor trauma. Reproducibility of chest wall pain is generally a good marker for costochondritis or chest wall pain. However, the absence of this finding does not always exclude a musculoskeletal cause. The duration of musculoskeletal chest pain can be relatively long. In differentiating between costochondritis and idiopathic chest pain, an early study found that the former had a mean duration of pain of 96.8 days, but that idiopathic chest pain was still significantly longer in duration (797.8 days) (LOE 2).[4] The studies indicate that a musculoskeletal etiology should always be considered when evaluating a patient with chest pain simply based on the frequency of this diagnosis. One might assume that palpitations associated with chest pain would point to a cardiac etiology for pain. However, one study showed that in patients who presented to the cardiology clinic with chest pain, palpitations were actually significantly associated with both chest wall pain (83% of all etiologies) and cardiac-related diagnoses (LOE 2).[1] Diagnostic studies usually do not help identify musculoskeletal chest pain.

Idiopathic

Idiopathic chest pain is perhaps the most common diagnosis for children who present with chest pain. Despite a careful history and physical examination, in 21% to 45% of cases of pediatric chest pain, evaluated in two studies in a prospective manner, no diagnosis could be determined with certainty (LOE 2).[2,4] The child's pain was then labeled as idiopathic in these cases. Nonorganic disease including idiopathic chest pain was more likely if pain persisted more than 6 months ($P = .0009$)[2] (LOE 2). Driscoll and colleagues[4] (LOE 2) also found children with idiopathic pain had symptoms longer than other diagnostic groups (mean 798 days). The more chronic the complaint of pain, the less likely it is that a specific etiology will be found.

Precordial catch syndrome is sometimes diagnosed in children with chest pain. This condition, also called Texidor's twinge, was first described by Miller and Texidor[14] in 1955 in a case series of adult patients (LOE 5). They noted patients had sudden, sharp, stabbing well-localized precordial pain. It is often worse with a deep breath, and examination findings are normal (LOE 5).[15] One study of 168 children with chest pain in the ED included precordial catch syndrome in the musculoskeletal category and found the incidence to be 64% (LOE 2).[1] They defined the category of musculoskeletal chest pain as "classically stabbing and exaggerated with respiration, [lasting] seconds to minutes... not associated with activity (or occurs after participation in sports activity) and sometimes, may be reproduced by palpation." Based on this definition and forward selection analysis these authors found that a "lack of cough, previous trauma, stressful event, dyspnea, meal-related pain, fever, pathologic cardiac auscultation, palpitations, and anxiety predicted the adherence of 97% of [chest wall] patients to that category" (LOE 2).[1] However, Selbst and colleagues[2] included patients with precordial catch syndrome in their "idiopathic" category, because the etiology is unknown (LOE 2).

Studies have shown that if the history and examination are unrevealing, diagnostic studies such as CXR and EKG are also unlikely to pinpoint a diagnosis. Abnormal laboratory studies usually reveal previously known or clinically suspected problems from the history and physical examination (LOE 2).[2,4] It is thus recommended that laboratory studies should not be obtained empirically, but rather be based on history and physical examination findings.

Pulmonary

Although most parents are concerned about a cardiac etiology for chest pain, clinicians should not overlook pulmonary causes of chest pain, as these are often readily treatable. Pulmonary causes of chest pain include common disease processes such as pneumonia and asthma, as well as less frequent diagnoses—pneumothorax, pneumomediastinum, pleural effusion, pleurodynia, foreign body aspiration, and pulmonary embolism. Pulmonary causes of chest pain have been estimated between 13% and 19% based on two prospective studies from the ED setting (LOE 2).[1,3] When the pulmonary etiology was further delineated, 10% of patients had chest pain because of persistent cough, 7% because of asthma, and 4% because of pneumonia (LOE 2).[2]

These prospective studies were naturally not designed to assess the frequency of more rare and serious diagnoses such as pneumothorax or pulmonary embolism. However, chest pain is thought to be a prominent feature in almost all patients with pneumothorax. One 12-year retrospective study of 17 pediatric patients with pneumothorax found that 100% of children had chest pain on initial presentation (LOE 4).[16] Chest pain may be less common in children with pneumomediastinum. According to a 10-year retrospective study of 29 patients in Ohio, neck pain and sore throat were the most common (38%) presenting symptoms in patients with this condition (LOE 4).[17] Chest pain was not discussed as a specific symptom in this study, and the most common presenting finding was subcutaneous emphysema. Pneumothorax and pneumomediastinum are generally found in children with asthma or lower respiratory tract disease such as bronchiolitis, cystic fibrosis, and Marfan syndrome (see section on Marfan syndrome later in this article). However, previously healthy children may rupture an unrecognized subpleural bleb with minimal precipitating factors and present with respiratory distress and chest pain as a result of a spontaneous pneumothorax. Decreased breath sounds on the affected side are likely if the pneumothorax is significant. Case reports indicate that patients who snort cocaine are also at risk for barotraumas and may present with sudden severe chest pain, anxiety, respiratory distress, and tachycardia (LOE 5).[18]

There are few studies describing chest pain and pulmonary embolism (PE) in children. A recent retrospective case series of 14 patients with PE noted that all children were symptomatic (LOE 5).[19] All patients either had chest pain (71%) or dyspnea on exertion (79%). Screening with D-dimer was normal in 40% and this inconsistency may have delayed diagnosis in some cases (LOE 5).[19] This condition is rare in the pediatric population and multicenter trials are needed to better evaluate clinical characteristics and risk factors for PE. However, this diagnosis should be considered in any pediatric patient with venous thromboembolism or with increased likelihood of clotting. The latter can be seen in nephrotic syndrome, systemic lupus erythematosis, malignancy, inflammatory bowel disease, postoperative state, hypercoagulable states, recent abortion, or leg injury (LOE 4).[20] Patients with pulmonary embolism are likely to have acute onset of pleuritic chest pain as well as dyspnea or cough.

History of fever and signs of tachypnea, shortness of breath, or pathologic auscultation of the lungs should prompt further evaluation for a pulmonary cause of chest pain. In addition, in a patient with a known history of asthma, one should always consider chest pain could be secondary to this underlying diagnosis. While this may seem self-evident, asthma exacerbation as a cause of chest pain may be underdiagnosed. Massin and colleagues[1] (LOE 2) in their study of chest pain in the ED setting observed that five patients who were categorized as having chest wall pain did, in fact, have a history of asthma without signs of wheezing. They postulated that the lung examination might be normal in small airways hyperreactivity. Another study of 88 children with chest pain who underwent exercise-stress testing found significant improvement in symptoms as well objective measures of pulmonary function after bronchodilator treatment (LOE 4).[21] The frequency of asthma in patients who present with chest pain was found in 15% in one study (LOE 2).[3] Given this relatively high incidence, it is reasonable in clinically stable patients with a prior history of asthma to try bronchodilator therapy in the office or ED setting to try to relieve symptoms regardless of the presence of wheezing on examination.

Fever associated with chest pain should also raise suspicion of pulmonary disease such as pneumonia or other organic disease (rare cardiac infections as noted above). Selbst and colleagues[2] (LOE 2) found that fever with chest pain was significantly associated (P<.001) with a diagnosis of pneumonia, documented on CXR, in their prospective study of 407 pediatric patients. Similarly, Massin and colleagues[1] found that fever was significantly correlated (*P*<.05) with respiratory or cardiac disease (LOE 2). Cough was also significantly correlated with respiratory conditions (*P*<.05). Cough and fever predicted 99% of patients with a respiratory cause of chest pain (LOE 2).[1] In addition, one retrospective study of 368 patients showed that chest pain was significantly associated with complicated pneumococcal pneumonia compared with uncomplicated pneumonia (LOE 3).[22] An obvious limitation of this study is that all patients may not have been asked about chest pain specifically because it was a retrospective study. It is important to note that chest pain alone is generally not enough to diagnose pneumonia. In one study designed to look at clinical decision making regarding diagnosis and treatment of pneumonia, the prevalence of pleuritic pain was found to be only 8% (LOE 5).[23] However, given the evidence, we would recommend obtaining a chest radiograph if chest pain is present with either fever or cough.

CHEST WALL DEFORMITIES

Chest wall deformities in children are sometimes correlated with chest pain. They can also lead to restricted lung function, and many are related to psychologic problems in children because of the associated cosmetic defects.

Pectus Excavatum

Pectus excavatum (chest depression) is the most common congenital deformity of the anterior chest wall. The condition is generally present at birth or shortly after, but is usually asymptomatic initially. It may become more marked during childhood and teenage growth (LOE 3).[24] Problems such as chest pain and adverse physiologic effects like decreased exercise tolerance may be noted over time (LOE 3, LOE 5, LOE 4).[25–27] Significant psychologic stress related to the cosmetic defect is common (LOE 5).[26] It is believed that cardiac filling is reduced in pectus excavatum as a result of compression of the sternum on the right heart chambers, thereby lowering exercise cardiac output. In a study of 13 patients with pectus excavatum, Zhao and colleagues[25] (LOE 3) showed reduced oxygen uptake and stroke volume when subjects were exercising in the sitting position, but this was equal to controls during supine exercises. The supine advantage in patients with pectus excavatum suggests that upright exercise capacity is affected by reduced filling of the heart in the nonsupine position.

Children with pectus excavatum may become short of breath during strenuous exercise and complain that they are easily fatigued (LOE 3).[24] However, it is not clear if this is clinically significant as the complaints are subjective. Pulmonary function tests may be normal or may show a restrictive defect in children with this deformity. Haller and Loughlin[24] studied 36 teenage patients with pectus excavatum who underwent surgical correction (LOE 3). Before surgery, pectus subjects had significantly lower forced vital capacity (FVC) than controls (81% ± 14% versus 98% ± 9% predicted, *P*<.001). Mean values fell within normal range. Postoperative exercise pulmonary stress tests showed a significant increase in duration of exercise in patients with the pectus deformity but not in controls. The absolute FVC was increased after surgery in patients with pectus excavatum, but when expressed as a percent predicted, it did not change significantly. There were no differences in preoperative respiratory function during exercise between controls and patients with the pectus deformity. After surgery, patients with pectus excavatum exercised for longer and had improved cardiac function during exercise, as shown by an elevated oxygen and a decrease in heart rate for the same workload. Many also had subjective improvement. In summary, a few patients with pectus excavatum have mild restrictive pulmonary function tests at rest. This restrictive disease is not improved significantly by surgery. There is a statistically signif-icant improvement in exercise duration and cardiac function following surgery (LOE 3).[24]

Patients with pectus excavatum often have EKG abnormalities. An EKG usually shows right axis deviation and depressed ST segments (LOE 5).[26] Cardiac arrhythmias such as supraventricular tachycardia (SVT) and atrial fibrillation have been reported, presumably as a result of impingement of the sternum on the heart. Wolff-Parkinson-White (WPW) syndrome is found in 4% of patients with this deformity,[28] whereas the incidence is about 0.5% in the general population. One study found that patients with severe pectus deformity are less likely to have WPW and SVT, suggesting cardiac im-pingement is not the mechanism (LOE 4).[28]

The diagnosis of pectus excavatum is clinical, although a chest radiograph may demonstrate the depression. Standard anterior/posterior (AP) and lateral chest radio-graphs show sternal depression and cardiac displacement. Pectus excavatum is con-sidered severe if the defect is greater than 2.5 cm (ie, the child's sternum is 2.5 cm or more below the chest wall) (LOE 3)[24] Park recommends an EKG to evaluate children with a pectus deformity, as it is inexpensive and noninvasive (LOE 4).[28] An EKG may show right axis deviation or mitral valve prolapse (MVP). Echocardiograms may also demonstrate MVP, but the clinical significance of this is unclear (LOE 4).[29] A CT scan of the chest is no longer recommended for children with pectus excavatum. The CT scan demonstrates the depression and can quantitate the extent of the defor-mity. However, a study of 12 adolescents showed that the Haller index, used to mea-sure the severity of the deformity, could be measured just as accurately using a chest radiograph as with a CT scan (LOE 4).[27] The CT scan offered no additional information for operative planning. In children with pain or other symptoms, a CT may be consid-ered (LOE 4).[27]

There is not clear evidence to support a best management practice for children with pectus excavatum. Surgery may be done for cosmetic reasons. Haller and Loughlin[24] recommends surgery for those with shortness of breath, fatigue during exercise, abnor-mal breathing dynamics in which the sternum retracts paradoxically instead of expand-ing during inspiration, or for a CT scan that shows a pectus index greater than 3 and a range of 3.2 to 6.0 (LOE 3). Whether surgical correction halts progression of cardiovas-cular compromise and improves exercise tolerance is debated. A meta-analysis of eight studies (169 patients with pectus excavatum) found that surgical repair of the chest wall defect significantly improved cardiovascular function (LOE 1).[30] However, a more recent study criticized that meta-analysis. In their review of 1600 reports from 1965 to 2007, the authors found five papers with primary data on cardiac function before and after surgery. There was no convincing evidence of improvement in pulmonary or cardiac function after thoracic surgery for pectus excavatum (LOE 5).[31]

Pectus Carinatum

Pectus carinatum (pigeon chest) is the second most common congenital defect of the anterior chest wall, but it is much less common than pectus excavatum (LOE 5).[32] It is usually not noticed until early school years and progression at puberty is common. Symptoms (chest pain, dyspnea with exertion) are less likely than with pectus excava-tum, and some report no physical limitations related to this condition (LOE 5).[33] A pec-tus carinatum deformity often leads to psychologic issues for a child because of the unsightly protuberant chest. In some instances, chest pain is noted. It is theorized that this is because of compression of intercostal nerves between adjacent costo-chondral cartilages. The pain is said to be sharp and brief in quality, and radiates to the epigastrium (LOE 5).[33] The diagnosis of pectus carinatum is clinical, but chest radiographs and CT scans add details (LOE 5).[32]

Surgical correction of this deformity has been the mainstay of treatment. However, there is no evidence of changes between preoperative and postoperative pulmonary or cardiac function tests for these patients (LOE 5).[33] A retrospective review of 100 patients with pectus carinatum showed a custom fitted, unobtrusive chest compression brace (worn for 14 to 16 hours/day for 2 years) was just as effective as surgery. In this study, 29 patients were fitted for a brace and 22 of those were followed more than 6 months. Another 17 patients underwent surgery. Outcomes were successful for all and there were no significant complications in either group. This study was not well controlled and 57 patients had no specific treatment. Those children with no therapy were monitored during the 7-year study period, but their outcome is not reported (LOE 4).[34]

Marfan Syndrome

Chest wall deformities are common in Marfan syndrome and these patients are at risk for serious complications, which could lead to chest pain and death. Marfan syndrome is an autosomal dominant disorder of connective tissue with an incidence of 1 in 10,000 in the general population (LOE 5).[35] In approximately 15% of cases, there is no family history for Marfan syndrome, indicating a new mutation. Patients with Marfan syndrome have clinical findings involving three major organ systems: skeletal, cardiac, and ocular. Some of the skeletal abnormalities associated with this syndrome include increased height and arm span, scoliosis, thoracic lordosis, and disorders of the anterior chest, including pectus deformities (LOE 5).[26] Approximately 66% of patients with Marfan syndrome have pectus excavatum or pectus carinatum (LOE 5).[36] Severe pectus excavatum may impact on subsequent cardiothoracic procedures that many patients with Marfan syndrome require. Also, a severe pectus deformity, in association with scoliosis or lordosis may compromise the patient's respiratory status by reducing lung capacity in children with Marfan syndrome. Because of these potential problems, Arn and colleagues[37] recommends surgical repair of pectus excavatum in patients with Marfan syndrome after the patient becomes skeletally mature (LOE 3).

Patients with Marfan syndrome may present with chest pain because the connective tissue defect puts them at risk for spontaneous pneumothorax. These patients are also at risk for dissection of the aorta. Progressive aortic root dilatation occurs in 80% to 100% of cases. Because both such conditions may be life threatening, the complaint of chest pain in a patient with suspected Marfan syndrome must be taken seriously. Echocardiography facilitates detection of patients with cardiac complications and is recommended for all patients with this condition (LOE 2).[38]

Summary

When a child presents with chest pain:

1. Take a careful *history* and focus on:
   - Onset of pain—acute pain is more likely to have an organic etiology
   - Pain wakes child from sleep—more likely to have an organic etiology
   - Pain associated with exertion, syncope—more likely to be cardiac in nature, or exercise-induced asthma
   - Report of fever—more likely to be pneumonia; consider myocarditis, pericarditis
   - Description of midsternal burning pain, worsens when recumbent—consider gastroesophageal reflux
   - History of heart disease—pain is sometimes related to underlying condition (often just anxiety about the underlying condition)

- Serious associated conditions (long-standing diabetes mellitus, Kawasaki disease, asthma, Marfan syndrome, lupus)—these children are at risk for serious complications like ischemia, pneumothorax, pleural effusion
- Stressful life events that correlate with onset of pain—consider psychogenic pain (anxiety)

Grade: Moderate
Level of evidence: Mostly prospective or cohort studies, some retrospective studies

2. Perform a complete *physical examination* and focus on:
   - Respiratory distress, abnormal vital signs—consider transfer to ED
   - Decreased breath sounds, palpable subcutaneous air—consider pneumonia, pneumothorax
   - Wheezing—consider asthma and pain related to complications like pneumomediastinum, pneumothorax
   - Abnormal auscultation of the heart (pathologic murmur, rub, arrhythmia)—consider pericarditis, myocarditis, SVT, structural heart disease
   - Fever—consider pneumonia, myocarditis, pericarditis
   - Evidence of trauma—consider pneumothorax, chest wall injury
   - Reproducible pain—consider musculoskeletal pain, costrochondritis
   - Drooling in a young child—consider foreign body (coin) ingestion
   - Tall, thin patient—consider pneumothorax

Grade: Moderate
Level of Evidence: Prospective studies, retrospective studies, case series, case reports

3. Consider a *chest radiograph* if (see **Table 2**):
   - Unexplained pain of acute onset
   - Respiratory distress, abnormal chest examination
   - Abnormal cardiac examination
   - Significant cough
   - Fever
   - Drooling, gagging, young child
   - Underlying heart disease or serious medical problems

Grade: Moderate
Level of Evidence: Prospective studies, retrospective studies, case series, case reports

4. Consider an *electrocardiogram* if (see **Table 2**):
   - Pain associated with exercise, syncope
   - Abnormal cardiac examination
   - Fever
   - Underlying serious medical problems (Kawasaki disease, long-standing diabetes mellitus, congenital heart disease)

Grade: Moderate
Level of Evidence: Retrospective studies, case series, case reports

5. Consider further testing:
   - D-dimer, chest CT scan—if patient has increased risk for pulmonary embolism (coagulation disorder, recent abortion, trauma, takes oral contraceptives)

- Drug screen for cocaine—if anxious adolescent, hypertension, tachycardia present
- Echocardiogram—if cardiac disease suspected
- Holter monitor—if arrhythmia suspected
- Exercise stress test, pulmonary function tests—if pain is related to exercise

Grade: Low
Level of Evidence: Retrospective studies, case series, case reports

6. Begin *treatment* directed at underlying etiology:
   - Bronchodilators for asthma-related pain
   - Antibiotics for suspected pneumonia
   - H-2 blocker or proton pump inhibitor for midsternal burning pain
   - Analgesics for musculoskeletal pain

Grade: Low
Level of Evidence: Prospective studies, retrospective studies, case series, case reports

7. Treat idiopathic or undiagnosed pain:
   - Analgesics for all (acetaminophen or ibuprofen)
   - Consider H-2 blocker or proton pump inhibitor as a therapeutic trial
   - Arrange follow-up care

Grade: Low
Level of Evidence: Prospective studies, retrospective studies, expert opinion

8. *Refer* patients if:
   - Significant distress, trauma—direct referral to ED
   - Pleural effusion, pneumothorax—direct referral to ED
   - Significant anxiety, depression—consider referral to a psychologist, psychiatrist
   - Associated syncope, dizziness, exercise induced—consider referral to a cardiologist
   - Abnormal cardiac examination—consider referral to cardiologist
   - History of heart disease—consider referral to cardiologist
   - Underlying illness that puts the patient at risk for cardiac disease—consider referral to cardiologist
   - Esophageal foreign body—refer to a specialist for prompt removal
   - Abdominal pain, burning midsternal pain—consider referral to a general pediatrician or gastroenterologist
   - Persistent wheezing—consider referral to a general pediatrician or pulmonologist

Grade: Moderate
Level of Evidence: Prospective studies, retrospective studies, expert opinion

SUMMARY

Chest pain and chest wall deformities are common in children. Chest pain is often a recurrent, chronic symptom. Although most children with chest pain have a benign diagnosis, some have a serious etiology for pain, so the complaint must be addressed carefully. Unfortunately, there are few prospective studies to evaluate this complaint in children. **Table 3** summarizes the prospective studies on pediatric chest pain. Most available studies involve small numbers and are not well controlled. Serious causes for chest pain are rare, making it difficult to develop clear guidelines for

Table 3
Summary of prospective studies on chest pain

Name	Setting	Patients Included	Etiology of Chest Pain	Follow-Up	Limitations
Driscoll DJ, et al. (1976)	Outpatient, ED, or Cardiac Clinic at Milwaukee Children's Hospital	43 (40 agreed to participate) patients in 9 weeks with a primary complaint of chest pain	Idiopathic 18/40 (45%) Costochondritis 9/40 (23%) Bronchitis/cough 5/40 (13%) Muscle strain 2/40 (5%) Direct trauma 2/40 (5%) Miscellaneous (10%): Sickle cell disease 1/40 (3%) Lobar pneumonia 1/40 (3%) Viral syndrome 1/40 (3%) Disc space narrowing 1/40 (3%)	Telephone follow-up at 4 to 8 weeks, contacted 31/40 patients	(1) 3 patients not included. (2) Small number from various settings (none fully represented). (3) Were categories established in advance or for convenience based on results?
Massin MM, et al. (2004)	ED and Cardiac Clinic in Liege, Belgium	168 ED patients with primary complaint of chest pain and 69 patients referred to cardiac clinic for primary complaint of chest pain	ED Chest wall pain 108/168 (64%) Pulmonary 21/168 (13%) Psychologic 15/168 (9%) Cardiac 9/168 (5%) Traumatic 8/168 (5%) Gastrointestinal 6/158 (3%) Herpes zoster 1/168 (1%) Cardiac Clinic Chest Wall pain 61/69 (81%) Cardiac / SVT 5/69 (7%) Respiratory 3/69 (4%)	"Passive" follow-up through medical records available, unclear for what time period	(1) ED patients only examined by a resident physician? (2) Idiopathic pain lumped with chest wall pain so cannot distinguish the two with statistical markers. (3) 23% of patients from outside the EU, so may have included many travelers?

Study	Setting	Population	Diagnoses	Follow-up	Comments
Rowe BH, et al. (1990)	ED at Children's Hospital of Eastern Ontario, Ottawa, Canada	336 patients with complaint of chest pain over 1 year	Chest wall pain 90/325 (28%) Pulmonary 60/325 (19%) Traumatic 49/325 (15%) Idiopathic 39/325 (12%) Psychogenic 17/325 (5%) Miscellaneous (21%) Upper respiratory tract 30/325 (99%) Abdominal pain referred 27/325 (89%) Cardiac 5/325 (29%)	No formal follow-up, but authors felt that adverse outcomes would be made known to them because of the nature of the common health system and their role as a referral center for serious pediatric conditions.	(1) Physical examination in 325/336 (others only had surveys). (2) Authors assumed that they would know about adverse outcomes because children always come to their hospital from the specific referral area.
Selbst SM, et al. (1988)	ED at Children's Hospital of Philadelphia	407 children with complaint of chest pain over 1 year	Idiopathic 21% Musculoskeletal 15% Cough 10% Costochondritis 9% Psychogenic origin 9% Asthma 7% Trauma 5% Pneumonia 4% Gastrointestinal disorders 4% Cardiac disease 4% Sickle cell crisis 2% Miscellaneous 9% (Including precordial catch, pneumothorax, pregnancy, thyroid disease, drugs, etc.)	Follow-up with EKG/Echo for ill-defined or cardiac chest pain. Also had follow-up of 147 patients for 6 months and 51 patients for 2+ years in separately published results.	(1) 23% of patients only seen by a resident physician. (2) Only patients in an ED, so more acute patients likely. (3) Diagnostic studies were not standardized—EKG and CXR were left to the discretion of the clinicians. (4) No patients had sudden death related to chest pain.

Abbreviations: CXR, chest radiograph; ED, emergency department; EKG, electrocardiogram; EU, European Union.

evaluation and management. Based on evidence available the following seems reasonable. A detailed history and physical examination are essential. Although diagnostic tools such as CXR and EKG are relatively inexpensive, it is not practical or necessary to obtain these for all children with chest pain. Laboratory tests should be reserved for those with concerning findings on the history or physical examination. The child with acute onset of pain, pain that is precipitated by exercise, associated with syncope, palpitations, or shortness of breath should be evaluated with diagnostic tests such as CXR and EKG. Also, pain related to a possible coin ingestion, trauma, previous heart disease, asthma, or Marfan syndrome deserves further study. In addition, any child with chest pain that also has abnormalities on physical examination (fever, respiratory distress, abnormal breath sounds, abnormal cardiac examination, obvious trauma, or concerning vital signs) should have a more thorough investigation. The child who appears well, has a normal physical examination, and lacks worrisome history noted above, deserves reassurance and careful follow-up rather than extensive studies.

The level of evidence backing many recommendations in this report is not of superior quality. Multicenter, controlled trials are needed to provide better evidence for diagnosis and management of chest pain and chest wall deformities.

REFERENCES

1. Massin MM, Bourguignont A, Coremans C, et al. Chest pain in pediatric patents presenting to an emergency department or to a cardiac clinic. Clin Pediatr 2004; 43(3):231–8.
2. Selbst SM, Ruddy RM, Clark BJ, et al. Pediatric chest pain: a prospective study. Pediatrics 1988;82:319–23.
3. Rowe BH, Dulberg CS, Peterson RQ, et al. Characteristics of children presenting with chest pain to a pediatric emergency department. CMAJ 1990;143(5):388–94.
4. Driscoll DJ, Glicklich LB, Gallen WJ. Chest pain in children: a prospective study. Pediatrics 1976;57:648–51.
5. Brenner JI, Ringel RE, Berman MA. Cardiologic perspectives of chest pain in childhood: a referral problem? To whom? Pediatr Clin North Am 1984;31:1241–58.
6. Swenson JM, Fischer DR, Miller SA. Are chest radiographs and electrocardiograms still valuable in evaluating pediatric patients with heart murmurs or chest pain? Pediatrics 1997;99(1):1–3.
7. Roodpeyma S, Sadeghian N. Acute pericarditis in childhood: a 10-year experience. Pediatr Cardiol 2000;21(4):363–7.
8. Desai A, Patel S, Book W, et al. "Myocardial infarction" in adolescents: do we have the correct diagnosis? Pediatr Cardiol 2005;26:627–31.
9. Lane JR, Ben-Shachar G. Myocardial infarction in healthy adolescents. Pediatrics 2007;120:e938–43.
10. Berezin S, Medow MS, Glassman MS, et al. Chest pain of gastrointestinal origin. Arch Dis Child 1988;63:1457–60.
11. Sabri MR, Ghavanini AA, Haghighat M, et al. Chest pain in children and adolescents: epigastric tenderness as a guide to reduce unnecessary work-up. Pediatr Cardiol 2003;24:3–5.
12. Lipsitz JD, Masia-Warner C, Apfel H, et al. Anxiety and depressive symptoms and anxiety sensitivity in youngsters with noncardiac chest pain and benign heart murmurs. J Pediatr Psychol 2004;29(8):607–12.
13. Selbst SM, Ruddy R, Clark BJ. Chest pain in children: follow-up of patients previously reported. Clin Pediatr 1990;29:374–7.

14. Miller A, Texidor TA. "Precordial catch": a neglected syndrome of precordial pain. J Am Med Assoc 1955;159:1364–5.
15. Reynolds JL. Precordial catch syndrome in children. South Med J 1989;82: 1228–30.
16. Wilcox DT, Glick PL, Karamanoukian HL, et al. Spontaneous pneumothorax: a single-institution, 12-year experience in patients under 16 years of age. J Pediatr Surg 1995;30(10):1452–4.
17. Damore DT, Dayan PS. Medical causes of pneumomediastinum in children. Clin Pediatr 2001;40:87–91.
18. Uva JL. Spontaneous pneumothoraces, pneumomediastinum and pneumoperitoneum: consequences of smoking crack cocaine. Pediatr Emerg Care 1997;13:24–5.
19. Rajpurkar M, Warrier I, Chitiur M, et al. Pulmonary embolism—experience at a single children's hospital. Thromb Res 2007;119(6):699–703.
20. Sirachainan N, Chuanswmrit A, Angchaisuksiri P, et al. Venous thromboembolism in Thai children. Pediatr Hematol Oncol 2007;24(4):245–56.
21. Weins L, Sabath R, Ewing L. Chest pain in otherwise healthy children and adolescents is frequently caused by exercise-induced asthma. Pediatrics 1992;90:350–3.
22. Tan TQ, Mason EO, Wald ER, et al. Clinical characteristics of children with complicated pneumonia caused by *Streptococcus pneumoniae*. Pediatrics 2002;110:1–6.
23. Grossman LK, Caplan SE. Clinical laboratory, and radiological information in the diagnosis of pneumonia in children. Ann Emerg Med 1988;17(1):43–6.
24. Haller JA, Loughlin GM. Cardiorespiratory function is significantly improved following corrective surgery for sever pectus excavatum. J Cardiovasc Surg 2000;41:125–30.
25. Zhao L, Feinberg MS, Gaides M, et al. Why is exercise capacity reduced in subjects with pectus excavatum? J Pediatr 2000;136:163–7.
26. Ellis DG. Chest wall deformities in children. Pediatr Ann 1989;18(3):161–5.
27. Mueller C, Saint-Vil D, Bouchard S. Chest x-ray as a primary modality for preoperative imaging of pectus excavatum. J Pediatr Surg 2008;43:71–3.
28. Park JM, Farmer AR. Wolff-Parkinson-White syndrome in children with pectus excavatum. J Pediatr 1988;112(6):926–8.
29. Shamberger RC, Welch KJ, Sanders SP. Mitral valve prolapse associated with pectus excavatum. J Pediatr 1987;111(3):404–6.
30. Malek MH, Berger DE, Housh TJ, et al. Cardiovascular function flowing surgical repair of pectus excavatum—a meta-analysis. Chest 2006;130:500–16.
31. Guntheroth WG, Spiers PS. Cardiac function before and after surgery for pectus excavatum. Am J Cardiol 2007;99:1762–4.
32. McGuigan RM, Azarow KS. Congenital chest wall defects. Surg Clin North Am 2006;86:353–70.
33. Golladay ES, Golladay GJ. Chest wall deformities. Indian J Pediatr 1997;64: 339–50.
34. Frey AS, Garcia VF, Brown RL, et al. Non-operative management of pectus carinatum. J Pediatr Surg 2006;41:40–5.
35. Giampietro PF, Raggio C, Davis JG. Marfan syndrome: orthopedic and genetic review. Curr Opin Pediatr 2002;14:35–41.
36. Pyeritz RE, McKusick VA. The Marfan syndrome: diagnosis and management. N Engl J Med 1979;300:772–7.
37. Arn PH, Scherer LR, Haller JA. Outcome of pectus excavatum in patients with Marfan syndrome and in the general population. J Pediatr 1989;115:954–8.
38. Van Karnebeek CDM, Naeff MSJ, Mulder BJM, et al. Natural history of cardiovascular manifestations in Marfan syndrome. Arch Dis Child 2001;84:129–37.

Recurrent Respiratory Infections

Andrew Bush, MBBS (Hons), MA, MD, FRCP, FRCPCH[a,b,*]

KEYWORDS

- Pneumonia • Croup • Otitis media • Immunodeficiency
- Cystic fibrosis • Primary ciliary dyskinesia
- Human immunodeficiency virus • Gastro-esophageal reflux

This article begins with a symptom-based approach to the diagnosis of the child who has recurrent infections of the upper or lower respiratory tract, or of both. Because the differential diagnosis is huge, it is summarized in tables, but no attempt is made to describe in detail every conceivable condition that can present (eg, multifocal consolidation). The second section discusses the presentation of a few specific respiratory conditions that may present as recurrent upper and/or lower respiratory tract infection (eg, cystic fibrosis [CF]). For reasons of space, this article does not discuss the details of specific therapies for these conditions. The problem in trying to provide an evidence-based review of this topic is that there is very little, if any, evidence to review. The methodology required would be to recruit prospectively a large cohort of children presenting with a particular condition (eg, multifocal consolidation), to investigate them in detail, to generate predictive indices for particular conditions or indices that would exclude the need for certain tests, and to validate these indices in at least one other population. Although a systematic approach has been described for cough,[1] it has not been validated in a second population, and in most cases there is not even a discovery population.

Most children experience one or more acute respiratory infections. The challenge is first to decide when the time has come to move from symptomatic therapy to performing diagnostic testing, then to determine which tests need to be done and when testing should be discontinued, and finally to institute specific therapies for the child's underlying condition.

The key decision, whether or not to investigate, is always made on the basis of clinical judgment and experience. Factors to be considered vary with the different specific conditions and are discussed later. General pointers are listed in **Boxes 1–3.**

[a] Imperial School of Medicine at National Heart and Lung Institute, London, UK
[b] Department of Paediatric Respiratory Medicine, Royal Brompton Hospital, Sydney Street, London SW3 6NP, UK
* Department of Paediatric Respiratory Medicine, Royal Brompton Hospital, Sydney Street, London SW3 6NP, UK.
E-mail address: a.bush@rbh.nthames.nhs.uk

Pediatr Clin N Am 56 (2009) 67–100
doi:10.1016/j.pcl.2008.10.004
0031-3955/08/$ – see front matter

Box 1
Pointers that suggest early investigation of a child with recurrent infection may be indicated

The acronym "*SPUR*" (*S*evere, *P*ersistent, *U*nusual, *R*ecurrent) may be a useful mnemonic.

Respiratory infection plus extrapulmonary infections or other disease (eg, arthropathy)

Positive family history: unexplained death, infections or multisystem disease

<u>S</u>evere infection

<u>P</u>ersistent infection and failure of expected recovery

<u>U</u>nusual organisms (eg, *Pneumocystis jiroveci*)

<u>R</u>ecurrent infection

Unless otherwise stated in this article, the level of evidence should be assumed to be low, based on informal consensus and case reports or series.

CLINICAL SCENARIOS: UPPER AIRWAY

Most children presenting with recurrent upper airway infection are normal. Immunodeficiency, however, can present with upper airway problems.[2,3] Particular triggers for further investigation include:[4]

Eight or more new ear infections within a year
Two or more serious sinus infections (eg, requiring intravenous antibiotic treatment) within a year
Persistent oral or cutaneous candidiasis
Two or more months of continuous antibiotics with no effect
The need for intravenous antibiotics to clear infections
Associated systemic features including recurrent deep-seated or skin abscesses or infections, recurrent pneumonia, failure to thrive, positive family history of immunodeficiency

Recurrent Viral Colds

A large, community-based study documented that in childhood the median number of viral colds is five per year, but more than 10% of children have 10 or more colds per

---

Box 2
Pointers in the history of a child presenting with respiratory symptoms that should lead to further investigation

Is the child/family in fact describing true wheeze?

Marked chronic upper airway symptoms: snoring, rhinitis, sinusitis

Symptoms from the first day of life

Very sudden onset of symptoms

Chronic moist cough/sputum production (differentiate from recurrent acute symptoms)

More severe symptoms (or irritability) after feeds and when the child is lying down (vomiting and choking on feeds suggests gastroesophageal reflux or aspiration syndrome)

Any feature of a systemic immunodeficiency

Continuous, unremitting, or worsening symptoms

Box 3
Pointers in the physical examination of a child presenting with respiratory symptoms that should lead to further investigation

Digital clubbing, signs of weight loss, failure to thrive

Upper airway disease: enlarged tonsils and adenoids, prominent rhinitis, nasal polyps

Unusually severe chest deformity (Harrison's sulcus, barrel chest)

Fixed monophonic wheeze

Stridor (monophasic or biphasic)

Asymmetric wheeze

Signs of cardiac or systemic disease

---

year.[5,6] A viral cold usually is a trivial illness. The mean duration of symptoms is around 8 days, but the normal range extends beyond 2 weeks.[6] Symptoms are nasal congestion, rhinorrhea, cough, sore throat, and fever. Thus a normal child may have symptoms of the common cold for nearly 6 months in the year. The misinterpretation of common symptoms as "wheeze"[7–10] may lead to an incorrect diagnosis of asthma. Not unexpectedly, attendance in child day care facilities early in life increases the risk of viral colds.[11] The frequency and duration of colds may come as a surprise, particularly to first-time parents, and misconceptions about the need for treatment are common.[12] The issue of virally induced wheezing is discussed under in the section devoted to the lower airway.

Recommendations
In the absence of any other worrying features on history and examination (**Boxes 2** and **3**), isolated recurrent viral colds do not require further investigation unless the frequency is more than 15 per year, and the duration habitually is more than 15 days per episode. Level of evidence: low.

Rhinitis

Intermittent acute rhinitis must be distinguished from chronic rhinitis, which has a wider differential diagnosis. The definitions of acute and persistent rhinitis are variably defined; one group defined persistent rhinitis as occurring at least 4 days a week for at least 4 weeks;[13] another group holds that acute rhinitis may last as long as 12 weeks.[14] The evidence base on the timing and nature of appropriate investigations in persistent rhinitis is scanty; however, recent combined adult and pediatric guidelines have listed potential investigations that may be useful.[14] The two common causes are infective and allergic rhinitis, and skin prick testing may be indicated. Unilateral rhinitis should lead to consideration of anatomic abnormalities such as unilateral choanal stenosis or the presence of a foreign body. The combination of persistent rhinitis and lower respiratory tract symptoms should prompt diagnostic consideration of allergic rhinitis and asthma (the most common cause); primary ciliary dyskinesia (PCD), especially with neonatal onset of rhinitis; CF (especially if there are nasal polyps); and Wegener's granulomatosis (seen in 21 of 25 patients in one series).[15]

Recommendations
Persistent rhinitis usually does not require detailed investigations. Evidence of allergic sensitization may be sought, and empiric therapeutic trials are reasonable, unless

there is evidence that rhinitis is part of a more generalized disease. Level of evidence: low.

Recurrent Tonsillitis and Pharyngitis

In childhood, significant tonsillar disease manifests commonly as either obstructive sleep apnea (not discussed here) or recurrent acute tonsillitis. Children are considered to have an episode of significant tonsillitis if they satisfy at least one of the following criteria: (1) an oral temperature of at least 38.3°C; (2) cervical lymphadenopathy (enlarged by > 2 cm or tender cervical nodes); (3) tonsillar or pharyngeal exudate; and (4) a positive culture for group A β-hemolytic streptococcus. Conventionally, tonsillectomy is indicated if there have been seven or more documented episodes in the preceding year, five or more in each of the 2 preceding years, or three or more in each of the preceding 3 years.[16] The other indication for tonsillectomy is obstructive sleep apnea. One study has suggested tonsillectomy is a cost-effective strategy for treating obstructive sleep apnea,[17] but in a randomized, controlled trial the risks of surgery were thought to outweigh any benefits.[18] Furthermore, about two thirds of operations are performed for less stringent and thus even less evidence-based criteria.[19] Usually no other investigations are performed for isolated recurrent tonsillitis in the absence of features listed in **Boxes 2** and **3**, but there is no good-quality evidence to inform the decision making about the need for further investigation.

Recommendations

Isolated recurrent tonsillitis and pharyngitis do not require further investigation in the absence of any other worrying features (see **Boxes 2** and **3**). Level of evidence: low.

Sinusitis

Acute sinusitis in children is common and usually a self-limiting disease that requires no investigation. Further investigation, usually in collaboration with an ear, nose, and throat surgeon, should be considered in children who have recurrent acute or severe chronic sinusitis. The differential diagnosis includes respiratory allergy, CF (particularly if nasal polyps or other features of this condition are present), PCD (nasal polyps are said to be common in this condition, but this has not been the author's experience), and systemic immunodeficiency.[14] Mechanical obstruction of the ostia should be considered; the most common isolated cause is an antrachoanal polyp. Gastroesophageal reflux also enters the differential diagnosis or may be a significant comorbidity.[20] Of note: laryngopharyngeal reflux disease may differ from the more usual patterns of reflux, being more common when the patient is upright, and extending into the hypopharynx.[21] Many patients are unaware of the extent of this problem.[22]

In a child who has recalcitrant sinusitis, allergy should be excluded with skin prick tests or radioallergosorbent tests to aeroallergens; the exact panel should be determined by the child's environment. In very young children, genuine allergy may be present, but the skin prick test may not have become positive. As discussed later, it may be necessary to exclude CF, PCD, and immunodeficiency. Imaging of the sinuses with CT or MRI may enable rare anatomic diagnoses to be made.[23] Endoscopy may need to be considered for unilateral disease. Endoscopy also can indicate the presence of reflux disease, which may be associated with one or more of the following observations;[24]

Cobblestoning of the mucosa of the larynx and pharynx
Inflammation of the upper respiratory tract
Sinus involvement
Rhinorrhea

Subglottic stenosis
Velopharyngeal insufficiency
Pharyngotracheitis
Tracheomalacia

Diagnosis may be confirmed by a pH study, or a therapeutic trial of medication may be given.

Recommendations

Most children who have sinusitis need no investigation. Unusually severe or chronic sinusitis may be the presenting feature of a local or systemic immunodeficiency or of gastroesophageal reflux. There is little evidence on which to make specific recommendations about the nature and timing of the most appropriate investigations for sinusitis. Level of evidence: low.

Recurrent Acute and Chronic Otitis Media with Effusion

Acute otitis media is common: one study reported 1.72 episodes per child per year between 6 months and 3 years of age.[6] Viral colds were complicated by acute otitis media (37%) and otitis media with effusion (24%).[24] Chronic otitis media with effusion may be a sign of respiratory allergy (for investigation, see the previous discussion of sinusitis) and immunodeficiency. Eight or more new ear infections per year should be considered a sign of potential immunodeficiency.[4] Curiously, middle ear disease is not increased greatly in CF but is an important feature of PCD. Particular features pointing to a diagnosis of PCD include early-onset and severe hearing loss and prolonged offensive otorrhea after tympanostomy tube insertion. Typically, there is chronic infection with *Pseudomonas aeruginosa* that can be eliminated only with quinolone eardrops. The child has an obvious smelly discharge running down the side of the face, and there is no improvement in hearing. Unfortunately, multiple procedures often are performed before the diagnosis is made.[25]

Recommendations

Most children who have otitis media with or without effusion need no investigation. The possibility of underlying immune deficiency, and in particular PCD, should be borne in mind. There is little evidence on which to make specific recommendations about the nature and timing of the most appropriate investigations for middle ear disease. Level of evidence: low.

Croup and other Causes of Acute Upper Airway Obstruction

Viral croup typically presents with the sudden onset of barking cough, stridor, and respiratory distress in the setting of a coryzal illness. The acute management and differential diagnosis are well described in two recent reviews.[26,27] Importantly, medical management with oral dexamethasone or another oral steroid and nebulized adrenaline should permit intubation to be avoided. Generally infants only have a single or very few episodes, but occasionally patients experience multiple episodes that extend into mid-childhood. In neither review is there any recommendation as to when and how to investigate further. The differential diagnosis includes spasmodic croup, an unsuspected congenital structural abnormality such as a web, subglottic hemangioma, and acquired laryngeal disorders such as a foreign body, subglottic stenosis secondary to previous intubation, or respiratory papillomatosis. Stridor caused by a subglottic hemangioma may present as croup and apparently respond to steroids, because they lead to shrinkage, only to recur subsequently as the hemangioma re-expands.[28]

Recommendations

A single episode of uncomplicated croup with rapid and complete recovery does not require further investigation. Croup should be investigated if

1. The episode is severe (prolonged intubation required).
2. There are atypical features in the history or on examination.
3. Symptoms or signs persist beyond an arbitrary time period (eg, 2 weeks). Croup can be complicated by subglottic stenosis if intubation has been required, and subglottic stenosis enters the differential diagnosis of persistent stridor in a previously well child.
4. There are recurrent episodes, particularly if severe.

There is, however, insufficient evidence to identify the point at which investigation is warranted. Level of evidence: low.

Further investigations in upper airway obstruction

Before any investigation is undertaken, a detailed history and examination should be performed. If the child is old enough, a flow–volume curve should be performed; the typical truncated shape of extrathoracic obstruction may be seen (**Fig. 1**). In younger infants, a tidal flow–volume loop may be suggestive of large airway obstruction.[29] A neck radiograph may reveal a radiopaque foreign body but generally is not helpful. The most useful investigations are a fiberoptic bronchoscopy, under general anesthesia using a pernasal approach via a facemask held by the anesthetist; and serum calcium levels (hypocalcemia may present as recurrent stridor) and C_1-esterase inhibitor levels (deficiency presents as recurrent subglottic swelling leading to stridor).

The relationship between croup, croup with wheeze, and recurrent croup with subsequent asthma is controversial. In one study[30] physician-diagnosed croup was inversely associated with atopy at school age. The Oslo study showed that atopic children who had a diagnosis of croup were less likely to have a subsequent diagnosis of asthma, whereas non-atopic children were more likely to have a later diagnosis of asthma.[31] Another study showed that the odds ratio for a diagnosis of asthma was increased by a diagnosis of croup and increased still further if croup was recurrent.[32] Croup with wheeze may be more predictive of subsequent asthma.[33] Overall, although croup may be a marker for future asthma in some children, for most children it is an

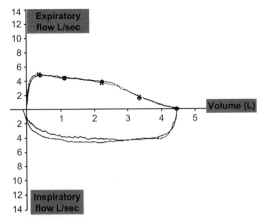

Fig. 1. Pulmonary function testing. Rigid tracheal obstruction is suggested by abrupt attenuation of flows in inspiration and expiration.

isolated illness with no long-term sequelae. Because the early institution of inhaled corticosteroids has not been shown to prevent recurrent croup and certainly does not prevent the progression of intermittent wheeze to multi-trigger wheeze,[34–38] the debate about the relationship between croup and asthma is not of practical clinical importance at the moment.

Recently, the most important infectious cause of stridor is bacterial tracheitis.[39] Immunization has almost completely abolished acute epiglottitis and laryngeal diphtheria, although these diseases should be considered in the nonimmunized child. Retropharyngeal abscess, which may be associated with a penetrating foreign body, is another rare cause of presentation with a crouplike illness, although the child usually is more toxic.

Recommendations for further investigations

There is no evidence on which to base guidelines for further investigation of children who have upper airway infections causing stridor not caused by viral laryngotracheitis. Most pediatricians would not investigate a single episode in an otherwise well child. Possibly, a single documented episode of type B *Haemophilus Influenzae* epiglottitis in a fully immunized child might merit further investigation. Level of evidence: low.

CLINICAL SCENARIOS: LOWER AIRWAY

This section is divided into three parts: chronic productive cough, recurrent wheezing lower respiratory tract infection, and recurrent radiologic shadowing. This approach has been found to be useful in personal practice, although some investigations that cut across clinical scenarios may be described inadequately or, conversely, there may be repetition. Specific conditions that are referred to in the differential diagnosis in these sections (eg, CF, PCD, and immunodeficiency) are discussed in the final sections of the article.

Many children are too young for pulmonary function testing, although increasingly techniques such as airway resistance using the interrupter technique (R_{INT})[40] and the lung clearance index[41–43] are applicable in preschool-age children. The shape of the tidal flow–volume loop may suggest an obstructive picture.[29] If there are facilities to carry out spirometry, lung volumes, and carbon monoxide transfer, and the child is able to perform these tests, much useful information can be obtained. Pulmonary function testing provides only part of the clinical information, however, and the only specific diagnoses that can be made in the pulmonary function laboratory are exercise-induced asthma and hyperventilation syndromes.

Airway disease is suggested by the combination of hyperinflation (raised residual volume, functional residual capacity, and total lung capacity) with reduced 1-second forced expiratory volume (FEV_1) and FEV_1 to forced vital capacity (FVC) ratio. Elevated carbon monoxide transfer (DL_{co}) is suggestive of asthma or bronchiectasis, whereas reduced DL_{co} suggests parenchymal destruction as well as airflow obstruction (eg, the sequelae of chronic lung disease of prematurity). Parenchymal disease is suggested by reduced FEV_1 and FVC, with a normal or elevated FEV_1:FVC ratio and reduced residual volume, functional residual capacity, and total lung capacity. A high DL_{co} per liter of accessible lung volume suggests chest wall restriction, such as scoliosis. An isolated reduction in DL_{co} suggests pulmonary vascular disease, such as recurrent pulmonary embolism or primary pulmonary hypertension. An isolated elevation in DL_{co} suggests recent pulmonary hemorrhage.

The shape of the flow–volume loop may give additional clues. Rigid tracheal obstruction is suggested by abrupt attenuation of flows in inspiration and expiration (see **Fig. 1**). Attenuation in only the expiratory limb suggests variable obstruction (eg, malacia) of the intrapulmonary trachea or large airways. Isolated attenuation of the inspiratory limb may be caused by variable obstruction of the extrathoracic trachea, inspiratory muscle (diaphragm) dysfunction, or stiff lungs. Marked variability, and in particular a very variably impaired inspiratory flow–volume curve, is highly suggestive of vocal cord dysfunction.[44]

Another important issue is the state of the child's immune system. In the following sections, it is assumed that the child does not have a known and diagnosed immune deficiency but is thought at presentation to have a normal immune system. The special problems of the immunodeficient child are discussed in a separate section or are referred to specifically where applicable. For example, recurrent infiltrates would be investigated very differently, and much more urgently, in a child who has pancytopenia after chemotherapy than in an otherwise well child who has similar radiologic appearances.

Chronic, Usually Productive Cough

It is important to distinguish recurrent, acute, productive-sounding cough, which usually is secondary to a series of viral colds, from a continuous productive cough, which needs investigation if it persists beyond a certain time period. In a group of children who had cough severe enough to be referred to a specialist pediatrician and who then were submitted to a detailed diagnostic algorithm after 3 weeks of cough (nearly 90% of which was productive), more than 20% got better spontaneously, suggesting this duration of cough is too short to merit referral.[1] The British Thoracic Society recommends 8 weeks as the definition of chronic cough,[45] but this recommendation is not based on any firm evidence. Clearly context is crucial: if the child is clinically unwell, investigation may need to begin at once, and it would be wrong to specify a duration that warrants investigation. In a hospital context, it is clear that parental report of a productive cough correlates well with the finding of secretions in the lower airway.[46] The largest study systematically investigating children who had chronic cough used a protocol of successively performing laboratory tests (sweat chloride, common CF mutations, serum *Mycoplasma pneumoniae* IgM, and *Bordetella pertussis* IgA serology, immunoglobulins G, A, M, and E and IgG subclasses), bronchoscopy (occasionally induced sputum), chest high-resolution CT (HRCT), and a pH probe. Finally, when necessary, blind trials of therapy were performed. A number of important lessons emerged. The first is that the adult causes of chronic cough (asthma, gastroesophageal reflux disease, and upper airway disease) are uncommon causes of chronic cough in children. Indeed, many lines of evidence support the view that isolated cough in children is rarely caused by asthma and should not be treated as such.[47,48] The most common cause identified was persistent bacterial bronchitis (PBB) in nearly 40% of children.[1] In this report the diagnostic criteria for confirmed PBB were a history of chronic moist cough, a positive bronchoalveolar lavage fluid (BAL) culture, and response to antibiotic treatment (amoxicillin/clavulanic acid suspension) with resolution of the cough within 2 weeks. Probable PBB was defined as a history of chronic moist cough and either positive BAL culture or immediate response to antibiotic therapy with resolution of the cough within 2 weeks. In most cases of probable PBB, the BAL culture reached only 10^3 or 10^4 colony-forming units (cfu)/mL rather than an arbitrary 10^5 cfu/mL, or the patients required additional antibiotic therapy before the cough disappeared. A subsequent article suggested that multiple courses of antibiotics were needed to resolve the cough,[49] and that the rapid response to a short course reported by Marchant and colleagues[1] might reflect the relatively short duration of symptoms in their group. It also is not clear whether it would be more cost effective to prescribe an empiric course of antibiotics before embarking on investigations.

PBB is undoubtedly a real and important entity, but most clinicians believe that the diagnostic criteria should be tighter than those listed in the previous paragraph. PBB is a diagnosis of exclusion; it should be suspected in the child who has chronic productive cough lasting longer than 8 weeks, and investigations should show a neutrophilic BAL with positive cultures (with normal BAL cytology, a positive culture may represent a contaminant) but also must eliminate bronchiectasis, gastroesophageal reflux disease, and local and systemic immunodeficiency as a cause for the symptoms. BAL findings alone are insufficient for the diagnosis. The relationship between PBB and subsequent idiopathic bronchiectasis is unclear. An attractive hypothesis is that untreated PBB can progress to idiopathic bronchiectasis, but at the moment there is no evidence that PBB is pre-bronchiectatic.[50] There also is no knowledge of the etiology; PBB may be the result of a congenital or acquired postinfective localized immune deficiency, which subsequently may improve. The presence of PBB in children older than age 10 years suggests that the abnormality is acquired.

Although asthma is not an infectious disease, the problem of cough-variant asthma is considered here because it is misdiagnosed so frequently. There is no doubt that cough-variant asthma does exist, but it is rare and is virtually unknown in non-atopic children. The author is reluctant to diagnose any form of asthma in the absence of significant breathlessness. Indeed, it is rare to find airway eosinophilia suggestive of asthma even in atopic children who have cough as their sole symptom.[48] In children old enough to perform pulmonary function tests, cough-variant asthma should not be diagnosed unless clear-cut evidence of variable airflow obstruction can be demonstrated. In the younger child, in whom pulmonary function testing is not be practical in most circumstances, a three-stage therapeutic trial is recommended:

1. Commence inhaled corticosteroids. There is some evidence that some children who seem not to respond to inhaled salbutamol respond to inhaled corticosteroids.[51,52] Oral steroids are not recommended because of potential systemic effects and also because of possible upper airway effects (eg, shrinking adenoidal tissue), which may confuse the issue. There is no evidence on which to base the dose and duration of inhaled corticosteroids; anecdotally, a moderately high-dose (800 µg/d) beclomethasone equivalent for 8 weeks is suggested.
2. Stop therapy after a period of time. The duration of the trial should be sufficient to ensure that any possible response is detected. If there is no response, the child does not have cough-variant asthma. An apparent response, however, may in fact be a spontaneous regression of cough, in which case treatment is not indicated.
3. Restart therapy only if the symptoms recur on stopping treatment. This precaution eliminates the possibility of labeling transient symptoms as cough-variant asthma. Treatment then is titrated down to the lowest dose needed to control symptoms.

It is convenient to consider what role, if any, exhaled nitric oxide measurements (FeNO) have in the diagnostic process. Nasal NO is discussed in the section devoted to PCD. In general, there is too much overlap between the FeNO measurements for CF, bronchiectasis, PCD, and asthma for this test to be of much use in diagnosing individuals.[53] A very high FeNO (twice the upper limit of normal) was reported only in children who had asthma. Some individuals, however, seem to have a constitutively high FeNO in the absence of symptoms,[54] and a high FeNO should not be equated uncritically with a diagnosis of asthma. At the present time, FeNO cannot be recommended as a diagnostic test in recurrent respiratory infections.

Recommendations

1. A child who has a true chronic cough (as opposed to recurrent acute cough) of several weeks' duration should be investigated systematically. The duration of symptoms before investigation is not clear but should not exceed 8 weeks and should be shorter in a child who is unwell. Systematic, protocol-driven evaluation leads to a high diagnostic yield. Level of evidence: moderate
2. Chronic isolated cough is rarely caused by asthma and should not be treated as such. Cough-variant asthma usually is a diagnosis of exclusion. Level of evidence: moderate
3. FeNO is not a useful test in the diagnosis of recurrent respiratory infections. Level of evidence: moderate to high

Recurrent Wheezing Lower Respiratory Tract Infection

In young children, recurrent wheezing in the lower respiratory tract almost always is caused by recurrent viral infection. It is important to note that patients' families often use the term "wheeze" imprecisely. Some European languages do not have such a term; in England, many different airway sounds may be described as "wheeze," including upper airway rattling and even stridor.[7–10] The use of a video questionnaire may help define the noise. In one study, physician assessment of wheeze correlated with objective measurements, but parents and nurses were not so accurate.[55] Furthermore, the nomenclature of this condition is confused: wheeze can be defined either by symptom pattern or by epidemiologic course. Symptom pattern is more useful prospectively, and the history should categorize the pattern as either episodic (viral) or multi-trigger wheeze. Epidemiologically, wheeze is either transient (disappearing after the first 3 years of life) or persistent (present throughout the first 6 years of life). It sometimes is assumed that the terms "viral" (episodic) and "transient," and "multi-trigger" and "persistent" can be used interchangeably, but there is no evidence that this is the case. Thus, further investigation should be considered in three scenarios:

1. Recurrent acute or chronic nonspecific airway sounds (not true wheeze)
2. Episodic (viral) wheeze
3. Multi-trigger wheeze (usually a combination of episodic, viral-associated symptoms and interval, multi-trigger wheeze)

There also has been interest in the role of bacterial coinfection in viral wheeze. The Copenhagen Prospective Study on Asthma in Childhood (COPSAC) study showed that positive upper airway cultures for bacterial pathogens in babies are associated with subsequent wheeze.[56] A smaller study showed that serologic investigation frequently revealed evidence of bacterial coinfection with respiratory virus–induced wheeze,[57] although features suggestive of a major infection, such as systemic toxicity and elevation in C-reactive protein, were rare. The most likely hypothesis is that the propensity for viral wheeze and low-grade mucosal bacterial infection are both manifestations of a subtle and probably maturational mucosal immune deficiency,[58] which may be related to antenatal events such as maternal smoking[59–61] and possibly to epigenetic mechanisms.[62] Further discussion of this possibility is beyond the scope of this article.

Airway sounds that are not true wheeze

Commonly the child has viral colds with relatively prolonged symptoms or nonspecific upper airway noises that require no treatment other than reassurance of the family. Symptoms may persist beyond the third birthday. Occasionally, stridor may be misdiagnosed as wheeze and should be investigated along standard lines; most would advocate an early bronchoscopy.

Episodic (viral) wheeze

Wheeze with viral colds is common, often is not severe (ie, is not life threatening), but frequently is a cause of considerable morbidity and loss of time from work for the child's care givers. In some children, however, the attacks really may be severe. In an otherwise well child who has mild to moderate episodic wheeze, investigation is not necessary. If the wheezing illness really is severe, investigation may be indicated, as discussed later.

Multi-trigger wheeze

In older children, multi-trigger wheeze usually is associated with demonstrable variable airflow obstruction and responds to standard asthma therapy. When no other feature of the history or examination suggests an alternative diagnosis, no further investigation is required. One group used a detailed protocol to investigate severely affected wheezy (episodic and multi-trigger) preschool children.[63] Measurements included immunoglobulins and subclasses, a sweat test, nasal ciliary brushings, a pH probe, HRCT, and bronchoscopy. There was a high yield of abnormal findings, including gastroesophageal reflux, PBB, and airway eosinophilia, often despite oral or inhaled steroid therapy. What this group could not demonstrate was whether this aggressive approach leads to an improved outcome; a prospective clinical trial is required for this issue to be resolved.

Recommendations

1. Most children who have true wheezing caused by lower respiratory tract infections do not require further investigation. Level of evidence: moderate
2. Aggressive, protocol-driven investigation of severe wheeze will lead to new diagnoses, but the clinical relevance of these diagnoses often is not clear. Level of evidence: moderate.

Recurrent Radiologic Shadowing

The vague term "radiologic shadowing" is used because many of these conditions can cause either consolidation or atelectasis. Although radiologic patterns may give a clue to the diagnosis, the patterns often are nonspecific, and detailed further investigation usually is indicated.

"Recurrent chest infection" in lay parlance usually means recurrent episodes of a productive cough, generally in association with viral colds, and is not the same as recurrent shadowing on chest radiographs. Recurrent bouts of coughing may require investigation, as discussed previously, but cough is normal,[64] and the frequency of cough is notoriously poorly evaluated by parents and children.[65–68] At least two episodes of documented radiologic shadowing are required to merit investigation for possible recurrent lower respiratory tract infection. A single episode of uncomplicated lobar pneumonia in an otherwise well and thriving child does not require investigation. Indeed, if the child is seen by an experienced clinician and is thought to have made a complete recovery, even a follow-up chest radiograph is not necessary.[69,70] Further investigation is mandated, however, if the child has had a previous history of unusual infections, there is a family history of an immune problem or an unexplained death from infection, there are any features to suggest a systemic illness, or the pneumonia is at all atypical in its course.

The child with recurrent shadowing on the chest radiograph should not be assumed to be having repeated infections, particularly if there is not complete radiologic clearing between episodes. The differential diagnoses and investigation of recurrent shadowing in the same area and of multifocal recurrent shadowing are described here in turn. The reader will need to consult standard texts for the further detailed investigation of many of these conditions.

Recurrent radiologic shadowing in the same place

A child with two or more radiologically documented episodes of shadowing in the same lobe or segment, particularly if there is incomplete clearing between episodes or with a single episode that does not clear should be investigated further. The differential diagnosis is summarized in **Box 4**. The radiologic changes of acute pneumonia may take 6 to 12 weeks or even longer to resolve, depending on the causative

---

Box 4
Differential diagnosis of recurrent or chronic localized radiographic changes

Right middle lobe syndrome

Localized airway obstruction

  Within the lumen

    Congenital webs

    Endobronchial foreign body

    Mucus plug

    Carcinoid or other pedunculated tumor

    Inflammatory pseudotumor secondary to previous intubation

  Within the airway wall

    Localized malacia

    Localized bronchiectasis (underlying cause must be sought)

    Complete cartilage rings

    Intramural tumor

  Extrinsic compression

    Congenital thoracic malformation

    Enlarged cardiac chamber caused by right to left shunting, cardiomyopathy

    Vascular ring, pulmonary artery sling

    Lymph nodes: tuberculosis, lymphoma, other

    Mediastinal or lung tumor

    Fibrosing mediastinitis

Pulmonary parenchymal disease

  Congenital: cystic congenital thoracic malformation

  Acquired: infection in residual cystic change after a cavitating pneumonia or tuberculosis (tumor will be focal and progressive)

*First manifestation of a cause of recurrent fluctuating multifocal consolidation (see **Box 5**)*

organism.[71,72] Determining when to investigate thus becomes a matter of clinical judgment, depending on the history, whether the child is improving clinically, and whether there are any other features suggestive of another condition. There are no evidence-based recommendations to guide the clinician.

Right middle lobe syndrome probably is the most common clinically encountered focal consolidation for which there is some evidence to base recommendations. It is the most common recurrent focal investigation encountered in clinical practice and thus merits a separate section. Right middle lobe syndrome also may be related to the conditions listed in **Box 4**. The definition of right middle lobe syndrome is clinical: atelectasis of the right middle lobe or lingula persisting for more than 1 month or recurring twice or more despite treatment.[73] The author's experience is that the lingula is affected only rarely in comparison with the right middle lobe, although others report right middle lung disease being as only twice as common as lingula disease.[74] The likely explanation of the frequency of right middle lobe disease is the anatomy: every bronchoscopist is familiar with the acute take-off and often slitlike orifice of the right middle lobe bronchus, which intuitively makes it likely to be vulnerable to occlusion. A pathologic study of 21 resected specimens (adults and children) showed bronchiectasis (n = 10), chronic bronchitis and bronchiolitis with lymphoid hyperplasia (n = 7), patchy organizing pneumonia (n = 6), atelectasis (n = 5), granulomatous inflammation (n = 5), and abscess formation (n = 4).[75] These findings obviously represent the most severe cases but suggest that infection is important, and thus early diagnosis and aggressive treatment of infection may be beneficial. Studies in which BAL was performed documented infection in one third to one half of cases; *H. influenzae* was the most common pathogen. Only 2 of 53 subjects had an endobronchial obstruction seen at bronchoscopy. More than 25% had bronchiectasis, and, unsurprisingly, their outcome after treatment was less good.[73]

The relationship between right middle lobe syndrome and atopy and asthma is controversial. One group made the diagnosis more commonly in atopic patients.[74] Another group showed an increase in bronchial responsiveness, but not atopy, in children who had right middle lobe syndrome.[76] By contrast, De Boeck and colleagues[77] showed that one third of the children who had been diagnosed with right middle lobe syndrome had subsequent chronic asthmalike symptoms. It seems likely (but is unproven) that any hypersecretory respiratory syndrome such as asthma may be complicated by right middle lobe syndrome, but the series are too small to pick up such an effect (eg, in the largest recent series only 5 of 53 subjects had an eosinophilic lavage).[73,76] It would be wise to follow these children carefully.

Recommendations
1. Children who have right middle lobe syndrome may have underlying chronic infection and bronchiectasis. If radiologic changes have not cleared within 1 month, or if they recur after treatment, further investigation with bronchoscopy and perhaps HRCT scanning is indicated. The diagnostic yield of these tests probably is high, but there are no outcome data to show that aggressive investigation is beneficial. Level of evidence: moderate
2. The families of children who have right middle lobe syndrome should be advised that these children are at risk of chronic respiratory symptoms and asthma and should be followed carefully or should return for re-evaluation at the first signs of recurrent symptoms. Level of evidence: moderate.

Other recurrent focal abnormalities in a single site
Important steps in the investigation of focal abnormalities are a fiberoptic bronchoscopy to rule out focal airway disease and HRCT scanning to exclude focal

parenchymal disease. Other imaging modalities that may help include endobronchial ultrasound to demonstrate complete cartilage rings and CT reconstruction of the airway anatomy. It always is good practice to try to obtain previous imaging, to see if the abnormality is new or might be congenital. Ideally HRCT should be performed when the child is not acutely infected, because acute changes may complicate the interpretation of the scans. It is worth considering giving intravascular contrast with the HRCT to delineate vascular anatomy: if the abnormality has an arterial supply from the abdominal aorta or drains into the systemic circulation, a congenital thoracic malformation is likely. If mediastinal disease is thought to be an issue, an MRI scan may be indicated; the lack of radiation makes this modality attractive, but the current requirement for general anesthesia for small children in most centers militates against its use unless essential. An echocardiogram is a simple investigation which is often forgotten and which may show an enlarged cardiac chamber compressing the bronchus. The differential diagnosis is wide and is summarized in **Box 4**. If HRCT and bronchoscopy have not established the diagnosis, a more invasive approach, including surgical excision or lymph node biopsy, may be indicated. The possibility that a single-site change may be the first presentation of a generalized illness should not be forgotten.

Recommendations
1. The differential diagnosis of recurrent or chronic shadowing in a single site is wide, and investigation is indicated. There is no evidence base to inform the clinician of the optimal timing of investigation or the optimal sequence of tests. Level of evidence: low
2. If simple investigations have not yielded a diagnosis, aggressive investigation of recurrent or chronic shadowing in a single site, including surgical excision or mediastinoscopy as appropriate, is justified. Level of evidence: low.

Recurrent multifocal radiologic shadowing
Again, the differential diagnosis for recurrent multifocal shadowing, as for recurrent radiologic shadowing in a single site, is wide (**Box 5**), and details of specific conditions are given elsewhere. Fixed or relentlessly progressing pulmonary shadowing (eg, caused by malignancy or interstitial lung disease) is not discussed here. This section suggests a few, perhaps less obvious, points that may be valuable in elucidating this problem, without attempting to all possibilities in detail.

As always, a detailed history is essential. Because international travel is common, a detailed history of where the child has been is vital. A medication history is important and should not be limited to prescription drugs.[78] Nervous system disease may affect the lung through many mechanisms. Neurologic incoordinate swallowing may be overlooked easily. Specific questions about choking and swallowing must be asked, and if there is any doubt, the child should be evaluated by an experienced speech therapist. Another cause of swallowing problems is a laryngeal cleft, which may be overlooked unless a rigid bronchoscope is used to examine the upper airway. Laryngeal cleft may coexist with esophageal atresia and enters the differential diagnosis of recurrent aspiration after surgical repair of the atresia.[79] Cough is a fundamental defense mechanism, requiring both inspiratory and especially expiratory muscle strength. Disease such as spinal muscular atrophy may present first in the respiratory muscles and typically affects the expiratory muscles preferentially, leading to recurrent infection and mucus plugging.

Gastroesophageal reflux and respiratory disease have a complex relationship. There is no doubt that respiratory disease can worsen aspiration by multiple mechanisms. Also, reflux can cause respiratory disease, both by direct aspiration and by an esophagobronchial reflex,[80] or reflux can be an incidental finding of no consequence. The diagnosis of reflux also is controversial. The reference standard for a diagnosis of acid reflux is 24-hour pH-metry. This technique has been refined by the use of an upper and lower esophageal electrode, to try to determine the significance of any esophageal acid,[81] but, as pointed out previously, acid reflux confined to the lower esophagus is not necessarily benign. The significance of non-acid reflux has been debated. Although non-acid reflux now can be detected, its measurement between 24-hour periods is more variable than that of pH-metry,[82] and currently the evidence that this measurement adds anything of clinical importance to the standard test is, at best, controversial.[83]

If reflux is difficult to identify, is it possible to diagnose direct aspiration of gastric contents into the respiratory tract? This finding would be unequivocal evidence of harm. The use of lipid-laden macrophages measured on BAL has long been popular, but this test lacks specificity.[84] Perhaps the best evidence is negative: if there are no lipid-laden macrophages in the BAL, significant aspiration is unlikely. Measurement of BAL pepsin may be more specific,[85] but this test is not widely available. Finally, simultaneous measurement of intra-esophageal and intratracheal pH has been described,[86] but this tool is unlikely to be practical in children.

Late-presenting congenital H-type fistula may be difficult to diagnose.[87] A tube esophagram is the usual investigation, but in the author's experience a normal test does not exclude a fistula, and direct visualization at bronchoscopy may be needed. For suspected esophageal dysmotility defects, sophisticated manometry may be needed.

Pulmonary hemorrhagic syndromes may result in a diagnostic challenge if the child swallows rather than expectorates blood. Presentation then may be with iron deficiency anemia, and an extensive gastroenterologic work-up must be performed.[88] Iron-laden macrophages on the BAL are pathognomonic of pulmonary hemorrhage but cannot distinguish between the various causes of primary and secondary bleeding. Generally, if there is no evidence of a systemic disease or secondary cause of pulmonary hemorrhage, the condition is considered to be idiopathic pulmonary hemosiderosis, and a confirmatory lung biopsy is not performed. If the child bleeds repeatedly, however, open lung biopsy to exclude a neutrophilic capillaritis should be considered,[89] because this diagnosis may prompt treatment with cyclophosphamide. If a connective tissue disease is suspected, the help of a pediatric rheumatologist should be sought. If immunodeficiency is suspected (discussed later), the author performs simple screening investigations but refers the patient for more sophisticated testing. A reasonable series of screening tests for the pediatric pulmonologist who suspects a connective tissue disease consists of an erythrocyte sedimentation rate, anti-neutrophil cytoplasmic antibody studies, double-stranded DNA, rheumatoid factor, complement studies, anti-glomerular basement membrane antibody (for children who have pulmonary hemorrhage and renal disease), and circulating immune complexes.

Recommendations

1. Children who have recurrent multifocal chest radiographic changes should be investigated, but there is no evidence base to guide the clinician as to the most appropriate timing or sequence of investigations. Level of evidence: low
2. The differential diagnosis of recurrent multifocal chest radiographic changes is so wide, and the number of possible tests is so great, that a targeted approach, based on clinical suspicion driven by history and physical examination, is recommended. Level of evidence: low.

Box 5
Differential diagnosis of recurrent fluctuating multifocal radiographic changes

Recurrent respiratory infection

    Local immunodeficiency

        Cystic fibrosis

        Primary ciliary dyskinesia

        Other subtle abnormalities of mucosal defense also likely

    Systemic immunodeficiency (most require investigation by immunologic specialist)

        Congenital (see **Box 7**)

        Acquired (see **Box 7**)

    Structural abnormality

        Postinfective or idiopathic bronchiectasis

    Neurologic disease causing weakness of particularly expiratory muscles

    Unusual non-granulomatous infections

        Hydatid disease (usually but not inevitably nonfluctuating)

Recurrent aspiration syndromes

    Bulbar and pseudobulbar palsy

        Central neurologic disease, peripheral nerve or muscle disease

    Laryngeal cleft

    Isolated, late-presenting H-type fistula

    Esophageal dysmotility syndromes

        After tracheoesophageal fistula repair

        Achalasia

        Others

    Severe gastroesophageal reflux

        Primary or secondary to respiratory disease

        Anatomic defects: hiatus hernia

        Delayed gastric emptying

    Lipid inhalation

        Oily medication and nose drops

Recurrent pulmonary edema

    Left to right shunting (eg, ventricular septal defect, patent arterial duct)

    Heart failure (eg, cardiomyopathy}

Major airway obstruction (trachea, carina, large bronchi)

    Vascular rings and slings (look for a right-sided aortic arch on the chest radiograph)

    Generalized bronchomalacia (Williams Campbell syndrome, others)

    Multiple complete cartilage rings

    Airway compression by an enlarged heart or great vessels (eg, absent pulmonary valve syndrome)

Iatrogenic

    Direct pulmonary drug toxicity

    Indirect effects of medications (eg, on the heart)

Hypersecretory syndromes

    Hypersecretory asthma

    Plastic bronchitis syndromes

Pulmonary hemorrhagic syndromes

    Secondary pulmonary hemorrhage

        Pulmonary venous hypertensive syndromes

        Coagulopathy

        Bronchial circulatory hypertrophy of any cause

    Isolated pulmonary syndromes

        Idiopathic pulmonary hemosiderosis

        Isolated pulmonary vasculitic syndromes

        Pulmonary arteriovenous malformation

    Part of a systemic disease

        Goodpasture's syndrome

        Other autoimmune diseases and vasculitis

Autoimmune disease unrelated to pulmonary hemorrhage

    Systemic lupus erythematosus

    Rheumatoid syndromes

    Others

Allergic lung disease

    Allergic bronchopulmonary aspergillosis (usually secondary to cystic fibrosis)

    Extrinsic allergic alveolitis

Granulomatous disease

    Sarcoidosis

    Tuberculosis

    Other chronic infections

DIAGNOSING SPECIFIC CONDITIONS PRESENTING AS CHRONIC OR RECURRENT ACUTE ON CHRONIC PRODUCTIVE COUGH

Cystic Fibrosis

Increasingly, most cases of CF are diagnosed by newborn screening. Even in areas where screening is routine, however, mild atypical cases are missed. In areas where the prevalence is thought to be a low, the diagnosis may be forgotten. The respiratory phenotype suggestive of CF as against other causes of recurrent infection is chronic productive cough with positive cultures for typical CF-related organisms, especially when combined with suggestive extrapulmonary features. Typical CF organisms include *Staphylococcus aureus*, *Pseudomonas aeruginosa* (especially mucoid strains), other gram-negative rods such as *Burkholderia cepacia* and *Stenotrophomonas maltophilia,* and nontuberculous *Mycobacteria. H. influenzae* also is found in CF but is not particularly specific to that disease. Extrapulmonary manifestations that must be sought actively include pancreatic insufficiency, rectal prolapse, electrolyte disorders (heat exhaustion, hyponatremia), liver disease (which occurs only if the child has pancreatic insufficiency), very severe sinus disease, and particularly nasal polyps, which in childhood are almost pathognomonic of CF.

Once CF is suspected, diagnosis usually is straightforward. The sweat test is diagnostic in more than 98% of cases.[90] For practical purposes, a properly performed sweat test with a chloride concentration of more than 60 mmol in duplicate can be considered diagnostic. The most common cause of a false-positive finding is operator inexperience, followed by eczema. Although a number of extremely rare conditions are reported to elevate sweat chloride,[91] this writer has never encountered them in practice. Although most cases are diagnosed easily, a small minority presents a very vexatious problem. The diagnosis of CF has undergone a revolution in the last 20 years: whereas the sweat test previously was considered the reference standard for the diagnosis of CF, it has become clear that patients who have CF may have normal sweat electrolytes. These cases often, but not invariably, have a mild or atypical phenotype. A study in adults suggested that in equivocal cases, giving fludrocortisone, 3 mg/m^2, on two successive days, and repeating the sweat test on the third day may be helpful; healthy persons who had an equivocal sweat sodium then present in the normal range.[92] In the absence of pediatric data, however, this test should be used with caution.

Genetic testing may be helpful; however, at least 1300 variants of the CF transmembrane conductance regulator (*CFTR*) gene have been described, and routine laboratory testing detects the only most common 90% to 95%. There are marked ethnic differences in *CFTR* gene frequencies, and if the genetic laboratory is to be used most efficiently, race-specific panels should be used. Even with this approach, in many cases only a single gene or no gene is detected, leaving the diagnosis still in doubt. Complete gene sequencing may be helpful but is not widely available.

There are a number of potential problems with genetic testing.[93] First, it is essential to distinguish harmless polymorphisms from disease-producing mutations. At least in theory, a second *CFTR* mutation can cancel out the effects of the first. Even with normal exon amino acid sequences, CF may be produced by intron modifications. Finally, phenotypic CF has been described with completely normal *CFTR* gene sequences.[94] The explanation of these findings is unknown, but a likely possibility comes from consideration of the biology of CFTR. CTFR is a multifunctional protein that interacts with many other proteins at the cell surface and also requires interaction with many other proteins to traverse to the cell surface.[95] It may be that CF with a normal *CFTR* gene sequence is caused by a mutation in one of these interacting proteins. There is precedent for such an idea: the histologic pattern of pulmonary alveolar proteinosis may be produced by mutations in either the surfactant B or C genes but also occurs without abnormality in these genes but with mutations in a surfactant protein-processing gene, *ABCA3*.[96]

A further direct test of CFTR function is the measurement of electrical potential differences in the nose,[97] the lower airway,[98] or on rectal biopsy in an Ussing chamber.[99] All these tests require sophisticated apparatus and operator skill and experience and are not widely available. The nasal test requires cooperation from the patient and is difficult in unsedated young children. Protocols usually involve making baseline measurements referenced to a peripheral electrode, then perfusing the nose with amiloride to block sodium transport, and then stimulating CFTR by perfusion with isoproterenol and low-chloride solution.[97] Compared with unaffected persons, the CF patient has a more negative baseline PD, a bigger positive deflection with amiloside, and no negative deflection with low-chloride/isoproterenol, this last being the most discriminatory test. Lower airway potentials measured during bronchoscopy are a research technique that probably will find a place as an end point in clinical trials of novel therapies. Rectal biopsy and in vitro measurement of CFTR function is available in only a very few centers.

Ancillary testing may be helpful in the diagnosis. Human fecal elastase 1 can be measured in a small sample of stool and is sensitive and specific for pancreatic insufficiency,[100] which supports a diagnosis of CF. In males, absence of the vas deferens (which may be diagnosed on ultrasound) or azoospermia also is supportive. The complete absence of upper airway disease on HRCT scanning would be very unusual in CF.

Where does this discussion leave the diagnosis of CF in the twenty-first century? Most cases are obvious, but how should the clinician proceed in the gray areas? The question has been reviewed,[93] and the conclusion was almost paradoxical: despite the advent of ever-more-sophisticated testing, the diagnosis of CF must be a clinical one. The two main difficult situations are (1) the child who has positive tests but no symptoms, and (2) the child who has clinical indications of CF (eg, bronchiectasis with chronic infection with *S. aureus* and mucoid *P. aeruginosa*) but negative tests. For the well child in whom tests are positive, the term "pre-CF" has been proposed but has not been uniformly accepted. The chances of progression to full-blown clinical CF depend on the nature of the tests, progression being inevitable for the asymptomatic child who is homozygous for ΔF_{508} but less certain for an asymptomatic elevation in sweat chloride with no or mild genetic mutations discovered on testing. These children, who are well, certainly cannot be said to have a disease, but they should be monitored carefully to ensure that the earliest signs of disease are detected. For the second group, the diagnostic tests should be reviewed in detail, and other possibilities should be considered. If a different diagnosis is not found, these children should be followed and treated exactly as if they had CF, with treatment of any complication such as *P. aeruginosa* infection along standard lines. The alternative, of reassuring the family that the tests are negative, the child does not have CF, and therefore no follow-up is needed, can have catastrophic consequences. In a proportion of children, the sweat test or other test may be positive when repeated, and the child then is found to have CF after all; even if the child only has a CF-like illness, the consequences may be as bad as for CF itself.[101] The management of CF, once diagnosed, is described in standard texts and reviews and is beyond the scope of this article.

Recommendations

1. The diagnosis of CF should be suspected, particularly if the child has a chronic infection with typical CF-associated organisms and associated with extrapulmonary features of CF, but CF also enters the differential diagnosis in many less specific scenarios. Level of evidence: high
2. In most cases the diagnosis of CF can be made by a properly performed sweat test, but rare and atypical cases may need more sophisticated testing. Both false-positive and false-negative CF diagnoses have been described. Level of evidence: high
3. If the diagnosis of CF is in doubt, the patient still should be followed carefully, because in a proportion of cases either the diagnosis will become clear, or, while

still undiagnosed, the child may develop significant complications. Level of evidence: moderate.

Primary Ciliary Dyskinesia

The management of PCD in the lower airway is similar to that of bronchiectasis from any other cause, but it is important to make the diagnosis because the disease in the upper airway is managed in a different way,[25] and there are genetic implications. PCD usually is inherited as an autosomal recessive, occasionally X-linked, condition. Cilia are complex structures formed from more than 250 different proteins. The complexity of the various genes discovered has been reviewed recently.[102] The prevalence is not known but is estimated to be 1 in 15,000. Particular features that should alert the clinician to the possibility of the diagnosis are given in **Table 1**. Typically, the child has a combination of upper and lower airway symptoms; isolated dry cough is unlikely to be caused by PCD. It is important to be alert to the diagnosis; it is missed frequently, probably because many of the symptoms of PCD (rhinitis, cough, otitis media with effusion) are common in normal children,[103] and diagnosis is delayed.[104] Diagnostic testing is a sequential process.[102] Unless the clinical features are highly suggestive (for example, mirror image arrangement with neonatal onset of respiratory distress and chronic rhinorrhea), in which case direct diagnostic testing is indicated, other, more common conditions such as CF are excluded first. In vivo mucociliary clearance may be tested in the older, cooperative child by using the saccharine test or a variant thereof.[105] A small saccharine tablet is placed on the inferior turbinate. The child is asked to lean forward without coughing, sneezing, or sniffing and should be able to taste saccharine within 60 minutes. If the child does not taste the saccharine, further testing is required; PCD cannot be diagnosed using this test alone. There also is a danger that PCD may be excluded wrongly, if the child tastes the saccharine because he has sniffed the microtablet into the pharynx. Nasal nitric oxide (nNO) measurements may be a more useful screening test. A normal nNO virtually excludes PCD, and if the history is not typical and nNO is normal, further testing may not be needed.[106] There is much less experience with nNO in infants than in older children,[107,108] and measurements in uncooperative younger children should be interpreted with caution.

Table 1
Features leading to the diagnosis of primary ciliary dyskensia

Presenting Feature	Number of Cases (%) (n = 55)
Significant neonatal respiratory distress	37 (67)
Abnormal situs	38 (69)
Cough most days	46 (84)
Sputum production	24 (44)
Rhinorrhea from the newborn period	42 (76)
"Wheeze"	16 (29)
Sinusitis	6 (11)
Serous otitis media	28 (51)
Hearing loss	14 (25)
Diagnosis made in a sibling	6 (11)

Most children had multiple symptoms, typically a combination of upper and lower airway disease.
Data from Coren ME, Meeks M, Buchdahl RM, et al. Primary ciliary dyskinesia (PCD) in children—age at diagnosis and symptom history. Acta Paediatr 2002;91:667–9.

If nNO is low, further testing is mandated; low nNO is reported in CF[109] and also in diffuse panbronchiolitis.[110]

The test that usually is most specific is obtaining nasal brushings to study the function and morphology of cilia in vitro.[102] This test is an out-patient procedure. Strips of ciliated epithelial cells are examined by light microscopy, and beat frequency and pattern are reported. The findings also are recorded digitally, and the sample is examined under an electron microscope. The most common finding is the absence of either or both of the inner and outer dynein arms, but many others have been described. Whether primary ciliary disorientation exists is controversial; disoriented cilia more usually are secondary to chronic infection. Key to the diagnosis is to distinguish primary (congenital) abnormalities from secondary ciliary dysfunction caused by a viral or other infection. Secondary postviral abnormalities may take many weeks to reverse, and if there is any doubt, the brushing should be repeated. It may be difficult to obtain an adequately ciliated sample if the child has chronic infective rhinitis, even after energetic medical treatment. In such cases, culture of the ciliary biopsy is useful. Secondary ciliary abnormalities disappear in culture, whereas primary ones persist. Genetic testing may be useful in some cases, although this service is far from being routinely available. Sophisticated immunofluorescence staining also may be helpful[111] but is not widely available.

Recommendations

1. A diagnosis of PCD should be suspected if there is a combination of upper and lower airway symptoms, particularly with onset in the neonatal period. Although mirror image arrangement and heterotaxy are seen in nearly 50% of patients who have PCD,[112] their absence does not exclude the condition. Level of evidence: moderate

2. Although simple screening tests such as the saccharine test and nNO may be useful to exclude the need for further testing for PCD, the diagnosis always should be confirmed by detailed examination of ciliary function and structure in an experienced center. If clinical suspicion is high, screening tests may be omitted, and the child should proceed directly to definitive testing. Level of evidence: high

3. PCD may be confused with secondary ciliary dysfunction caused by a viral infection; if there is any doubt, the tests must be repeated after a few months. Alternatively, cilia can be examined from another site or cultured in vitro. Level of evidence: high

Idiopathic Bronchiectasis

Bronchiectasis has been described as an "orphan disease." It is much more common and more severe in the developing world,[113] but one group has estimated its prevalence to be at least 1 in 15,000 in a developed-world setting.[114] The key symptom that should prompt consideration of the diagnosis is chronic productive cough lasting without remission for at least 8 weeks. Other diagnostic clues are summarized in **Box 6**. Suspicion should be particularly high if there also is an unexplained suggestive family history or if there are extrapulmonary features of a specific condition such as CF, PCD, or immunodeficiency.

There is no evidence base to guide the clinician in the sequence and timing of the investigation. When the diagnosis is suspected, the author first confirms that bronchiectasis is present with a HRCT scan. Although the distribution of any bronchiectasis offers some diagnostic clues (eg, CF initially is an upper lobe disease, and PCD predominantly affects the lower lobes), in general the distribution is not a reliable basis for

---

Box 6

Diagnostic pointers to the presence of bronchiectasis in the child in whom the diagnosis is suspected for the first time

Chronic unremitting productive cough lasting more than 8 weeks

Atypical "asthma" that does not respond to therapy

A single positive sputum culture for an unusual organism (eg, *S. aureus, P. aeruginosa, B. cepacia*)

Nonresolving pneumonia

Recurrent or persistent radiographic changes

Prior infection with known predisposing organisms (eg, *B. pertussis,* adenovirus serotype 7, 14, and 21)

Palpable secretions on coughing, persistent over time

Persistent crackles on auscultation

Severe esophageal disease

Localized bronchial obstruction including right middle lobe syndrome

---

diagnosis. Even if the HRCT does not demonstrate frank bronchiectasis, the clinician should not be lulled into a false sense of security but should continue to investigate the child (as discussed previously in the section, "Chronic, Usually Productive, Cough") and should institute appropriate treatment to prevent airway damage. The next series of investigations is to determine the underlying cause. A detailed protocol applied in two tertiary referral centers in the United Kingdom determined the cause in about two thirds of patients, and the diagnosis led to a management change in more than half the patients.[114] A specific cause may have consequences for the airway management (eg, recombinant human deoxyribonuclease is very effective in many children who have CF[115] but not in children who have idiopathic bronchiectasis)[116] and for extrapulmonary management (chronic secretory otitis media in PCD is managed very differently from the same condition in otherwise healthy children).[25] There may be specific treatments, such as immunoglobulin replacement therapy; and there may be genetic implications for the extended family, as in CF, PCD, and immunodeficiency. The diagnostic protocol should be very different in a developed-world setting, where tuberculosis and other infections are a major cause. (The diagnosis of tuberculosis is discussed in detail in a later section.)

There are numerous causes of bronchiectasis, and hence there are many possible investigations. The author's practice is to exclude CF and PCD, to screen for immunodeficiency (as described later), and to exclude reflux and aspiration (as described previously) in all cases. The need for more sophisticated testing is determined by the history, examination, and the initial test results. Finally, the consequences of bronchiectasis should be assessed. If the disease is severe, nocturnal hypoxemia may lead to pulmonary hypertension; if in doubt, it is wise to perform an overnight oximetry study and a baseline echocardiogram.

Recommendations

Children suspected of having bronchiectasis should be investigated in detail to determine the cause. In more than 50% of cases, this investigation leads to a change in management. Level of evidence: moderate.

The Special Problems of Congenital and Acquired Immunodeficiency

The number of immunodeficiencies is large, and the diagnosis and management of many of these conditions requires the expertise of a specialist pediatric immunologist (**Box 7**). Many immunodeficiencies, however, are seen first by a pediatric pulmonologist. The clinical picture and simple tests may indicate the presence of an underlying immunodeficiency. The acronym "SPUR" was introduced in the opening section of this article. Additional pointers to immunodeficiency include hepatosplenomegaly, arthropathy, failure to thrive, and a family history of immunodeficiency.

The initial investigations may contain clues that often are overlooked. Neutropenia is always sought on a full blood cell count, but lymphopenia (<2.8) often is overlooked and may be a clue to the diagnosis of severe combined immunodeficiency. In one series, 28 (88%) of 32 infants would have been diagnosed before 6 months of age if the possibility of immunodeficiency had investigated after the first low lymphocyte count.[117] In this report, the first symptoms occurred at a median of 5 weeks (range, 1 day to 8 months) and included respiratory infection (91%), vomiting and diarrhea (81%), failure to thrive (88%), candidiasis (50%), and skin lesions (28%). The median delay between the first abnormal lymphocyte count and diagnosis was 7 weeks (range 1 day to 13 months). This report and others highlight unusually severe mucocutaneous candidiasis as a sign of possible immunodeficiency. The chest radiograph may yield clues. Bronchial situs should be determined, because right isomerism (bilateral right lung morphology, Ivemark's syndrome) and hence susceptibility to overwhelming pneumococcal sepsis is associated with asplenia in around 80% of cases.[118]

The type of infection may give a clue to the nature of the immunodeficiency. In one series,[2] pneumonia was diagnosed in 92%, 81%, and 77% of patients who had antibody, combined, and cellular deficiencies, respectively. Other major illnesses such as bronchiolitis, acute gastroenteritis, otitis media, and bacteremia did not differ in prevalence. Skin abscess, pneumonia, and lymphadenitis (in 55%, 45%, and 27% of cases, respectively) were the most common infections in patients who had phagocyte defects. Age at onset of infection was around 3 years in common variable immunodeficiency but was as early as 4 months in the hypogammaglobulinemias. Combined deficiencies presented at around 6 months of age. Sixty percent of all patients were hospitalized initially for infection. A specific microbiologic diagnosis could be made in a little more than half the episodes. Patients who have antibody deficiencies have a propensity for infection with capsulated organisms, *Pneumocystis jiroveci* and enterovirus; intracellular pathogens are a feature of cellular deficiency. Chronic granulomatous disease may present with *B. cepacia* or catalase-positive infection, whereas disseminated nontuberculous *Mycobacterial* infection suggests a defect of the interferon gamma/interleukin-12 axis.[119] A large study of common variable immunodeficiency[3] reported that respiratory presentations, especially bronchitis, sinusitis, pneumonia and bronchiectasis, are very common. Associated diarrhea was a feature in more than one third of cases. Although there is evidence that diagnostic delays are lessening over time, they still are unacceptably long in many children, underscoring the need for the respiratory pediatrician to be alert to the possibility of immunodeficiency.

The investigation of the immunocompromised child who has single or multiple infiltrates is likely to be much more urgent than in the otherwise well child. The differential diagnosis includes the full spectrum of infectious disease (bacterial, viral, fungal, parasitic, and mycobacterial, depending on the nature of the immunodeficiency, and, in a transplanted child, on the time from transplantation), iatrogenic complications such as pulmonary drug toxicity, pulmonary edema caused by iatrogenic

Box 7
Important congenital and acquired immunodeficiencies that may have a respiratory presentation

Congenital immunodeficiencies

Antibody deficiency

    X-linked

    Common variable immunodeficiency

    IgA deficiency (not invariably significant)

    Hyper IgM (CD40 deficiency)

    IgG subclass deficiency (may be insignificant)

Complement disorders

    C3 deficiency

    Mannose-binding lectin deficiency

Neutrophil disorders

    Autoimmune neutropenia of infancy

    Cyclical neutropenia

    Shwachman-Diamond syndrome

    Kostman syndrome

    Chronic granulomatous disease

Other syndromes

    Di George syndrome (T-cell deficiency)

    Down syndrome

    Heterotaxic syndromes with asplenia (right isomerism, Ivemark's syndrome)

    Ataxia telangiectasia

    Wiskott-Aldrich syndrome

    Hyper-IgE (STAT-3 mutations)

    Interferon gamma receptor mutations (suspect if disseminated mycobacterial disease)

    Interleukin-12 pathway mutations (suspect if disseminated mycobacterial disease)

Acquired

Infective

    HIV

Iatrogenic

    Steroids or immunosuppressant medication

    Postradiotherapy

    Post bone marrow and solid organ transplantation

Malignancy (often also associated with iatrogenic)

    Leukemia and lymphoma

    Solid organ

Miscellaneous

    Acquired hyposplenism (trauma, sickle cell anemia)

    Malnutrition of any cause

    Chronic renal or liver failure

    Diabetes

    Burns

cardiomyopathy or as part of the spectrum of acute lung injury, and recurrence of leukemia or lymphoma, if that was the primary cause of the immunodeficiency. HRCT scanning may be suggestive of specific diagnoses (for example, the halo sign suggests invasive aspergillosis) or may guide the site of BAL. In most children, early bronchoscopy and BAL are performed. The author's practice is not to perform a transbronchial biopsy in this setting because of the risk of bleeding and pneumothorax. The diagnostic yield varies with the underlying condition and with the duration and nature of any anti-infection prophylaxis and blind therapy. There are no satisfactory evidence-based guidelines to determine the optimal timing of bronchoscopy. If no diagnosis is made on the initial BAL, and the child is continuing to deteriorate, it is preferable to proceed straight to an open-lung biopsy rather than perform further BAL.[120]

Tuberculosis

This section summarizes a huge topic very briefly, and the reader is referred to a recent evidence-based guideline.[121] Readers in the developing world may need to modify the

---

Box 8
Potential diagnostic tests for tuberculosis

Obtaining an organism

  Gastric aspirate

  Spontaneously expectorated sputum (older child)

  Induced sputum

  String test

  Bronchoscopy

  Early-morning urine (disseminated tuberculosis)

  Bone marrow biopsy (disseminated tuberculosis)

  Lymph node aspiration or biopsy (lymph node tuberculosis)

Imaging (nondiagnostic)

  Chest radiograph

  CT scan (more sensitive for nodal involvement, but false positives likely)

Molecular test on infected material

  PCR for Mycobacterium tuberculosis

  PCR for genes encoding drug resistance

Skin tests

  Heaf test

  Mantoux test

Serologic tests

  Specific T-cell interferon-γ synthesizing cells

Other tests

  Organ biopsy

Box 9
Summary of potential investigations in the child who has recurrent infections

Suspected CF

    Sweat test

    CF genotype

    Electrical potentials (nasal, bronchial, rectal biopsy)

    Supportive tests (eg, human fecal elastase-1)

Suspected PCD

    Screening: saccharine test, nasal nitric oxide

    Ciliary structure and function: high-speed videomicroscopy, electron microscopy

    Culture of ciliary biopsy

    Genetic studies

    Immunostaining of specific dynein proteins

Screening for suspected immune deficiency (referral to a pediatric immunologist mandatory for most specific immunodeficiencies)

    Full blood cell count (neutropenia, lymphopenia)

    T-cell subsets

    Immunoglobulins

    Immunoglobulin subclasses

    Vaccine antibody responses

    Complement studies

    HIV test

Suspected gastroesophageal reflux

    pH-metry

    Impedance probe

    Isotope milk scan

    Barium swallow (exclude anatomic causes such as hiatus hernia)

    Esophageal manometry

Suspected incoordinated swallowing

    Videofluoroscopy

    Rigid endoscopy to exclude laryngeal cleft

Suspected aspiration

    HRCT scan: dependant bronchocentric consolidation (not specific)

    Lipid-laden macrophages (absence probably excludes significant aspiration)

    BAL pepsin (gastric contents)

Suspected structural esophageal disease

    Tube esophagram

    Bronchoscopy (H-type fistula)

    Barium swallow

Suspected structural airway disease

    Bronchoscopy

    Endobronchial ultrasound

    CT reconstruction

Suspected bronchiectasis

    HRCT scanning

    Exclude CF, PCD, immunodeficiency, tuberculosis (see other sections)

    Consider excluding esophageal disease, incoordinated swallowing, reflux, and aspiration

    Echocardiogram, overnight saturation studies

Suspected tuberculosis

    See **Box 8**

Suspected cardiovascular disease

    Echocardiogram (enlarged cardiac chambers caused by left-to-right shunt, vascular ring)

    Barium swallow (vascular ring)

    CT or MRI with vascular reconstruction (vascular ring)

Suggested vasculitis or connective tissue disease (referral to pediatric rheumatologist probably is advisable)

    Erythrocyte sedimentation rate, C-reactive protein

    Double-stranded DNA

    Rheumatoid factor

    Antineutrophil cytoplasmic antibody studies

    Circulating immune complexes

    Anti-glomerular basement membrane antibodies

recommendations substantially in the light of resources available to them. In developing countries, tuberculosis should be considered in almost all clinical settings. In the developed world, particularly in these days of easy international travel, the possibility of tuberculosis should not be overlooked. Most work on the symptoms that should lead to a suspicion of pulmonary tuberculosis has come from the developing world. These symptoms may be very nonspecific, but highly suggestive in a high-prevalence area is the combination of persistent, unremitting cough lasting longer than 2 weeks, documented failure to thrive for 3 months, and fatigue.[122] This combination was less reliable in children under 3 years of age and in HIV-positive children (a minority of tuberculosis-infected children, even in regions where HIV is common). In other studies, weight loss, fatigue, and chest pain were fairly specific for tuberculosis but were poorly sensitive.[123] In general, a high index of suspicion is needed, especially in young children (in whom treatment legitimately may be started on clinical suspicion alone, because of the horrific potential consequences of miliary and, in particular, central nervous system and meningeal tuberculosis) and in those who are HIV infected.

The particular diagnostic algorithms used depend on the setting and available resources (**Box 8**).

Combinations of tests may be better than the individual tests alone; for example, the diagnostic yield with both gastric aspirates and induced sputum tests is better than that of either test alone. In the past, gastric aspirates were reported to be more sensitive than bronchoscopy, but with the use of PCR technology the differences are not great,[124] although with bronchoscopy direct visualization of endobronchial tuberculosis may allow immediate confirmation of the diagnosis. The chest radiograph is used widely in children and has a sensitivity of 39% and a specificity of 74%,[125] but interobserver agreement is not good, at least for the detection of lymphadenopathy.[126] HRCT scan reveals more lymphadenopathy than a chest radiograph,[127] although whether these nodes are always tuberculous is conjectural, and in most parts of the world, HRCT may not be readily available.

The use of serologic tests to diagnose tuberculosis is a current hot topic, and the place of these tests has yet to be determined, particularly in young children and those who are HIV infected. Two serologic tests currently are available.[121] One measures the release of interferon-γ from whole blood after stimulation with early secreted antigenic target (ESAT)-6 and culture filtrate protein (CFP)-10, which are relatively specific for *Mycobacterium tuberculosis*. In the other test, individual ESAT-6 and CFP-10 T cells are delineated with enzyme-linked immunosorbent spot methodology. In the past, robust guidelines have been produced on the basis of skin tests and chest radiography; whether and how these newer tests can improve the diagnosis of tuberculosis has yet to be worked out fully.

In summary, it can be seen that the diagnosis of tuberculosis can be challenging even with newer investigations. The timeless principles remain: a high index of suspicion is essential, and when in doubt, particularly in high-risk situations such as very young children, blind treatment is safer than a prolonged period of diagnostic havering.

SUMMARY

The child who has recurrent infections poses one of the most difficult diagnostic challenges in pediatrics. The outcome may be anything from reassurance that the child is normal to the diagnosis of a life-threatening condition. A huge range of tests is available (**Box 9**).

The clinician faces a twofold challenge in determining:

1. Is this child normal? (This question may be the most difficult in all clinical practice.)
2. If this child seems to have a serious disease, how can the diagnosis be confirmed or excluded with the minimum number of the least-invasive tests?

It is hoped that, in the absence of good-quality evidence for most clinical scenarios, the experience-based approach described in this article may prove a useful guide to the clinician.

REFERENCES

1. Marchant JM, Masters IB, Taylor SM, et al. Evaluation and outcome of young children with chronic cough. Chest 2006;129:1132–41.
2. Chang SH, Yang YH, Chiang BL. Infectious pathogens in pediatric patients with primary immunodeficiencies. J Microbiol Immunol Infect 2006;39:503–15.
3. Oksenhendler E, Gérard L, Fieschi C, et al. DEFI Study Group. Infections in 252 patients with common variable immunodeficiency. Clin Infect Dis 2008;46:1547–54.

4. Primary Immodeficiency Resource Center home page. Available at: http://www. info4pi.org. Accessed November 15, 2008.

5. Chonmaitree T, Revai K, Grady JJ, et al. Viral upper respiratory tract infection and otitis media complication in young children. Clin Infect Dis 2008;46:815–23.

6. Grüber C, Riesberg A, Mansmann U, et al. The effect of hydrotherapy on the incidence of common cold episodes in children: a randomised clinical trial. Eur J Pediatr 2003;162:168–76.

7. Cane RS, Ranganathan SC, McKenzie SA. What do parents of wheezy children understand by "wheeze"? Arch Dis Child 2000;82:327–32.

8. Elphick HE, Ritson S, Rodgers H, et al. When a "wheeze" is not a wheeze: acoustic analysis of breath sounds in infants. Eur Respir J 2000;16:593–7.

9. Cane RS, McKenzie SA. Parents' interpretations of children's respiratory symptoms on video. Arch Dis Child 2001;84:31–4.

10. Saglani S, McKenzie SA, Bush A, et al. A video questionnaire identifies upper airway abnormalities in preschool children with reported wheeze. Arch Dis Child 2005;90:961–4.

11. Ball TM, Holberg CJ, Aldous MB, et al. Influence of attendance at day care on the common cold from birth through 13 years of age. Arch Pediatr Adolesc Med 2002;156:121–6.

12. Lee GM, Friedman JF, Ross-Degnan D, et al. Misconceptions about colds and predictors of health service utilization. Pediatrics 2003;111:231–6.

13. Bousquet J, Van Cauwenberge P, Khaltaev N. Allergic rhinitis and its impact on asthma. J Allergy Clin Immunol 2001;108:S147–334.

14. Scadding GK, Durham SR, Mirakian R, et al. British Society for Allergy and Clinical Immunology. BSACI guidelines for the management of allergic and non-allergic rhinitis. Clin Exp Allergy 2008;38:19–42.

15. Akikusa JD, Schneider R, Harvey EA, et al. Clinical features and outcome of pediatric Wegener's granulomatosis. Arthritis Rheum 2007;57:837–44.

16. Paradise JL, Bluestone CD, Bachman RZ, et al. Efficacy of tonsillectomy for recurrent throat infection in severely affected children. Results of parallel randomized and nonrandomized clinical trials. N Engl J Med 1984;310:674–83.

17. Tarasiuk A, Simon T, Tal A, et al. Adenotonsillectomy in children with obstructive sleep apnea syndrome reduces health care utilization. Pediatrics 2004;113: 351–6.

18. Paradise JL, Bluestone CD, Colborn DK, et al. Tonsillectomy and adenotonsillectomy for recurrent throat infection in moderately affected children. Pediatrics 2002;110:7–15.

19. van den Akker EH, Schilder AG, Kemps YJ, et al. Current indications for (adeno)tonsillectomy in children: a survey in The Netherlands. Int J Pediatr Otorhinolaryngol 2003;67:603–7.

20. Jecker P, Orloff LA, Wohlfeil M, et al. Gastroesophageal reflux disease (GERD), extraesophageal reflux (EER) and recurrent chronic rhinosinusitis. Eur Arch Otorhinolaryngol 2006;263:664–7.

21. Ford CN. Evaluation and management of laryngopharyngeal reflux. JAMA 2005; 294:1534–40.

22. Bercin S, Kutluhan A, Yurttas V, et al. Evaluation of laryngopharyngeal reflux in patients with suspected laryngopharyngeal reflux, chronic otitis media and laryngeal disorders. Eur Arch Otorhinolaryngol 2008;265:1539–43.

23. Scadding GK, Durham SR, Mirakian R, et al. British Society for Allergy and Clinical Immunology. BSACI guidelines for the management of rhinosinusitis and nasal polyposis. Clin Exp Allergy 2008;38:260–75.

24. Barbero GJ. Gastro-esophageal reflux and upper airway disease. Otolaryngol Clin North Am 1996;29:27–38.

25. Hadfield PJ, Rowe-Jones JM, Bush A, et al. Treatment of otitis media with effusion in children with primary ciliary dyskinesia. Clin Otolaryngol Allied Sci 1997; 22:302–6.

26. Bjornson CL, Johnson DW. Croup. Lancet 2008;371:329–39.

27. Cherry JD. Clinical practice. Croup. N Engl J Med 2008;358:384–91.

28. Kiff KM, Mok Q, Dunne J, et al. Steroids for intubated croup masking airway haemangioma. Arch Dis Child 1996;74:66–7.

29. Reiterer F, Eber E, Zach MS, et al. Management of severe congenital tracheobronchomalacia by continuous positive airway pressure and tidal breathing flow-volume loop analysis. Pediatr Pulmonol 1994;17:401–3.

30. Ramsey CD, Gold DR, Litonjua AA, et al. Respiratory illnesses in early life and asthma and atopy in childhood. J Allergy Clin Immunol 2007;119:150–6.

31. Nafstad P, Brunekreef B, Skrondal A, et al. Early respiratory infections, asthma, and allergy: 10-year follow-up of the Oslo Birth Cohort. Pediatrics 2005;116:e255–62.

32. Van Bever HP, Wieringa MH, Weyler JJ, et al. Croup and recurrent croup: their association with asthma and allergy. An epidemiological study on 5–8-year-old children. Eur J Pediatr 1999;158:253–7.

33. Castro-Rodríguez JA, Holberg CJ, Morgan WJ, et al. Relation of two different subtypes of croup before age three to wheezing, atopy, and pulmonary function during childhood: a prospective study. Pediatrics 2001;107:512–8.

34. van Essen-Zandvliet EE, Hughes MD, Waalkens HJ, et al. Effects of 22 months of treatment with inhaled corticosteroids and/or beta-2-agonists on lung function, airway responsiveness, and symptoms in asthma. The Dutch Chronic Nonspecific Lung Disease Study Group. Am Rev Respir Dis 1992;146:547–54.

35. Waalkens HJ, van Essen-Zandvliet EE, Hughes MD, et al. Cessation of long-term treatment with inhaled corticosteroid (budesonide) in children with asthma results in deterioration. The Dutch CNSLD Study Group. Am Rev Respir Dis 1993;148:1252–7.

36. Murray CS, Woodcock A, Langley SJ, et al. Secondary prevention of asthma by the use of inhaled fluticasone dipropionate in wheezy Infants (IWWIN): double-blind, randomised controlled study. Lancet 2006;368:754–62.

37. Guilbert TW, Morgan WJ, Zeiger RS, et al. Long-term inhaled corticosteroids in preschool children at high risk for asthma. N Engl J Med 2006;354:1985–97.

38. Bisgaard H, Hermansen MN, Loland L, et al. Intermittent inhaled corticosteroids in infants with episodic wheezing. N Engl J Med 2006;354:1998–2005.

39. Hopkins A, Lahiri T, Salerno R, et al. Changing epidemiology of life-threatening upper airway infections: the reemergence of bacterial tracheitis. Pediatrics 2006;118:1418–21.

40. Pao CS, Healy MJ, McKenzie SA. Airway resistance by the interrupter technique: which algorithm for measuring pressure? Pediatr Pulmonol 2004;37:31–6.

41. Gustafsson PM, Aurora P, Lindblad A. Evaluation of ventilation maldistribution as an early indicator of lung disease in children with cystic fibrosis. Eur Respir J 2003;22:972–9.

42. Aurora P, Bush A, Gustafsson P, et al. Multiple breath washout as a marker of lung disease in preschool children with cystic fibrosis. Am J Respir Crit Care Med 2005;171:249–56.

43. Lum S, Gustafsson P, Ljungberg H, et al. Early detection of cystic fibrosis lung disease: multiple-breath washout vs. raised volume tests. Thorax 2007;62:341–7.

44. Goldman J, Muers M. Vocal cord dysfunction and wheezing. Thorax 1991;46:401–4.

45. Shields MD, Bush A, Everard ML, et al. British Thoracic Society guidelines. Recommendations for the assessment and management of cough in children. Thorax 2008;63(Suppl 3):iii1–15.
46. Chang AB, Gaffney JT, Eastburn MM, et al. Cough quality in children: a comparison of subjective vs. bronchoscopic findings. Respir Res 2005;6:3.
47. Kelly YJ, Brabin BJ, Milligan PJ, et al. Clinical significance of cough and wheeze in the diagnosis of asthma. Arch Dis Child 1996;75:489–93.
48. Ferreira de A, Filho LV, Rodrigues JC, et al. Comparison of atopic and nonatopic children with chronic cough: bronchoalveolar lavage cell profile. Pediatr Pulmonol 2007;42:857–63.
49. Donnelly D, Critchlow A, Everard ML. Outcomes in children treated for persistent bacterial bronchitis. Thorax 2007;62:80–4.
50. Eastham KM, Fall AJ, Mitchell L, et al. The need to redefine non-cystic fibrosis bronchiectasis in childhood. Thorax 2004;59:324–7.
51. Chavasse RJ, Bastian-Lee Y, Richter H, et al. Persistent wheezing in infants with an atopic tendency responds to inhaled fluticasone. Arch Dis Child 2001;85:143–8.
52. Chavasse RJ, Bastian-Lee Y, Richter H, et al. Inhaled salbutamol for wheezy infants: a randomised controlled trial. Arch Dis Child 2000;82:370–5.
53. Narang I, Ersu R, Wilson NM, et al. Nitric oxide in chronic airway inflammation in children: diagnostic use and pathophysiological significance. Thorax 2002;57:586–9.
54. Pijnenburg MW, Bakker EM, Lever S, et al. High fractional concentration of nitric oxide in exhaled air despite steroid treatment in asthmatic children. Clin Exp Allergy 2005;35:920–5.
55. Levy ML, Godfrey S, Irving CS, et al. Wheeze detection in infants and pre-school children: recordings versus assessment of physician and parent. J Asthma 2004;41:845–53.
56. Bisgaard H, Hermansen MN, Buchvald F, et al. Childhood asthma after bacterial colonization of the airway in neonates. N Engl J Med 2007;357:1487–95.
57. Lehtinen P, Jartti T, Virkki R, et al. Bacterial coinfections in children with viral wheezing. Eur J Clin Microbiol Infect Dis 2006;25:463–9.
58. von Mutius E. Of attraction and rejection—asthma and the microbial world. N Engl J Med 2007;357:1545–7.
59. Devereux G, Barker RN, Seaton A. Antenatal determinants of neonatal immune response to allergens. Clin Exp Allergy 2002;32:43–50.
60. Noakes PS, Holt PG, Prescott SL. Maternal smoking in pregnancy alters neonatal cytokine responses. Allergy 2003;58:1053–8.
61. Noakes PS, Hale J, Thomas R, et al. Maternal smoking is associated with impaired neonatal toll-like-receptor-mediated immune responses. Eur Respir J 2006;28:721–9.
62. Miller RL, Ho SM. Environmental epigenetics and asthma: current concepts and call for studies. Am J Respir Crit Care Med 2008;177:567–73.
63. Saglani S, Nicholson A, Scallan M, et al. Investigation of young children with severe recurrent wheeze. Any clinical benefit? Eur Respir J 2006;27:29–35.
64. Munyard P, Bush A. How much coughing is normal? Arch Dis Child 1996;74:531–4.
65. Archer LNJ, Simpson H. Night cough counts and diary card scores in asthma. Arch Dis Child 1985;60:473–4.
66. Falconer A, Oldman C, Helms P. Poor agreement between reported and recorded nocturnal cough in asthma. Pediatr Pulmonol 1993;15:209–11.

67. Munyard P, Busst C, Logan-Sinclair R, et al. A new device for ambulatory cough recording. Pediatr Pulmonol 1994;18:178–86.
68. Hamutcu R, Francis J, Karakoc F, et al. Objective monitoring of cough in children with cystic fibrosis. Pediatr Pulmonol 2002;34:331–5.
69. Gibson NA, Hollman AS, Paton JY. Value of radiological follow up of childhood pneumonia. Br Med J 1993;307:1117.
70. Surén P, Try K, Eriksson J, et al. Radiographic follow-up of community-acquired pneumonia in children. Acta Paediatr 2008;97:46–50.
71. Geppert EF. Chronic and recurrent pneumonia. Semin Respir Infect 1992;7: 282–8.
72. Stein RT, Marostica PJC. Community-acquired bacterial pneumonia. In: Chernick V, Boat TF, Wilmott RW, et al, editors. Kendig's disorders of the respiratory tract in children. 7th edition. Philadelphia: Saunders; 2006.
73. Priftis KN, Mermiri D, Papadopoulou A, et al. The role of timely intervention in middle lobe syndrome in children. Chest 2005;128:2504–10.
74. Sekerel BE, Nakipoglu F. Middle lobe syndrome in children with asthma: review of 56 cases. J Asthma 2004;41:411–7.
75. Kwon KY, Myers JL, Swensen SJ, et al. Middle lobe syndrome: a clinicopathological study of 21 patients. Hum Pathol 1995;26:302–7.
76. Priftis KN, Anthracopoulos MB, Mermiri D, et al. Bronchial hyperresponsiveness, atopy, and bronchoalveolar lavage eosinophils in persistent middle lobe syndrome. Pediatr Pulmonol 2006;41:805–11.
77. De Boeck K, Willems T, Van Gysel D, et al. Outcome after right middle lobe syndrome. Chest 1995;108:150–2.
78. Gattuso JM, Kamm MA. Adverse effects of drugs used in the management of constipation and diarrhoea. Drug Saf 1994;10:47–65.
79. Ratan SK, Ratan J. Laryngotracheo-esophageal cleft in a neonate with esophageal atresia and tracheo-esophageal fistula: report of a case. Surg Today 2001; 31:59–61.
80. Wilson NM, Chudry N, Silverman M. Role of the oesophagus in asthma induced by the ingestion of ice and acid. Thorax 1987;42:506–10.
81. Mitchell DJ, McClure BG, Tubman TR. Simultaneous monitoring of gastric and oesophageal pH reveals limitations of conventional oesophageal pH monitoring in milk fed infants. Arch Dis Child 2001;84:273–6.
82. Dalby K, Nielsen RG, Markoew S, et al. Reproducibility of 24-hour combined multiple intraluminal impedance (MII) and pH measurements in infants and children. Evaluation of a diagnostic procedure for gastroesophageal reflux disease. Dig Dis Sci 2007;52:2159–65.
83. Vandenplas Y, Salvatore S, Devreker T, et al. Gastro-oesophageal reflux disease: oesophageal impedance versus pH monitoring. Acta Paediatr 2007;96:956–62.
84. Rosen R, Fritz J, Nurko A, et al. Lipid-laden macrophage index is not an indicator of gastroesophageal reflux-related respiratory disease in children. Pediatrics 2008;121:e879–84.
85. Farrell S, McMaster C, Gibson D, et al. Pepsin in bronchoalveolar lavage fluid: a specific and sensitive method of diagnosing gastro-oesophageal reflux-related pulmonary aspiration. J Pediatr Surg 2006;41:289–93.
86. Jack CI, Calverley PM, Donnelly RJ, et al. Simultaneous tracheal and oesophageal pH measurements in asthmatic patients with gastro-oesophageal reflux. Thorax 1995;50:201–4.
87. Ng J, Bartram J, Antao B, et al. H-type tracheoesophageal fistula masquerading as achalasia cardia in a 13-year-old child. J Paediatr Child Health 2006;42:215–6.

88. Yao TC, Hung IJ, Jaing TH, et al. Pitfalls in the diagnosis of idiopathic pulmonary haemosiderosis. Arch Dis Child 2002;86:436–8.
89. Jennings CA, King TE Jr, Tuder R, et al. Diffuse alveolar hemorrhage with underlying isolated, pauciimmune pulmonary capillaritis. Am J Respir Crit Care Med 1997;155:1101–9.
90. Cystic Fibrosis Foundation. Patient registry 1996 annual data report. Bethesda (MD): National Institutes of Health; 1997.
91. Wallis C. Diagnosis of cystic fibrosis. In: Hodson M, Geddes DM, Bush A, editors. Cystic fibrosis. 3rd edition. London: Publ Edward Arnold; 2007. p. 99–108.
92. Hodson ME, Beldon I, Power R, et al. Sweat tests to diagnose cystic fibrosis in adults. Br Med J (Clin Res Ed) 1983;286:1381–3.
93. Bush A, Wallis C. Time to think again: cystic fibrosis is not an "all or none" disease. Pediatr Pulmonol 2000;30:139–44.
94. Groman JD, Meyer ME, Wilmott RW, et al. Variant cystic fibrosis phenotypes in the absence of CFTR mutations. N Engl J Med 2002;347:401–7.
95. Wang X, Venable J, LaPointe P, et al. Hsp90 cochaperone Aha1 downregulation rescues misfolding of CFTR in cystic fibrosis. Cell 2006;127:803–15.
96. Doan ML, Guillerman RP, Dishop MK, et al. Clinical, radiological and pathological features of ABCA3 mutations in children. Thorax 2008;63:366–73.
97. Middleton PG, Geddes DM, Alton EW. Protocols for in vivo measurement of the ion transport defects in cystic fibrosis nasal epithelium. Eur Respir J 1994;7:2050–6.
98. Davies JC, Davies M, McShane D, et al. Potential difference measurements in the lower airway of children with and without cystic fibrosis. Am J Respir Crit Care Med 2005;171:1015–9.
99. Veeze HJ, Sinaasappel M, Bijman J, et al. Ion transport abnormalities in rectal suction biopsies from children with cystic fibrosis. Gastroenterology 1991;101:398–403.
100. Cohen JR, Schall JI, Ittenbach RF, et al. Fecal elastase: pancreatic status verification and influence on nutritional status in children with cystic fibrosis. J Pediatr Gastroenterol Nutr 2005;40:438–44.
101. Lebecque P, Leal T, De Boeck C, et al. Mutations of the cystic fibrosis gene and intermediate sweat chloride levels in children. Am J Respir Crit Care Med 2002;165:757–61.
102. Bush A, Chodhari R, Collins N, et al. Primary ciliary dyskinesia. Arch Dis Child 2007;92:1136–40.
103. Bush A, O'Callaghan C. Primary ciliary dyskinesia. Arch Dis Child 2002;87:363–5.
104. Coren ME, Meeks M, Buchdahl RM, et al. Primary ciliary dyskinesia (PCD) in children—age at diagnosis and symptom history. Acta Paediatr 2002;91:667–9.
105. Deitmer T. A modification of the saccharine test for nasal mucociliary clearance. Rhinology 1986;24:237–40.
106. Karadag B, James AJ, Gultekin E, et al. Nasal and lower airway level of nitric oxide in children with primary ciliary dyskinesia. Eur Respir J 1999;13:1402–6.
107. Franklin PJ, Turner SW, Mutch RC, et al. Measuring exhaled nitric oxide in infants during tidal breathing: methodological issues. Pediatr Pulmonol 2004;37:24–30.
108. Gabriele C, van der Wiel EC, Nieuwhof EM, et al. Methodological aspects of exhaled nitric oxide measurements in infants. Pediatr Allergy Immunol 2007;18:36–41.
109. Balfour-Lynn IM, Laverty A, Dinwiddie R. Reduced upper airway nitric oxide in cystic fibrosis. Arch Dis Child 1996;75:319–22.

110. Nakano H, Ide H, Imada M, et al. Reduced nasal nitric oxide in diffuse panbronchiolitis. Am J Respir Crit Care Med 2000;162:2218–20.
111. Fliegauf M, Olbrich H, Horvath J, et al. Mislocalization of DNAH5 and DNAH9 in respiratory cells from patients with primary ciliary dyskinesia. Am J Respir Crit Care Med 2005;171:1343–9.
112. Kennedy MP, Omran H, Leigh MW, et al. Congenital heart disease and other heterotaxic defects in a large cohort of patients with primary ciliary dyskinesia. Circulation 2007;115:2814–21.
113. Twiss J, Stewart AW, Byrnes CA. Longitudinal pulmonary function of childhood bronchiectasis and comparison with cystic fibrosis. Thorax 2006;61:414–8.
114. Li AM, Sonnappa S, Lex C, et al. Non-CF bronchiectasis: does knowing the aetiology lead to changes in management? Eur Respir J 2005;26:8–14.
115. Fuchs HJ, Borowitz DS, Christiansen DH, et al. Effect of aerosolized recombinant human DNase on exacerbations of respiratory symptoms and on pulmonary function in patients with cystic fibrosis. The Pulmozyme Study Group. N Engl J Med 1994;331:637–42.
116. Wills PJ, Wodehouse T, Corkery K, et al. Short-term recombinant human DNase in bronchiectasis. Effect on clinical state and in vitro sputum transportability. Am J Respir Crit Care Med 1996;154:413–7.
117. Hague RA, Rassam S, Morgan G, et al. Early diagnosis of severe combined immunodeficiency syndrome. Arch Dis Child 1994;70:260–3.
118. Cesko I, Hajdú J, Tóth T, et al. Ivemark syndrome with asplenia in siblings. J Pediatr 1997;130:822–4.
119. Glosli H, Stray-Pedersen A, Brun AC, et al. Infections due to various atypical mycobacteria in a Norwegian multiplex family with dominant interferon-gamma receptor deficiency. Clin Infect Dis 2008;46:e23–7.
120. Stefanutti D, Morais L, Fournet JC, et al. Value of open lung biopsy in immunocompromised children. J Pediatr 2000;137:165–71.
121. National Institute for Health and Clinical Excellence. Tuberculosis guidelines. Available at: http://www.nice.org.uk/guidance/index.jsp?action=byID&o=10979. Accessed November 15, 2008.
122. Marais BJ, Gie RP, Hesseling AC, et al. A refined symptom-based approach to diagnose pulmonary tuberculosis in children. Pediatrics 2006;118:e1350–9.
123. Marais BJ, Obihara CC, Gie RP, et al. The prevalence of symptoms associated with pulmonary tuberculosis in randomly selected children from a high burden community. Arch Dis Child 2005;90:1166–70.
124. Chierakul N, Anantasetagoon T, Chaiprasert A, et al. Diagnostic value of gastric aspirate smear and polymerase chain reaction in smear-negative pulmonary tuberculosis. Respirology 2003;8:492–6.
125. De Villiers RV, Andronikou S, Van de Westhuizen S. Specificity and sensitivity of chest radiographs in the diagnosis of paediatric pulmonary tuberculosis and the value of additional high-kilovolt radiographs. Australas Radiol 2004;48:148–53.
126. Du Toit G, Swingler G, Iloni K. Observer variation in detecting lymphadenopathy on chest radiography. Int J Tuberc Lung Dis 2002;6:814–7.
127. Swingler GH, du Toit G, Andronikou S, et al. Diagnostic accuracy of chest radiography in detecting mediastinal lymphadenopathy in suspected pulmonary tuberculosis. Arch Dis Child 2005;90:1153–6.

Upper Respiratory Tract Infections (Including Otitis Media)

Peter S. Morris, MBBS, PhD, FRACP[a,b,c,*]

KEYWORDS

- Evidence based • Rhinosinusitis • Pharyngitis
- Otitis media • Management

Upper respiratory tract infections (including otitis media) are the most common illnesses affecting children.[1] On average, children experience around six to eight upper respiratory tract infections (URTIs) each year.[2] Although these infections usually are mild and self limiting, they occasionally lead to complications that can be life threatening. Most URTIs can be placed within three main categories of infection: rhinosinusitis, pharyngitis, and otitis media. Within each category of illness there is a range of related conditions that may have similar or overlapping clinical presentations.[3] Some judgment is required in determining which part of the respiratory mucosa is most affected. In this article, the term "rhinosinusitis" is used to describe illnesses with predominantly nasal symptoms (including the common cold, nasopharyngitis, and sinusitis). The term "pharyngitis" is used to describe illnesses when sore throat is most prominent (including tonsillitis). The term "otitis media" is used to describe illnesses with predominantly middle ear symptoms (including acute otitis media [AOM], otitis media with effusion [OME], and chronic suppurative otitis media [CSOM]). Children who have cough as the predominant symptom are considered to have bronchitis (a lower respiratory tract infection). To make matters more complicated, all areas of the respiratory mucosa may be affected, simultaneously or at different times, during one illness.

The cause of these respiratory mucosal infections most commonly is viral but can be bacterial (**Table 1**),[4] and many infections involve both viruses and bacteria.[5] In developed countries, both viral and bacterial infections are likely to be self limited. Persistent disease is most likely to indicate a bacterial infection.

---

[a] Child Health Division, Menzies School of Health Research, P.O. Box 41096, Casuarina, NT 0811, Darwin, Australia
[b] Institute of Advanced Studies, Charles Darwin University, Darwin, Australia
[c] Northern Territory Clinical School, Flinders University, Darwin, Australia
* Menzies School of Health Research, Child Health Division, P.O. Box 41096, Darwin, Casuarina, NT 0811, Australia.
E-mail address: peterm@menzies.edu.au

Pediatr Clin N Am 56 (2009) 101–117
doi:10.1016/j.pcl.2008.10.009
0031-3955/08/$ – see front matter © 2009 Published by Elsevier Inc.

pediatric.theclinics.com

Table 1
Spectrum of disease, accepted terminology, and etiology of the common upper respiratory tract infections in children

Condition	Related Diagnoses	Etiology
Rhinosinusitis	Common cold, nasopharyngitis, infective rhinitis, acute rhinosinusitis, acute sinusitis, chronic sinusitis	Viral: rhinovirus, coronavirus, enterovirus, parainfluenza, influenza, respiratory syncytial virus, adenovirus, metapneumovirus Bacterial: *Streptococcus pneumoniae, Haemophilus influenzae, Moraxella catarrhalis, Staphylococcus aureus, Streptococcus pyogenes*
Pharyngitis	Pharyngitis, tonsillitis, recurrent tonsillitis	Viral: adenovirus, respiratory syncytial virus, Epstein-Barr virus, cytomegalovirus, parainfluenza, influenza Bacterial: *Streptococcus pyogenes*, Group C and G *Streptococci, Mycoplasma pneumoniae*
Otitis media	Acute otitis media without perforation, acute otitis media with perforation, otitis media with effusion, chronic suppurative otitis media.	Viral: respiratory syncytial virus, influenza, adenovirus, rhinovirus, coronavirus, enterovirus, parainfluenza, metapneumovirus Bacterial: *Streptococcus pneumoniae, Haemophilus influenzae, Moraxella catarrhalis, Streptococcus pyogenes*

The frequency of infection and association with fever and constitutional symptoms creates significant distress for the child and the family. By understanding the evidence available from high-quality studies, the clinician can advise the families on appropriate action.[6] The goal of this article is to support clinicians in answering the following questions:

1. What happened to children with these conditions when no additional treatment was provided?
2. Which interventions have been assessed in well-designed studies?
3. Which interventions have been shown to improve outcomes?
4. How large is the overall benefit?

THE APPROACH TO EVIDENCE USED IN THIS ARTICLE

URTIs are extremely common in children, and there is a long list of potential interventions. Because URTIs are common illnesses, there is no reason why high-quality randomized, controlled trials (RTCs) should not be conducted.[7] In addition, all families experience these conditions and may have strong personal preferences about treatment. The challenge for the clinician is to make an accurate diagnosis and then to match the effective treatment options with the preferences of the family.

This article initially considers the effects of an intervention compared with no intervention. Because each condition covers a spectrum of disease, the acute presentation of the initial URTI is discussed first and then, when appropriate, interventions for persistent disease or complications of the initial complaint are addressed. Because of the focus on trial evidence, not all the information relevant to an individual decision may be discussed. Furthermore, because the clinical course of participants enrolled in RCTs may be different from the clinical course observed in one's own practice, the overall effects of an intervention may need to be adjusted. Despite these limitations, clinicians using this article should be confident that they understand which interventions have been rigorously assessed and the overall findings of these assessments.

The GRADE Working Group has described the steps required to review evidence.[8,9] Ideally, explicit criteria should be used. Although this process has many advantages in terms of transparency, it does not guarantee that recommendations will be consistent across different sets of evidence-based guidelines (although this consistency is the long-term aim).[10] The GRADE Working Group proposes that a recommendation should indicate the decision that the majority of well-informed individuals would make.[8] It is difficult to be dogmatic about interventions for self-limited conditions with a low risk of complications. Therefore, the author has tried to provide a summary of evidence to assist discussions with families (**Tables 2–4**). The author's approach (informed by the best available evidence) is described in **Box 1**.

IMPORTANT HEALTH OUTCOMES AND TREATMENT EFFECTS

The self-limiting nature of these conditions is of the utmost importance in determining which treatments are indicated. The outcomes the author considers important are (1) persistent disease (short term, $\leq$ 14 days; medium term, >2 weeks to 6 months; and long term >6 months), (2) time to cure, and (3) complications arising from progressive disease. The author considered interventions to have very large effects if they were associated with a reduction in the outcome of interest of more than 80%; large effects were associated with a reduction in outcome of interest of at least 50%.[11] Reductions in outcome of interest between 20% and 50% were considered modest, and reductions of less than 20% were considered slight (or small). Because only a proportion of children who have URTIs experience bad outcomes, even large relative effects may not translate to clinically significant absolute benefits.

SEARCH STRATEGY

The author's search targeted evidence-based guidelines, evidence-based summaries, systematic reviews, and RCTs of interventions for rhinosinusitis, pharyngitis, and otitis media (**Box 2**). Even this simple strategy identified more than 6500 sources using PubMed alone. Inclusion as an evidence-based guideline, summary, or systematic review required an explicit search strategy and criteria for study inclusion. Inclusion as a clinical trial required randomization. The author used three primary sources to identify relevant information: *Clinical Evidence*;[11] the Cochrane library[12] and Medline (last accessed via PubMed on June 16, 2008). The evidence-based summaries in *Clinical Evidence* have links to major guidelines and use the GRADE Working Group approach to assess quality of evidence and strength of recommendations.[11]

RESULTS OF SEARCH

The search identified more than 50 evidence-based guidelines, evidence summaries, and systematic reviews (and many more additional RCTs) published since 2000. This

Table 2
Treatment effects of interventions for rhinosinusitis in children that have been assessed in randomized, controlled trials

Intervention	Evidence	Effect
Prevention		
Vitamin C	30 studies (11,350 participants)	No significant reduction in proportion of participants experiencing the common cold (48%)
Echinacea	Three studies (498 participants)	No significant reduction in proportion of participants experiencing the common cold (45%)
Treatment of initial rhinosinusitis		
Antihistamines	Five studies (3492 participants)	No significant reduction in proportion of participants with persistent symptoms at 1 to 2 days (55%)
Vitamin C	Seven studies (3294 participants)	No significant reduction in median duration of symptoms
Antibiotics	Six studies (1147 participants)	No significant reduction in persistent symptoms at 7 days (35% versus 31%); significant reduction in persistence of purulent rhinitis from 42% to 24%
Decongestants	Six studies (643 participants)	Subjective assessment of congestion reduced by 6% after one dose. Effect persisted with repeated doses over 3 days
Zinc lozenges	13 studies (516 participants)	No consistent effects on symptoms
Echinacea	Two studies (200 participants)	Proportion experiencing "full" cold reduced by 12% to 23% but no effect in other studies of different outcomes
Treatment of persistent rhinosinusitis/clinical sinusitis		
Intranasal corticosteroids	Three studies (1792 participants)	Persistent disease reduced from 27% to 19%.
Antibiotics	14 studies (1309 participants)	Persistent disease at around 2 weeks reduced from 60% to 46% in adults and from 46% to 35% in children

article does not include interventions that have been assessed in nonrandomized studies, interventions that have been assessed in studies with fewer than 200 participants (sparse data),[11] or studies of interventions that are available only experimentally.

RHINOSINUSITIS

Rhinosinusitis is an URTI that predominantly affects the nasal part of the respiratory mucosa.[13–15] Common cold infections are caused mainly by viruses (typically rhinovirus, but also coronavirus, respiratory syncytial virus, metapneumovirus, and others).[2] For many colds, no infecting organism can be identified. Common colds usually have a short duration. Symptoms peak within 1 to 3 days and generally clear by 7 to 10 days, although an associated cough (bronchitis) often persists.[2] Most people who have acute rhinosinusitis are assessed and treated in a primary-care setting.

Table 3
Treatment effects of interventions for pharyngitis in children that have been assessed in randomized, controlled trials

Intervention	Evidence	Effect
Treatment of initial pharyngitis		
Antibiotics	15 studies (3621 participants)	Pain at 3 days reduced from 66% to 48%
	13 studies (2974 participants)	Pain at 7 days reduced from 18% to 12%
	15 studies (3621 participants)	Median time to cure reduced from 4 days to 3 days
	Eight studies (2443 participants)	Peritonsillar abscess within 2 months reduced from 2.3% to 0.1%
	16 studies (10,101 participants)	Rheumatic fever within 2 months reduced from 1.8% to 0.7%
	11 studies (3760 participants)	Otitis media within 14 days reduced from 2% to 0.5%
Analgesics	17 studies (1742 participants)	Pain scores reduced by 25% to 80% within 4 hours; benefits persisted with regular treatment over 2 o 5 days
Corticosteroids	Five studies (421 participants)	Pain reduced by 12 to 24 hours but effects inconsistent
Treatment of recurrent pharyngitis		
(Adeno)Tonsillectomy	Six studies (1618 participants)	Sore throat episodes over 3 years reduced from 2.4 to 1.2 episodes per year

A preceding viral URTI often is the trigger for acute sinusitis; about 0.5% to 5% of common colds become complicated by the development of acute sinusitis.[16] Acute sinusitis is defined pathologically by transient inflammation of the mucosal lining of the paranasal sinuses lasting less than 30 days.[17,18] Clinically, acute sinusitis is characterized by nasal congestion, nasal discharge, and facial pain.[19] The diagnosis of acute sinusitis in infants and children usually is made in children who have purulent nasal drainage persisting beyond 10 days.[17] In straightforward cases, no investigations are required.[17] In more complicated (or frequent) presentations, possible underlying factors include nasal airway obstruction, immunodeficiencies, ciliary dysfunction, cystic fibrosis, and allergic rhinitis. The usual pathogens in acute bacterial sinusitis are *Streptococcus pneumoniae* and *Haemophilus influenzae*, with occasional infection with *Moraxella catarrhalis* and *Staphylococcus aureus*. Rarely, bacterial sinusitis in children leads to rare, life-threatening complications, such as meningitis, cavernous venous thrombosis, and orbital cellulitis.[4]

Options for Interventions

Most children who have rhinosinusitis improve spontaneously within 14 days, and complications from this illness are uncommon. There is evidence about the preventive effects of vitamin C and Echinacea on the onset of the illness.[20,21] Neither of these interventions has been proven to be effective. There is evidence about the treatment effects of antihistamines, vitamin C, antibiotics, decongestants, zinc lozenges, and Echinacea (see **Table 2**).[20–28] Of these interventions, only decongestants have been proven to be effective, but their beneficial effect is small.[26] Decongestants have not

Table 4
Treatment effects of interventions for otitis media in children that have been assessed in randomized, controlled trials

Intervention	Evidence	Effect
Prevention		
Conjugate pneumococcal vaccine	Three studies (39,749 participants)	Acute otitis media episodes reduced by 6% (eg, from 1.0 to 0.94 episodes per year); insertion of tympanostomy tubes reduced from 3.8% to 2.9%
Influenza vaccine	11 studies (11,349 participants)	Inconsistent results; modest protection against otitis media during influenza season in some studies
Treatment of initial acute otitis media		
Antihistamines and decongestants	12 studies (2300 participants)	No significant difference in persistent acute otitis media at 2 weeks
Antibiotics	Eight studies (2287 participants)	Persistent pain on day 2 through 7 reduced from 22% to 16%
	Six studies (1643 participants)	Persistent reduced from 55% to 30% in children younger than 2 years old who had with bilateral acute otitis media and from 53% to 19% in children who had acute otitis media with perforation
Myringotomy	Three studies (812 participants)	Early treatment failure increased from 5% to 20%
Analgesics	One study (219 participants)	Persistent pain reduced from 25% to 9% on day 2
Treatment of recurrent acute otitis media		
Antibiotics	16 studies (1483 participants)	Episodes of acute otitis media reduced from 3.0 to 1.5 episodes per year
Adenoidectomy	Six studies (1,060 participants)	No significant reduction in rates of acute otitis media
Tympanostomy tubes	Five studies (424 participants)	Episodes of acute otitis media reduced from 2.0 to 1.0 episodes per year
Treatment of persistent otitis media with effusion		
Antibiotics	Nine studies (1534 participants)	Persistent otitis media with effusion at around 4 weeks reduced from 81% to 68%
Tympanostomy tubes	11 studies (~1300 participants)	Modest improvement in hearing (9 dB at 6 months and 6 dB at 12 months); no improvement in language or cognitive assessment
Antihistamines and decongestants	Seven studies (1177 participants)	No difference in persistent otitis media with effusion at 4 weeks (75%)
Autoinflation	Six studies (602 participants)	Inconsistent results; modest improvement in tympanometry at 4 weeks in some studies
Antibiotics plus steroids	Five studies (418 participants)	Persistent otitis media with effusion at 2 weeks reduced from 75% to 52%
Treatment of chronic suppurative otitis media		
Topical antibiotics	Seven studies (1074 participants)	Persistent chronic suppurative otitis media at 2 to 16 weeks reduced from around 75% to 20% to 50%
Ear cleaning	Two studies (658 participants)	Inconsistent results; no reduction in persistent chronic suppurative otitis media at 12 to 16 weeks (78%) in a large African study

Box 1
Suggested approach for assessing and managing a child who has an upper respiratory infection

1. Take a history of the presenting complaint to elicit the primary symptom: nasal discharge (rhinosinusitis), sore throat (pharyngitis) ear pain, ear discharge, or hearing loss (otitis media). Ask about the frequency and severity of previous URTIs. Clarify the duration of illness and the presence of any associated features, including cough (bronchitis), fever, respiratory distress, cyanosis, poor feeding, or lethargy. Determine the concerns, expectations, and preferences of the child and the caregivers. (Grade: very low; level of evidence: cohort studies and other evidence)

2. Examine the child to confirm whether investigation and management should be directed at rhinosinusitis, pharyngitis, or AOM. Assess temperature, pulse and respiratory rate, presence and color of nasal discharge, nasal obstruction, facial tenderness, tonsillar enlargement, tonsillar exudate, cervical lymphadenopathy, presence of cough, presence of middle ear effusion (using pneumatic otoscopy or tympanometry), position and integrity of tympanic membrane, and proptosis. Ensure normal hydration, perfusion, conscious state, and no meningism, periorbital swelling, limitation of eye movements, upper airway obstruction, respiratory distress, or mastoid tenderness. (Grade: very low; level of evidence: cohort studies and other evidence)

3. Investigations
   - Rhinosinusitis: none required unless patient is febrile and less than 3 months of age or danger signs (respiratory distress, cyanosis, poor feeding, or lethargy) are present.

   (Grade: low; level of evidence: cohort studies)

   - Pharyngitis: none required unless patient is febrile and less than 3 months of age or danger signs (respiratory distress, cyanosis, poor feeding, or lethargy) are present.

   (Grade: low; level of evidence: cohort studies)

   - AOM: none required unless patient is febrile and less than 3 months of age or danger signs (respiratory distress, cyanosis, poor feeding, or lethargy) are present.

   (Grade: low; level of evidence: cohort studies)

4. Management
   - Rhinosinusitis: Provide symptomatic pain relief if indicated during watchful waiting with advice to parents on likely course and possible complications. Antibiotics can be considered if there is persistent nasal discharge for more than 10 days or purulent nasal discharge. Decongestants may be used in an older child who has significant nasal obstruction. (Grade: moderate; level of evidence: RCTs)

   - Pharyngitis: Provide symptomatic pain relief if indicated during watchful waiting with advice to parents on likely course and possible complications. Antibiotics can be used if pain is severe and does not respond to analgesics, if there is tonsillar exudate plus cervical lymphadenopathy and no nasal discharge or cough, or if the patient is at high risk of complications (especially rheumatic fever or peritonsillar abscess). (Grade: moderate; level of evidence: RCTs)

   - AOM: Provide symptomatic pain relief if indicated during watchful waiting with advice to parents on likely course and possible complications. Antibiotics can be used if the patient has AOM with perforation or is younger than 2 years old and has bilateral AOM, if there has been no improvement after 48 hours of watchful waiting, or if the patient is at high risk of suppurative complications (especially perforation of the tympanic membrane). (Grade: high; level of evidence: RCTs)

Box 2

A simple PubMed search strategy to identify evidence-based guidelines, evidence-based summaries, systematic reviews, and randmoized controlled trials on common upper respiratory tract infections

"rhinitis"[MeSH Terms] OR "nasopharyngitis"[MeSH Terms] OR "common cold" [MeSH Terms] OR "sinusitis"[MeSH Terms] OR "pharyngitis"[MeSH Terms] OR "tonsillitis"[MeSH Terms] OR "otitis"[MeSH Terms] AND (practice guideline[pt] OR systematic[sb] OR clinical evidence[jour] OR clinical trial[pt]).

---

been tested in young children. Antibiotics seem to be effective in individuals who have purulent rhinosinusitis, but the beneficial effect is modest.[24]

Given the available evidence from RCTs, most well-informed individuals choose a course of watchful waiting. Symptomatic relief using analgesic agents has not been assessed in RCTs but would be a reasonable in children who have pain or discomfort. Antibiotics are an option for children who have purulent nasal discharge but provide only a modest benefit. Decongestants are an option for older children who have nasal obstruction. It probably is worth persisting with decongestants only when there is symptomatic relief with the first dose.

A small proportion of children go on to develop persistent rhinosinusitis or classic sinusitis. There is evidence about the treatment effects of intranasal corticosteroids (from adult studies) and antibiotics.[17,18,29–33] Both of these interventions seem to be beneficial, but the beneficial effects are modest. If antibiotics are to be used, there no consistent evidence that a longer course of treatment ($\geq$ 7 days) is more effective than a shorter course.[32] There is no evidence to support the belief that any one of the commonly used antibiotics is more effective than the others (although the cephalosporin class of antibiotics does seem to be inferior to amoxicillin-clavulanate).[32] Given the available evidence from RCTs, most well-informed individuals choose either watchful waiting or a trial of antibiotics. Intranasal corticosteroids are a reasonable option in older children, particularly those who have any features of atopy.

PHARYNGITIS

Pharyngitis is an acute URTI that affects the respiratory mucosa of the throat, resulting in a predominant symptom of pain that may be associated with headache, fever, and general malaise.[3,34,35] In the United States, acute pharyngitis accounts for about 1% of primary care consultations and ranks in the top 20 diagnoses.[34] Infections leading to pharyngitis can be viral or bacterial (**Table 5**). It is difficult to distinguish bacterial infections from viral infections clinically. Studies have found that tonsillar or pharyngeal exudate, tender cervical lymphadenopathy, and recent exposure to streptococcal throat infection are most useful in predicting bacterial infection.[36] A useful clinical prediction rule found that streptococcal infection was present in 50% of children if three of the following features were positive: fever higher than 38°C; tonsillar swelling or exudate; tender cervical lymphadenopathy; and absence of cough. Even without treatment, sore throat resolves in 40% of cases by 3 days and in 85% of cases by 1 week.[3] A small proportion of children experience progression of the illness. Suppurative complications include peritonsillar abscess (quinsy), AOM, and acute sinusitis. Nonsuppurative complications include acute rheumatic fever and acute glomerulonephritis.

Options for Interventions

Most children who have pharyngitis improve spontaneously within 14 days, and complications from this illness are uncommon. There is evidence about the

Table 5
Typical clinical features of the common upper respiratory infections in children that have been assessed in randomized, controlled trials

Condition	Typical Clinical Features
Rhinosinusitis	Febrile illness associated with nasal discharge
Persistent rhinosinusitis	Persistent nasal discharge plus abnormalities on sinus radiographs
Pharyngitis	Febrile illness associated with sore throat plus localizing signs on examination
Recurrent tonsillitis	Recurrent febrile illnesses (more than three per year) associated with sore throat plus localizing signs on examination
Acute otitis media	Clinical diagnosis of acute otitis media with red tympanic membrane and ear pain
Recurrent acute otitis media	Recurrent clinical diagnosis of acute otitis media (three or more episodes in 6 months) with red tympanic membrane and ear pain
Otitis media with effusion	Asymptomatic persistent middle ear effusion confirmed by tympanometry
Chronic suppurative otitis media	Discharge through a perforated tympanic membrane for 2 to 6 weeks

treatment effects of antibiotics, analgesics, and corticosteroids on the onset of illness (see **Table 3**).[3,35,37–41] The beneficial effect of analgesics is large and persists over several days of treatment.[3,40] Antibiotics also have been proven to be effective,[3,37,38] with large to very large beneficial effects for preventing complications (peritonsillar abscess, rheumatic fever, and otitis media). These complications generally affect less than 2% of children, however. Antibiotics have a modest, short-term beneficial effect in improving the sore throat itself. If oral penicillin is used for treatment, there is evidence that a full 10-day course is more effective than shorter courses.[39] There is some evidence that systemic corticosteroids reduce pain within 12 to 24 hours.[3,41]

Given the available evidence from RCTs, most well-informed individuals choose symptomatic relief with analgesics and either watchful waiting or antibiotics. Antibiotics would be most appropriate in children at increased risk of complications, those who have features more consistent with a bacterial infection (fever higher than 38°C, tonsillar exudate, enlarged tender cervical nodes, and absence of nasal discharge and cough), and those who have severe pain that does not respond to analgesics. Corticosteroids are an option for children who have severe pain not responding to analgesics or who have very large tonsils that may lead to obstruction.

A small proportion of children go on to develop recurrent tonsillitis. There is evidence on the treatment effects of tonsillectomy.[35,42,43] Tonsillectomy has a large beneficial effect, but the rates of tonsillitis also reduce spontaneously without treatment, so absolute benefits are modest. In addition, the operation itself is associated with postoperative pain and some risk of complications. High-quality trials of prophylactic antibiotic treatment have not been done, but this treatment would be a reasonable option for families who want treatment but decide against surgery. Surgery is likely to be most beneficial in children who have very frequent severe infections. If surgery is the chosen treatment option, cold steel tonsillectomy is associated with less postoperative pain and bleeding than operation by diathermy.[35,44]

OTITIS MEDIA

Otitis media is an acute URTI that affects the respiratory mucosa of the middle ear cleft. It is a common illness in young children and occurs much less frequently in children more than 6 years old.[45,46] In developed countries, otitis media is the most common indication for antibiotic prescribing and surgery in young children. In the United States, annual costs associated with otitis media were estimated to be $3 to $5 billion in the 1990s.[45]

Otitis media is best regarded as a spectrum of disease. The most important conditions are OME, AOM without perforation (AOMwoP), acute otitis media with perforation (AOMwiP), and CSOM. Unfortunately, there currently is a lack of consistency in definitions of different forms of otitis media (especially AOM).[47] Generally, AOM is defined as the presence of a middle ear effusion plus the presence of the symptoms (especially pain) or signs (especially bulging of the tympanic membrane or fresh discharge). The diagnostic criteria used in studies of AOM vary. Some use symptomatic criteria, some use otoscopic criteria, and some require that both symptomatic and otoscopic criteria be met. OME usually is defined as the presence of a middle ear effusion without symptoms or signs of an acute infection. CSOM usually is defined as discharge through a perforated tympanic membrane for longer than 2 to 6 weeks.

Children who have immunodeficiency or craniofacial abnormalities (eg, cleft palate, Down's syndrome) are at increased risk of otitis media. Other risk factors that have been identified in epidemiologic studies include recent respiratory infection, family history, siblings, child care attendance, lack of breast feeding, passive smoke exposure, and use of a pacifier.[48]

Most children experience at least one episode of AOM.[45] The peak incidence of infection occurs between 6 and 12 months. Although the pathogenesis of AOM is multifactorial, both viruses and bacteria are implicated.[45] Bacteria infection with the common respiratory pathogens (S. pneumoniae, H. influenzae, and M. catarrhalis) often is preceded by a viral infection. Viruses (especially respiratory syntactical virus and influenza) can cause AOM without coinfection with bacteria.[45] The pain associated with AOM resolves within 24 hours in around 60% of cases and within 3 days in around 80%.[46] AOM is less likely to resolve spontaneously in children younger than 2 years.[49] Complications of AOM include CSOM, mastoiditis, labyrinthitis, facial palsy, meningitis, intracranial abscess, and lateral sinus thrombosis.[50] Mastoiditis was the most common life-threatening complication in the pre-antibiotic era. It occurred in 18% of children admitted to hospital with AOM in one study.[51] Mastoiditis and all other complications now are rare in developed countries.

CSOM is the most severe form of otitis media.[52] Although there is a lack of well-designed longitudinal studies, CSOM is the type of otitis media most likely to persist without treatment. In developing countries, CSOM occurs as a complication of AOM with perforation and can be a major health issue. The range of bacterial pathogens associated with CSOM is considerably broader than those seen in AOM. Pseudomonas, Staphylococcus, Proteus, and Klebsiella species are the most commonly isolated pathogens, and mixed infections are common.[52] Multidrug antibiotic resistance is seen often in Pseudomonas infections. The associated hearing loss usually is greater than seen in OME, and CSOM is the most important cause of moderate conductive hearing loss (>40 dB) in many developing countries.[53]

In developed countries, CSOM now is very uncommon. A recent risk factor study in Holland found that most cases of CSOM now occur as a complication of tympanostomy tube insertion.[54] Children who have immunodeficiency and some indigenous populations also are at greatly increased risk. In rural and remote communities in northern Australia, more than 20% of young children are affected.[55]

OME is the most common form of otitis media. The point prevalence in screening studies is around 20% in young children.[45] OME can occur spontaneously, as a component of rhinosinusitis, or following an episode of AOM. The same respiratory bacterial pathogens associated with AOM have been implicated in the pathogenesis of OME. Most children who have OME improve spontaneously within 3 months, and complications from this illness are uncommon.[45] The average hearing loss associated with OME is around 25 dB.[45] Despite large numbers of studies, a causal relationship between OME and speech and language delay has not been proven.[50,56]

Children who have otitis media usually present with features related to (1) pain and fever (AOM); (2) hearing loss (OME); or (3) ear discharge (AOMwiP or CSOM). In some children, otitis media is detected as part of a routine examination. Making an accurate diagnosis is not easy. Generally a good view of the whole tympanic membrane and the use of either pneumatic otoscopy or tympanometry are required to confirm the presence of a middle ear effusion.[47,57] Studies of diagnostic accuracy in AOM have found ear pain to be the most useful symptom, but it is not very reliable on its own. Bulging, opacity, and immobility of the tympanic membrane are highly predictive of AOM. Normal color (pearly gray) of the tympanic membrane makes AOM unlikely.[58]

Options for Interventions

Most children who have AOM improve spontaneously within 14 days, and complications from this illness are uncommon. There is evidence concerning the preventive effects of conjugate pneumococcal vaccine and influenza vaccine on the onset of illness (see **Table 4**).[46,59–61] Both these vaccines have been shown to be effective, but the beneficial effects in terms of overall rates of infection are slight. The beneficial effects of the conjugate pneumococcal vaccine in reducing the rate of insertion of tympanostomy tubes are modest.[62] Most children do not fall into this risk group. There also is evidence about the treatment effects of antihistamines and decongestants, antibiotics, myringotomy, and analgesics (see **Table 4**).[46,50,51,63] Regular analgesics (paracetamol or ibuprofen) provide a benefit (assessment on day 2), and the beneficial effects are large.[46] Antibiotics also are effective,[49,51] but in most children the short-term beneficial effects are slight. The beneficial effects are modest in children younger than 2 years old who have bilateral AOM and are large in those who have AOMwiP. Studies of initial treatment with antibiotics have not documented a long-term effect. If antibiotics are to be used, there is evidence that a longer course of treatment ($\geq$ 7 days) is more effective, but the beneficial effects are modest (persistent AOM reduced from 22% to 15%).[64] There is no evidence that any one of the commonly used antibiotics is more effective than the others. The use of antihistamines and decongestants has not been shown to be beneficial, and myringotomy seems to be harmful compared with no treatment or antibiotics (see **Table 4**).[46,50,63]

Given the available evidence from RCTs on AOM, most well-informed individuals choose symptomatic relief with analgesics and either watchful waiting or antibiotics. Antibiotics are most appropriate in children younger than 2 years who have bilateral AOM, children who have AOMwiP, children at high risk of complications, and children who already have had 48 hours of watchful waiting. If the child is not in a high-risk, group, but the family prefers antibiotic treatment, the clinician should discuss "wait and see" prescribing. Provision of a script for an antibiotic along with advice to use it only if the pain persists for 48 hours can reduce antibiotic use by two thirds (with no negative effect on family satisfaction).[65–67]

A small proportion of children who have AOM experience recurrent AOM (three episodes within 6 months or four episodes within 12 months).[45] There is evidence about the treatment effects of prophylactic antibiotics, adenoidectomy, and tympanostomy tube insertion.[46,50,68–70] Antibiotics have been proven to be effective, but the beneficial effects are modest. The rates of AOM also reduce spontaneously without treatment, so the absolute benefits are less impressive than anticipated. Insertion of tympanostomy tubes also seems to reduce rates of AOM, and the level of effect is similar to that of antibiotics. Either of these options could be considered in children who have very frequent severe infections, especially infections occurring before the peak of respiratory illness in winter. Children who have tympanostomy tubes may develop a discharging ear, however, so tympanostomy tubes are not a good option in children who are at increased risk of suppurative infections (including those who have immunodeficiency or persistent bacterial rhinosinusitis). In these children, prophylactic antibiotics or prompt antibiotic treatment of infections probably is a more appropriate choice. Adenoidectomy does not seem to be an effective treatment.[50,69,70]

A small proportion of children who have AOMwiP go on to develop CSOM. In developed countries, CSOM occurs most commonly as a complication of tympanostomy tube placement. There is evidence about the treatment effects of topical antibiotics, topical antiseptics, systemic antibiotics, and ear cleaning.[52,53,71–73] The interpretation of a large number of small studies is challenging, but topical antibiotics have been proven to be effective, although the beneficial effects vary from large to modest. Most studies have not documented a long-term effect. Topical antibiotics also seem to be more effective than antiseptics and systemic antibiotics.[53] The role of topical antibiotics plus systematic antibiotics is unclear.[74] Cleaning the middle ear discharge has not been proven to be effective in RCTs but generally is regarded as necessary before insertion of topical antibiotics (at least in children who have profuse discharge). Although not seen in RCTs, there also is a very small risk of ototoxicity associated with most topical antibiotics (except topical quinolones) and topical antiseptics.[50] For children who do not respond to prolonged courses of topical antibiotics, two small studies (85 participants) have documented high cure rates and large beneficial effects associated with 2 to 3 weeks of intravenous antipseudomonal antibiotics (such as ceftazidime).[75,76]

Given the available evidence from RCTs on CSOM, most well-informed individuals choose topical antibiotic treatment. Even though this treatment is effective, prolonged or repeated courses of treatment often are required. If prolonged or repeated courses of topical antibiotic are needed, topical quinolones provide a slight benefit in terms of risk of ototoxicity.

OME affects all children but usually is asymptomatic.[45] A small proportion of children have persistent OME with associated hearing loss. There is evidence that screening to identify young children who have OME or hearing loss associated with OME is not effective in developed countries.[77] There also is evidence on the treatment effects of antibiotics, insertion of tympanostomy tubes, autoinflation devices, antihistamines and decongestants, and antibiotics plus steroids (see **Table 4**).[49,51,78–85] Early insertion of tympanostomy tubes (compared with watchful waiting with the option of later insertion) improves hearing at 6 and 12 months, but the beneficial effect is modest.[78,79,81] This improvement in hearing has not been associated with improvement in language development or cognitive assessment scores.[81] Tympanostomy tubes usually last 6 to 12 months, and there is no evidence of any ongoing benefit after they have been extruded. Antibiotics also have been shown to be an effective treatment, but the beneficial effects are slight and do not seem to persist long term.[50,78,79] Combining antibiotics with steroids seems to provide short-term benefits, but again the beneficial effect is modest.[78,85] There is some evidence that autoinflation devices are effective.[78,83] but the benefits are modest and have been documented to be only short term. Antihistamines and decongestants provide no benefit (see **Table 4**).[78,79,84]

Given the available evidence from RCTs on OME, most well-informed individuals initially choose a course of watchful waiting. For children who have persistent OME in both ears associated with hearing loss despite watching waiting for 6 to 12 months, a trial of antibiotics is reasonable. Insertion of tympanostomy tubes is most appropriate in children when the primary concern is conductive hearing loss and communication difficulties. Children who have the most severe conductive hearing loss are most likely to benefit. Children who experience frequent suppurative infections (including those who have immunodeficiency or persistent bacterial rhinosinusitis) are at greatest risk of developing CSOM as a complication of tympanostomy tubes. Families should be informed that a small proportion of children suffer recurrent persistent OME when the tympanostomy tubes are extruded and may need a second operation. In these children, tympanostomy tubes plus adenoidectomy is a reasonable option.[79,80]

SUMMARY

URTIs are the most common illnesses affecting children. Most illnesses are mild and resolve completely without specific treatment. Multiple interventions have been assessed in the treatment of rhinosinusitis, pharyngitis, and otitis media. None of the interventions had substantial absolute benefits for the populations studied. Therefore, for most children, symptomatic relief and watchful waiting (including education of the parents about important danger signs) is the most appropriate treatment option. Antibiotics have a role in children who have persistent bacterial infection and those at risk of complications.

REFERENCES

1. Monto AS. Epidemiology of viral respiratory infections. Am J Med 2002; 112(Suppl 6A):4S–12S.
2. Heikkinen T, Jarvinen A. The common cold. Lancet 2003;361(9351):51–9.
3. Kenealy T. Sore throat. BMJ Clinical Evidence 2008. Available at: http://clinical evidence.bmj.com. Accessed June 27, 2008.
4. Behrman RE. Textbook of pediatrics. 15th edition. Philadelphia: W.B. Saunders Company; 1996.
5. Revai K, Dobbs LA, Nair S, et al. Incidence of acute otitis media and sinusitis complicating upper respiratory tract infection: the effect of age. Pediatrics 2007;119(6):e1408–12.
6. Irwig L, Irwig J, Sweet M, et al. Smart health choices: making sense of health advice. Sydney (Australia): Hammersmith Press; 2007.
7. Altman DG, Bland JM. Statistics notes. Treatment allocation in controlled trials: why randomise? BMJ 1999;318(7192):1209.
8. Atkins D, Best D, Briss PA, et al. Grading quality of evidence and strength of recommendations. BMJ 2004;328(7454):1490–7.
9. Guyatt GH, Oxman AD, Vist GE, et al. GRADE: an emerging consensus on rating quality of evidence and strength of recommendations. BMJ 2008;336(7650):924–6.
10. Atkins D, Briss PA, Eccles M, et al. Systems for grading the quality of evidence and the strength of recommendations II: pilot study of a new system. BMC Health Serv Res 2005;5(1):25–36.
11. Clinical evidence. Available at: http://clinicalevidence.bmj.com. Accessed June 27, 2008.
12. The Cochrane Library. Available at: http://www3.interscience.wiley.com/cgi-bin/mrwhome/106568753/HOME. Accessed June 16, 2008.

13. Gwaltney- JMJ, Phillips CD, Miller RD, et al. Computed tomographic study of the common cold [see comments]. N Engl J Med 1994;330(1):25–30.

14. Puhakka T, Makela MJ, Alanen A, et al. Sinusitis in the common cold. J Allergy Clin Immunol 1998;102(3):403–8.

15. Pratter MR. Cough and the common cold: ACCP evidence-based clinical practice guidelines. Chest 2006;129(1 Suppl):72S–4S.

16. Ramadan HH. Pediatric sinusitis: update. J Otolaryngol 2005;34(Suppl 1):S14–7.

17. American Academy of Pediatrics, Subcommittee on Management of Sinusitis and Committee on Quality Improvement. Clinical practice guideline: management of sinusitis. Pediatrics 2001;108(3):798–808.

18. Ioannidis JP, Lau J. Technical report: evidence for the diagnosis and treatment of acute uncomplicated sinusitis in children: a systematic overview. Pediatrics 2001; 108(3):E57–64.

19. Williams JW Jr, Simel DL. Does this patient have sinusitis? Diagnosing acute sinusitis by history and physical examination. JAMA 1993;270(10):1242–6.

20. Douglas RM, Hemila H, Chalker E, et al. Vitamin C for preventing and treating the common cold. Cochrane Database Syst Rev 2007;(3):CD000980.

21. Linde K, Barrett B, Wolkart K, et al. Echinacea for preventing and treating the common cold. Cochrane Database Syst Rev 2006;(1):CD000530.

22. Arroll B. Common cold. BMJ Clinical Evidence 2008. Available at: http://clinical evidence.bmj.com. Accessed June 27, 2008.

23. Sutter AI, Lemiengre M, Campbell H, et al. Antihistamines for the common cold. Cochrane Database Syst Rev 2003;(3):CD001267.

24. Arroll B, Kenealy T. Antibiotics for the common cold and acute purulent rhinitis. Cochrane Database Syst Rev 2005;(3):CD000247.

25. Arroll B, Kenealy T. Are antibiotics effective for acute purulent rhinitis? Systematic review and meta-analysis of placebo controlled randomised trials. BMJ 2006; 333(7562):279–82.

26. Taverner D, Latte J. Nasal decongestants for the common cold. Cochrane Database Syst Rev 2007;(1):CD001953.

27. Kollar C, Schneider H, Waksman J, et al. Meta-analysis of the efficacy of a single dose of phenylephrine 10 mg compared with placebo in adults with acute nasal congestion due to the common cold. Clin Ther 2007;29(6):1057–70.

28. Marshall I. Zinc for the common cold. Cochrane Database Syst Rev 1999;(2):CD001364.

29. Ah-See K. Sinusitis (acute). BMJ Clinical Evidence 2008. Available at: http://clini calevidence.bmj.com. Accessed June 27, 2008.

30. Zalmanovici A, Yaphe J. Steroids for acute sinusitis. Cochrane Database Syst Rev 2007;(2):CD005149.

31. Young J, De Sutter A, Merenstein D, et al. Antibiotics for adults with clinically diagnosed acute rhinosinusitis: a meta-analysis of individual patient data. Lancet 2008;371(9616):908–14.

32. Ip S, Fu L, Balk E, et al. Update on acute bacterial rhinosinusitis. Evid Rep Technol Assess 2005;124:1–3.

33. Morris P, Leach A. Antibiotics for persistent nasal discharge (rhinosinusitis) in children. Cochrane Database Syst Rev 2002;(4):CD001094.

34. Vincent MT, Celestin N, Hussain AN. Pharyngitis. Am Fam Physician 2004;69(6): 1465–70.

35. Georgalas CC, Tolley NS, Narula A. Recurrent throat infections (tonsillitis). BMJ Clinical Evidence 2008. Available at: http://clinicalevidence.bmj.com. Accessed June 27, 2008.

36. Ebell MH, Smith MA, Barry HC, et al. The rational clinical examination. Does this patient have strep throat? JAMA 2000;284(22):2912–8.

37. Del Mar CB, Glasziou PP, Spinks AB. Antibiotics for sore throat. Cochrane Database Syst Rev 2006;(4):CD000023.

38. Robertson KA, Volmink JA, Mayosi BM. Antibiotics for the primary prevention of acute rheumatic fever: a meta-analysis. BMC Cardiovasc Disord 2005;5(1):11–9.

39. Casey JR, Pichichero ME. Metaanalysis of short course antibiotic treatment for group a streptococcal tonsillopharyngitis. Pediatr Infect Dis J 2005;24(10): 909–17.

40. Thomas M, Del Mar C, Glasziou P. How effective are treatments other than antibiotics for acute sore throat? Br J Gen Pract 2000;50(459):817–20.

41. Olympia RP, Khine H, Avner JR. Effectiveness of oral dexamethasone in the treatment of moderate to severe pharyngitis in children. Arch Pediatr Adolesc Med 2005;159(3):278–82.

42. Burton MJ, Towler B, Glasziou P. Tonsillectomy versus non-surgical treatment for chronic/recurrent acute tonsillitis. Cochrane Database Syst Rev 2000;(2): CD001802.

43. van Staaij BK, van den Akker EH, van der Heijden GJ, et al. Adenotonsillectomy for upper respiratory infections: evidence based? Arch Dis Child 2005;90(1):19–25.

44. Leinbach RF, Markwell SJ, Colliver JA, et al. Hot versus cold tonsillectomy: a systematic review of the literature. Otolaryngol Head Neck Surg 2003;129(4):360–4.

45. Rovers MM, Schilder AG, Zielhuis GA, et al. Otitis media. Lancet 2004;363(9407): 465–73.

46. Bradley-Stevenson C, O'Neill P, Roberts T. Otitis media in children (acute). BMJ Clinical Evidence 2008. Available at: http://clinicalevidence.bmj.com. Accessed June 27, 2008.

47. American Academy of Pediatrics Subcommittee on Management of Acute Otitis Media. Diagnosis and management of acute otitis media. Pediatrics 2004;113(5): 1451–65.

48. Uhari M, Mantysaari K, Niemela M. A meta-analytic review of the risk factors for acute otitis media [see comments]. Clin Infect Dis 1996;22(6):1079–83.

49. Rovers MM, Glasziou P, Appelman CL, et al. Antibiotics for acute otitis media: a meta-analysis with individual patient data. Lancet 2006;368(9545):1429–35.

50. Rosenfeld RM, Bluestone CD. Evidence-based otitis media. Hamilton (UK): B.C. Decker Inc; 2003.

51. Glasziou PP, Del Mar CB, Sanders SL, et al. Antibiotics for acute otitis media in children. Cochrane Database Syst Rev 2004;(1):CD000219.

52. Verhoeff M, van der Veen EL, Rovers MM, et al. Chronic suppurative otitis media: a review. Int J Pediatr Otorhinolaryngol 2006;70(1):1–12.

53. Acuin J. Chronic suppurative otitis media. BMJ Clinical Evidence 2008. Available at: http://clinicalevidence.bmj.com. Accessed June 27, 2008.

54. van der Veen EL, Schilder AG, van Heerbeek N, et al. Predictors of chronic suppurative otitis media in children. Arch Otolaryngol Head Neck Surg 2006; 132(10):1115–8.

55. Leach AJ, Morris PS. The burden and outcome of respiratory tract infection in Australian and aboriginal children. Pediatr Infect Dis J 2007;26(10 Suppl):S4–7.

56. Roberts JE, Rosenfeld RM, Zeisel SA. Otitis media and speech and language: a meta-analysis of prospective studies. Pediatrics 2004;113(3 Pt 1):e238–48.

57. Takata GS, Chan LS, Morphew T, et al. Evidence assessment of the accuracy of methods of diagnosing middle ear effusion in children with otitis media with effusion. Pediatrics 2003;112(6 Pt 1):1379–87.

58. Rothman R, Owens T, Simel DL. Does this child have acute otitis media? JAMA 2003;290(12):1633–40.
59. Straetemans M, Sanders EA, Veenhoven RH, et al. Pneumococcal vaccines for preventing otitis media. Cochrane Database Syst Rev 2004;(1):CD001480.
60. Jefferson T, Rivetti A, Harnden A, et al. Vaccines for preventing influenza in healthy children. Cochrane Database Syst Rev 2008;(2):CD004879.
61. Manzoli L, Schioppa F, Boccia A, et al. The efficacy of influenza vaccine for healthy children: a meta-analysis evaluating potential sources of variation in efficacy estimates including study quality. Pediatr Infect Dis J 2007;26(2):97–106.
62. Fireman B, Black SB, Shinefield HR, et al. Impact of the pneumococcal conjugate vaccine on otitis media. Pediatr Infect Dis J 2003;22(1):10–6.
63. Flynn CA, Griffin GH, Schultz JK. Decongestants and antihistamines for acute otitis media in children. Cochrane Database Syst Rev 2004;(3):CD001727.
64. Kozyrskyj AL, Hildes-Ripstein GE, Longstaffe SE, et al. Short course antibiotics for acute otitis media. Cochrane Database Syst Rev 2000;(2):CD001095.
65. Spurling GK, Del Mar CB, Dooley L, et al. Delayed antibiotics for respiratory infections. Cochrane Database Syst Rev 2007;(3):CD004417.
66. Spiro DM, Tay KY, Arnold DH, et al. Wait-and-see prescription for the treatment of acute otitis media: a randomized controlled trial. JAMA 2006;296(10):1235–41.
67. Little P, Gould C, Williamson I, et al. Pragmatic randomised controlled trial of two prescribing strategies for childhood acute otitis media. BMJ 2001;322(7282):336–42.
68. Leach AJ, Morris PS. Antibiotics for the prevention of acute and chronic suppurative otitis media in children. Cochrane Database Syst Rev 2006;(4):CD004401.
69. Mattila PS, Joki-Erkkila VP, Kilpi T, et al. Prevention of otitis media by adenoidectomy in children younger than 2 years. Arch Otolaryngol Head Neck Surg 2003; 129(2):163–8.
70. Hammaren-Malmi S, Saxen H, Tarkkanen J, et al. Adenoidectomy does not significantly reduce the incidence of otitis media in conjunction with the insertion of tympanostomy tubes in children who are younger than 4 years: a randomized trial. Pediatrics 2005;116(1):185–9.
71. Macfadyen CA, Acuin JM, Gamble C. Topical antibiotics without steroids for chronically discharging ears with underlying eardrum perforations. Cochrane Database Syst Rev 2005;(4):CD004618.
72. Macfadyen CA, Acuin JM, Gamble C. Systemic antibiotics versus topical treatments for chronically discharging ears with underlying eardrum perforations. Cochrane Database Syst Rev 2006;(1):CD005608.
73. Acuin J, Smith A, Mackenzie I. Interventions for chronic suppurative otitis media. Cochrane Database Syst Rev 2000;(2):CD000473.
74. van der Veen EL, Rovers MM, Albers FW, et al. Effectiveness of trimethoprim/sulfamethoxazole for children with chronic active otitis media: a randomized, placebo-controlled trial. Pediatrics 2007;119(5):897–904.
75. Leiberman A, Fliss DM, Dagan R. Medical treatment of chronic suppurative otitis media without cholesteatoma in children—a two-year follow-up. Int J Pediatr Otorhinolaryngol 1992;24(1):25–33.
76. Dagan R, Fliss DM, Einhorn M, et al. Outpatient management of chronic suppurative otitis media without cholesteatoma in children. Pediatr Infect Dis J 1992; 11(7):542–6.
77. Simpson SA, Thomas CL, van der Linden MK, et al. Identification of children in the first four years of life for early treatment for otitis media with effusion. Cochrane Database Syst Rev 2007;(1):CD004163.

78. Williamson I. Otitis media with effusion. BMJ Clinical Evidence 2008. Available at: http://clinicalevidence.bmj.com. Accessed June 27, 2008.

79. American Academy of Family Physicians, American Academy of Otolaryngology-Head and Neck Surgery, American Academy of Pediatrics Subcommittee on Otitis Media With Effusion. Otitis media with effusion. Pediatrics 2004;113(5): 1412–29.

80. Rosenfeld RM. Surgical prevention of otitis media. Vaccine 2000;19(Suppl 1): S134–9.

81. Lous J, Burton MJ, Felding JU, et al. Grommets (ventilation tubes) for hearing loss associated with otitis media with effusion in children. Cochrane Database Syst Rev 2005;(1):CD001801.

82. Rovers MM, Black N, Browning GG, et al. Grommets in otitis media with effusion: an individual patient data meta-analysis. Arch Dis Child 2005;90(5):480–5.

83. Perera R, Haynes J, Glasziou P, et al. Autoinflation for hearing loss associated with otitis media with effusion. Cochrane Database Syst Rev 2006;(4):CD006285.

84. Griffin GH, Flynn C, Bailey RE, et al. Antihistamines and/or decongestants for otitis media with effusion (OME) in children. Cochrane Database Syst Rev 2006;(4):CD003423.

85. Thomas CL, Simpson S, Butler CC, et al. Oral or topical nasal steroids for hearing loss associated with otitis media with effusion in children. Cochrane Database Syst Rev 2006;3:CD001935.

Acute Bronchiolitis and Croup

Mark L. Everard, MB, ChB, FRCP, DM

KEYWORDS

• Acute bronchiolitis • Croup • Wheeze • Wheezy bronchitis

Respiratory viruses are responsible for an extremely high proportion of all disease in young children presenting to medical services. Preschool children infected by one of these pathogens usually exhibit clinical illness with one or more upper airways manifestations such as coryza, pharyngitis, or otitis media. Extension of infection into the lower airways below the larynx most commonly causes "bronchitis," adding cough to the symptoms associated with the previously mentioned conditions. If the virus induces airways obstruction (most commonly through the induction of increased airways secretions and mucosal edema and/or bronchospasm), this obstruction may be manifest by increased work of breathing resulting in tachypnea and subcostal recession, gas trapping as manifested by hyperinflation, and noisy breathing caused by turbulent airflow.

The clinical phenotype of disease induced by a viral lower respiratory tract infection is determined by a number of factors, including the site of maximal inflammation, which in turn depends in part on the virus, the age of the infant or young child, and the existence of comorbidities such as atopic asthma. Although certain viruses classically are associated with certain disease phenotypes, such as parainfluenza with croup, respiratory syncytial virus (RSV) with acute bronchiolitis, and rhinovirus with exacerbation of asthma, any of the viruses can induce any of the clinical phenotypes.[1–5] The acute bronchiolitis associated with rhinovirus is clinically indistinguishable from that caused by RSV; RSV also is an important cause of croup and is responsible for a significant proportion of exacerbations of asthma in young children. The number of viruses known to target the respiratory tract continues to grow; viruses such as human metpneumovirus and human bocavirus have been added to the list of proven and likely respiratory pathogens.[5] As **Fig. 1** indicates for RSV (see **Fig. 1**A) and rhinovirus (see **Fig. 1**B), any of the conditions can be caused by any of the viruses, but the relative likelihood if a particular virus causing a particular condition varies with the virus.

One of the great challenges for those dealing with lower respiratory tract disease in children is that the lungs have a very limited repertoire of responses to acute or chronic insults. Increased airways secretions and cough are common to many conditions, such as acute or persistent bacterial infections, acute viral infections, untreated

---

Department of Respiratory Medicine, Sheffield Children's Hospital, Western Bank, Sheffield S10 2TH, UK

E-mail address: m.l.everard@sheffield.ac.uk

Pediatr Clin N Am 56 (2009) 119–133
doi:10.1016/j.pcl.2008.10.007
0031-3955/08/$ – see front matter

pediatric.theclinics.com

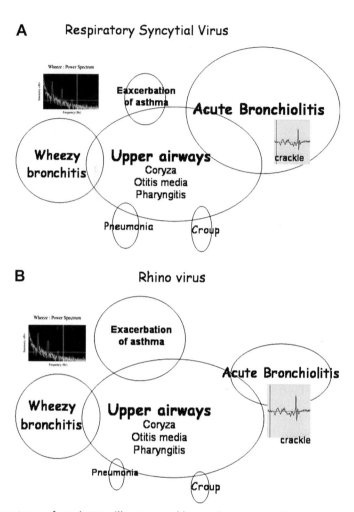

Fig. 1. Phenotypes of respiratory illness caused by respiratory syncytial virus and rhinovirus.

asthma, and recurrent aspiration. In some individuals bronchoconstriction also can contribute to airways obstruction. Disease within the lower airways frequently leads to the generation of adventitial sounds. Secretions within the large airways can induce audible rattles and coarse airways noises[6,7] but also may contribute to the wheeze in patients experiencing an exacerbation of asthma or wheezy bronchitis. The lack of precision in using the term "wheeze" adds to the difficulties in this area. It is clear that parents and doctors use the term "wheeze" for a variety of respiratory, and indeed nonrespiratory, noises.[7–9] Because wheeze is a key symptom driving both diagnostic and therapeutic decisions, this imprecision is a major problem. Obstruction of distal airways with secretions may lead to the generation of inspiratory crackles (crepitations) heard on auscultation as units of alveoli pop open.

The lack of a simple test to distinguish conditions such asthma, wheezy bronchitis, and bronchiolitis means that care must be taken to describe accurately the phenotype of disease being experienced by an individual patient. This identification is a key step in ensuring that the patient receives optimal management. It must also be recognized that, even when the key clinical features have been considered carefully, it frequently is impossible to provide an accurate diagnostic label. A preschool-age child with a clinically apparent viral upper respiratory tract infection, cough, and initial episode of wheeze may have a viral bronchitis with associated wheezing (wheezy bronchitis) or an exacerbation of asthma (see **Fig. 1**). There is no test to distinguish between the two conditions. Adding to the confusion, many clinicians label such an episode "acute bronchiolitis." The use of the term "virally associated wheeze" to describe wheezing associated with a viral infection in a nonasthmatic patient adds further unnecessary confusion, because the term includes both patients experiencing an exacerbation of asthma and patients who have wheezy bronchitis. Similarly, the term "reactive airways disease" does not help the clinician arrive at a more accurate diagnostic label. Although phenotypically the 13-month-old patient who has asthma may be indistinguishable form the 13-month-old patent who has wheezy bronchitis, there may be very important differences in some of the inflammatory components and the degree of bronchoconstriction. Thus a child who has wheezy bronchitis may look phenotypically like a child who has the first exacerbation of asthma; the airways inflammation dominated by neutrophils is likely to be very similar to that in a young child who has acute bronchiolitis characterized by widespread crackles. Thus two children with an obvious viral infection and prominent wheeze may look very similar but may respond quite differently to therapeutic interventions.

The lack of a definitive test and the resulting reliance on a clinical diagnosis adds a level of complexity to the consideration of the literature addressing lower airways conditions such as bronchiolitis. This complexity is compounded by lack of agreement between countries and indeed among clinicians within countries as to the definition of "acute bronchiolitis."

The clinical entity referred to as "acute viral croup" (acute laryngotracheobronchitis)[10] is less fraught with ambiguity, and this clarity probably accounts for the relative lack of controversy concerning this condition. Acute viral croup is identified more readily because, although the inflammation tends to involve the larynx, trachea, and large bronchi, the site of maximal airways obstruction generally is just below the larynx and thus is effectively extrathoracic. This extrathoracic positioning leads to airways obstruction that is maximal during inspiration: the negative pressure generated during inspiration leads to narrowing of the upper airway and the extrathoracic portion of the trachea. As a result, a RSV infection causing significant edema in the upper trachea produces the clinical picture of croup. When the inflammation is predominantly distal, it may cause acute bronchiolitis or an exacerbation of asthma with airways obstruction being maximal during the expiratory phase of the respiratory cycle. The differential diagnosis of a child who has an apparent viral infection, barking cough, and inspiratory stridor is quite different from that of the many conditions causing obstruction in the distal airways, and it is a condition that is much easier to characterize on clinical grounds.

ACUTE BRONCHIOLITIS
Evidence-Based Guidelines

At least two comprehensive evidence-based guidelines covering the diagnosis, management, and prevention of acute bronchiolitis have been published in the past 18 months. Both the American Academy of Pediatrics (AAP)[11] and the Scottish Intercollegiate Guideline Network (SIGN) guidelines[12] from Scotland used rigorous evidence-based methodology, including a comprehensive review of the literature, the use of relevant systematic reviews, consultation, and peer review. Reassuringly, in most respects, they have reached the same conclusions and reflect the author's practice based on a review of the literature (**Table 1**). They state that diagnosis should be based

Table 1
Diagnosis and management of acute bronchiolitis and croup

Practice	Recommended/Not Recommended	Strength of Recommendation[a]	Quality of Supporting Evidence
Acute bronchiolitis			
Diagnosis and assessment			
Diagnosis on basis of history and examination	Recommended (see text)	Moderate	Low
Transcutaneous oxygen saturation	Recommended	Strong	Moderate
Admission based on severity and risk factors	Recommended	Strong	Moderate
Virologic testing (for infection control)	Recommended	Weak	Low
Hematology/biochemistry	Not recommended	Strong	Moderate
Chest radiograph	Not recommended	Strong	Moderate
Interventions			
Oxygen prescription for transcutaneous oxygen < 92%	Recommended	Weak	Low
Prevent dehydration and moderate fluid restriction	Recommended	Strong	Moderate
Beta-agonists	Not recommended	Strong	Moderate
Adrenaline	Not recommended	Strong	Moderate
Routine antibiotics	Not recommended	Strong	High
Inhaled corticosteroids	Not recommended	Strong	Moderate
Oral corticosteroids	Not recommended	Strong	Moderate
Physiotherapy	Not recommended	Strong	Low
Antiviral therapy (ribavirin)	Not recommended	Strong	Moderate
Antileukotriene therapy	Not recommended	Strong	Moderate
Infection control			
Hand decontamination	Recommended	Strong	Strong
Gloves and gowns	Recommended	Strong	Moderate
Croup			
Diagnosis and assessment			
Clinical diagnosis	Recommended	Strong	Moderate
Admission based on clinical assessment of severity and risk factors	Recommended	Strong	Moderate
Transcutaneous oxygen measurements	Not recommended	Weak	Low
Virology	Not recommended	Strong	Moderate
Hematology/biochemistry	Not recommended	Strong	Moderate
Radiology	Not recommended	Strong	Moderate
Interventions			
Systemic (or nebulized) corticosteroids for moderate and severe croup	Recommended	Strong	High

(continued on next page)

Practice	Recommended/Not Recommended	Strength of Recommendation[a]	Quality of Supporting Evidence
Table 1 *(continued)*			
Nebulized adrenaline for moderate to severe croup	Recommended	Strong	Moderate
Heliox	Not recommended	Weak	Low
Humidification/steam	Not recommended	Strong	Moderate

Quality of supporting evidence regarding treatment depends entirely on whether there are important subgroups within the spectrum of disease covered by the term "acute bronchiolitis."

[a] Grading is based on the GRADE approach in Guyatt GH, Oxman AD, Vist GE, et al. GRADE: an emerging consensus on rating quality of evidence and strength of recommendations. BMJ 2008;336:924–6.

on clinical assessment and that no test is helpful in making the diagnosis. Assessment of the severity and need for admission to hospital or intensive care also should be based on clinical grounds, including assessment of age and risk factors such as prematurity, chronic lung disease, or significant cardiac disease. Pulse oximetry is helpful in identifying hypoxia, but the two guidelines agree that there is little evidence to support the use of any one or group of features as a means of predicting progression of the illness. Investigations such chest radiographs and blood tests are not indicated unless the illness is atypical or particularly severe. Management consists of good supportive care, which may include intensive supportive care. Management has not changed essentially since Reynolds and Cook[13] stated in 1963 that "oxygen is vitally important and there is little evidence that any other therapy is consistently or even occasionally useful." Supportive care includes administration of fluids sufficient to prevent dehydration but restricted to prevent problems with hyponatremia caused by inappropriate antidiuretic hormone secretion. Both guidelines are clear that there is no proven pharmacologic treatment other than oxygen and that pharmacologic agents such as α- or β-agonists, inhaled or systemic corticosteroids, ribavirin, and antibiotics should not be used routinely. The use of good infection control measures is key to preventing nosocomial spread within pediatric units. Hand decontamination, preferably with an alcohol-based rub, is the most important measure. Gloves and gowns probably provide further benefit, and education of staff, relatives, and visitors has been shown to have value. Both guidelines state that monoclonal prophylaxis may be given to infants at risk, but pharmacoeconomic issues lead to differences in the strength of the recommendation. Neither set of guidelines mentions a role for interventions to prevent future morbidity, but at present there is no evidence that any treatment, including inhaled or systemic steroids[14] and antileukotriene antagonists administered during or immediately after the illness, has any impact on future morbidity.

The guidelines grade the strength of many of these recommendations as high because they are based on a number of systematic reviews, many of which were undertaken as part of the Cochrane Collaboration.[15–19] There are, however, some subtle, potentially important differences within this broad consensus that infants and young children should be managed conservatively, avoiding the unnecessary tests and therapies that do not have any effect. These differences include a trial of α- and β-agonists, the indications for using supplemental oxygen, the use of monoclonal antibodies in the prevention of RSV disease, the value of viral testing in helping prevent nosocomial spread, and, perhaps most important of all, the diagnosis of the condition. Indeed both sets of guidelines seem to have some internal contradictions relating to some of these issues.

It also is of interest that these guidelines do not reflect practice in many countries, and there is good evidence that the introduction of similar guidelines in a variety of countries has had little effect on practice, particularly recommendations relating to pharmacologic agents, which still are widely prescribed.[20–23] In part this lack of effect may result from the well-known difficulty of changing clinical practice, in part because clinicians feel that they should provide treatment even though there is little evidence to support the practice. Principally, however, this lack of effect probably results from the difficulties involved in agreeing about what "acute bronchiolitis" is. The following section considers possible reasons for the ongoing controversies that exist in this area.

Bronchodilators Should Not Be Used Routinely But Remain an Option

Although the AAP guideline states under recommendation 2a that bronchodilators should not be used routinely in the management of bronchiolitis (recommendation: evidence level B; randomized, controlled trials (RCTs) with limitations; preponderance of harm of use over benefit). It then almost immediately makes recommendation 2b: that a carefully monitored trial of α-adrenergic or β-adrenergic medication is an option. Inhaled bronchodilators should be continued only if there is a documented positive clinical response to the trial using an objective means of evaluation.

Although all national guidelines state that there is no evidence that any pharmacologic agent is useful in the treatment of acute bronchiolitis, the position advocated under recommendation 2b reflects the practice of many clinicians around the world, and many publications have noted that compliance with the recommendation not to use pharmacologic agents is poor.[20–23] This apparent discrepancy within a guideline (and the lack of compliance with guidelines) probably reflects the lack of consistency and specificity in the use of terms such as "acute bronchiolitis," "asthma," and "wheezy bronchitis" by clinicians, be they primary care physicians or tertiary specialists. As with all systematic reviews, the conclusions that can be drawn are only as good as the quality of data available for assessment. Reynolds and Cook13 noted more than 45 years ago that

> Much of the confusion about the management of bronchiolitis results from the fact that are probably two groups of patients: (1) those with obstructive disease resulting entirely from infection, thickening of the bronchiolar walls and intrabronchial secretions and (2) those with a pre-disposition to asthma who develop obstruction as a result of both inflammation and bronchospasm. The two groups cannot be readily distinguished on clinical grounds, it would appear that most patients fall in the first group.

If data are derived from different studies that have different population of patients or from studies that contain mixed populations, the results at best may be mixed and at worst are misleading.

Implications of the Lack of Precision in the Definition of Acute Bronchiolitis

When assessing the literature referring to infants who have acute bronchiolitis, it is important to understand that the publication may refer to one of at least two quite distinct phenotypes. In the United States and a number of European countries, the term is used to describe a young child or infant who has an apparent viral respiratory tract infection and a first episode of wheeze, but in the United Kingdom, Australia, and some parts of Europe, the term refers to an infant who has an apparent viral respiratory tract infection with lower airways obstruction accompanied by widespread crackles (crepitations). The later definition recognizes that such infants may wheeze occasionally or intermittently during the disease, but widespread crackles are the key diagnostic feature. The presence of crackles indicates that maximal obstruction is at the level of the distal airways (bronchiolitis) with terminal unit opening suddenly during inspiration and resulting in the discontinuous adventitial sounds. Interestingly, countries using this second definition have much better compliance with the guidelines suggesting that pharmacologic agents are of little value.[24]

Previous studies have indicated that the inflammatory process in patients who have RSV-induced "UK bronchiolitis" is dominated by an intense neutrophilic influx into the airways.[25] This influx seems to be driven by very high levels of cytokines such as interleukin-8[26] and inhibition of polymorphonuclear neutrophil (PMN) apoptosis.[27] A PMN response seems to be characteristic of the response to this and other respiratory viruses.[28] PMN products such as human neutrophil elastase and myeloperoxidase are potent inflammatory mediators driving mucus secretion, airways edema, and cough. At present it is not known whether the PMNs contribute significantly to elimination of the virus, and it is possible that the virus utilizes this response to assist in dissemination to other subjects. In such a context, standard interventions used to treat older patients who have asthma might well prove to be ineffective. Corticosteroids are believed to have little effect on neutrophilic airways inflammation, whereas β-agonists are unlikely to have much effect if bronchoconstriction is not a prominent feature.

As noted previously and as illustrated in **Fig. 1**, it is possible that a child who has an apparent viral infection with a first episode of wheezing ("American bronchiolitis") may be experiencing a first exacerbation of asthma or may have "wheezy bronchitis." Epidemiologic data suggest that, in patients who have "wheezy bronchitis," pre-existing factors, which may include relative airways size,[29] predispose these children to suffering one or more episodes of airways obstruction induced by a viral lower respiratory tract infection that is accompanied by wheeze. This tendency to wheeze with a viral lower respiratory tract infection declines in the preschool years. It is probable, but not proven, that these children have a pattern of inflammation similar to that seen in those who have "UK bronchiolitis" but that the manifestations are different because of lung growth and factors such as the development of pores of Kohn. Hence, phenotypically these patients may be indistinguishable from a child of similar age who has an exacerbation of asthma, but in terms of inflammation they are much closer to patients who have "UK acute bronchiolitis." Hence two children who look very similar may react very differently to pharmacologic agents.

Because the type of patient included in any cohort or therapeutic study influences the results obtained, this semantic issue may be key to understanding why there is such controversy in this field. A group selected on the presence of wheeze without crepitations is likely to include a sizable group of asthmatics, but epidemiologic data indicate that asthmatics still will represent a minority of the patients. Consequently any treatment effect that might be present if "pure" asthmatics were included might be lost if there is little or no benefit in the wheezy bronchitis groups. Similarly, if a substantial proportion of the recruited subjects are "asthmatics," this population might be sufficient for a study to show a statistically significant benefit, even if there is no clinical benefit in the "nonasthmatic" subjects. The danger is that such a conclusion might be generalized to the whole population of young, acutely wheezy children.

The AAP guidelines notes that

Overall, results of the meta-analysis indicated that, at most, 1 in 4 children treated with bronchodilators might have a transient improvement in clinical score of unclear clinical significance. This needs to be weighed against the potential adverse effects and cost of these agents and the fact that most children treated with bronchodilators will not benefit from their use. Studies assessing the impact of bronchodilators on long-term outcomes have found no impact on the overall course of the illness.

Such results would be consistent with the proposal that a significant minority of those in whom wheeze, in the absence of crackles, is the prominent symptom is likely to have a virally induced exacerbation of asthma. An alternative explanation, however, is that, as in any study, some patients will improve while others may remain static or indeed deteriorate before improving, and that post hoc subgroup analysis provides spurious evidence for a subgroup of responders.

Clinicians would not withhold β-agonists from an older child experiencing a virally induced exacerbation of asthma, even though the bronchodilation achieved is limited (in contrast to an asthmatic with poor control, in whom large changes in lung function may be observed)[30] and even though bronchodilator per se does not have a significant impact on the course of the illness or duration of hospitalization. The bronchodilator provides modest, temporary relief while waiting for the corticosteroids to take effect.

Acute Bronchiolitis—Diagnostic Recommendations from Guidelines

In their review Reynold and Cook[13] noted that pediatricians recognized that bronchiolitis is the most common acute lower respiratory tract infection necessitating hospitalization in infants less than 1 year of age, but the lack of a clear definition of the illness has been associated with a marked confusion concerning its management. This problem is reflected 45 years later in the AAP guidelines that define bronchiolitis as

a disorder most commonly caused in infants by viral lower respiratory tract infection. It is the most common lower respiratory infection in this age group. It is characterized by acute inflammation, edema, and necrosis of epithelial cells lining small airways, increased mucus production, and bronchospasm.

Although most of these features have been confirmed by histology in the most severely affected patients who die from the condition, the inclusion of bronchospasm is difficult to justify, particularly because a key recommendation is that "bronchodilators should not be used routinely in the management of bronchiolitis."

The guidelines recommend that the diagnosis and assessment should be based on history and physical examination. They note:

Most clinicians recognize bronchiolitis as a constellation of clinical symptoms and signs including a viral upper respiratory prodrome followed by increased respiratory effort and wheezing in children less than 2 years of age. Clinical signs and symptoms of bronchiolitis consist of rhinorrhea, cough, wheezing, tachypnea, and increased respiratory effort manifested as grunting, nasal flaring, and intercostal and/or subcostal retractions.

There is no mention of crackles in this section on diagnosis and assessment, although the introduction contains a similar paragraph that includes the sentence, "Signs and symptoms are typically rhinitis, tachypnea, wheezing, cough, crackles, use of accessory muscles, and/or nasal flaring."

Similarly, the SIGN guidelines are not entirely internally consistent with their definition of the condition stating that bronchiolitis is a condition characterized by "fever, nasal discharge, a dry wheezy cough and on examination there are widespread fine crackles and/or high pitched expiratory wheeze." The guidelines then comment that

In the UK, crackles on auscultation are considered to be the hall mark of the condition. Infants with no crackles and only transient early wheezing are usually categorised as having viral-induced wheezing and not bronchiolitis. American definitions place much greater emphasis on the inclusion of wheeze in the definition. This makes it difficult to extrapolate from American research. Or vice versa!

Does the Definition of Acute Bronchiolitis Matter?

A study of patients admitted to hospital with an RSV infection demonstrated that the host response is an important determinant of both the phenotype of the acute illness and subsequent respiratory morbidity.[31] At presentation the patients were ascribed the phenotypes "RSV acute bronchiolitis" (bilateral crepitation) or "RSV wheeze" (wheeze but no crepitations), and the children were followed to 3 years of age. The group with wheeze was older at the time of the acute illness and had significantly higher rates of personal atopy than either the controls or the patients who had RSV bronchiolitis. (The patients who had RSV bronchiolitis, in turn, had slightly lower levels of atopy than controls). At 3 years of age the wheezing group had much higher levels of respiratory morbidity and use of inhaled corticosteroids. This finding suggests that the wheezing cohort was made up of two different groups, despite their sharing the same phenotype. Although there was some increase in respiratory morbidity, mainly with viral infections, in the patients who had RSV bronchiolitis, they did not have higher levels of inhaled corticosteroid use. These data suggest that it is not the virus per se but host factors (including immunologic, inflammatory, and physiologic factors) that determine the phenotype of the acute illness and the pattern of subsequent respiratory morbidity. Other studies have tried to distinguish RSV bronchiolitis (crackles) from RSV wheeze prospectively and have found differences in the inflammatory process.[32] These factors also influence the therapeutic effect, if any, of pharmacologic agents.

Until there is a simple test to diagnose asthma other than its being a condition that improves significantly with asthma treatment (as manifested by objective bronchodilation in response to β-agonists or a significant change in morbidity in response to inhaled corticosteroids) and reoccurs if the treatment is withdrawn—a position advocated by both the British SIGN/British Thoracic Society[33] and GINA guidelines[34]—the AAP recommendation 2b is likely to remain reasonable, if wheeze is considered the key feature of bronchiolitis.

Potential Importance of Choosing the Appropriate End Points

As noted earlier, the inclusion of a mixed population in a study of a pharmacologic agent may result in missing valuable treatment effects in a minority. Under recommendation 2b, the reviews noted that a minority of patients seemed to have a "transient improvement in clinical score of unclear clinical significance." In this setting the clinical benefit may be missed because of the patient's inability to communicate. The use of β-agonists would not be recommended in older children if their use did not lead to more rapid discharge compared with systemic corticosteroids alone. The transient and often small improvement in lung function observed when treating a patient who has a significant exacerbation of asthma is still appreciated by the patient while waiting for the corticosteroids to take effect.

Another example of a potential problem in developing evidence-based guidelines is illustrated in a letter criticizing the AAP guidelines for its recommendation that supplemental oxygen be administered if the patient's transcutaneous oxygen readings fall consistently below 90%. In the SIGN guidelines, a threshold value of 92% is suggested. Neither level seems to be associated with adverse outcomes in the short term. Extrapolating from the treatment of other conditions, it has been suggested that accepting levels as low as 90% may be associated with subtle but possibly important long-term neurodevelopment problems.[35] Because no study has ever addressed this issue, there is no means of addressing this potential problem without undertaking a long-term study. Clearly long-term outcomes are very important, as illustrated by the concerns regarding the possible link between the use of postnatal corticosteroids to treat chronic lung disease and neurodevelopmental outcomes.

Summary

Two rigorous evidence-based guidelines have come to very similar conclusions, but there are important, if subtle, differences that seem to relate to the precision with which terms such as "acute bronchiolitis" are used. The strength of the recommendations depends entirely on the robustness of the entry criteria in the studies subject to systematic reviews. Although the guidelines grade the evidence behind most recommendations as "good," being based on RTCs, this grading presupposes that the subjects included are a homogeneous, "clean" population, an assumption that may not be valid.

Presumably because the AAP committee working on the guideline recognized that this is a definitive, evidence-based guideline with potential limitations beyond their control, they inserted the prudent statement,

> This clinical practice guideline is not intended as a sole source of guidance in the management of children with bronchiolitis. Rather, it is intended to assist clinicians in decision-making. It is not intended to replace clinical judgment or establish a protocol for the care of all children with this condition. These recommendations may not provide the only appropriate approach to the management of children with bronchiolitis.

CROUP

Viral croup is a common clinical illness most commonly seen in preschool children, generally between 6 months and 5 years of age. The incidence peaks in the second year of life, and around 15% of children experience at least one episode. Although the infection involves the larynx and large central airways, the airways obstruction, when present, occurs during inspiration with the maximal narrowing occurring in the upper, extrathoracic, trachea.[10] As with all viral infections, the severity ranges widely, from an irritating barking cough to severe, life-threatening airways obstruction. The management of croup has been transformed during the past 20 years, in large part because of a systematic review that reviewed earlier small studies assessing the potential role of steroids in the management of croup.[36] Many pediatric pulmonologists previously had conclude that steroids had no place in the management of this conditions. This conclusion was based on small, underpowered studies; some of these studies had found a trend toward benefit, but none had demonstrated any clear, statistically significant benefit. The meta-analysis undertaken by Kairys and colleagues,[36] however, showed clearly that this opinion should be reconsidered. A series of studies, first in the ICU[37] and then in the emergency room, followed, indicating that corticosteroids, administered orally, parentally, or inhaled, led to a rapid improvement in the clinical status of patients who had croup.[38] Many centers have reported that admissions to hospital and intensive care have fallen dramatically with this approach,[39] although the use of corticosteroids does not inevitably prevent progression and even death.[40] More recent studies have considered the use of corticosteroids even for milder disease managed in the community. Interestingly, despite the systematic review and evidence from the ICU, one of the first large emergency room studies was rejected by a major journal largely because one reviewer believed that such a study was "unethical as everyone knew steroids did not work in croup" (G. Geelhoed, personal communication, 1998).

Assessment

Diagnosis

The diagnosis of acute viral croup is based on clinical assessment. The differential diagnosis in patients who have moderate to severe airways obstruction with stridor includes any condition that might cause acute narrowing at the larynx or upper trachea.[10,40,41] Traditionally the most important differential diagnosis has been acute epiglottitis, although the incidence of this condition has fallen dramatically with the widespread use of vaccination against type b *Haemophilus influenzae.* It still is important, however, to consider the possibility that it a child may have epiglottitis, which can occur because of vaccine failure or infection with other organisms. Laryngeal foreign bodies, bacterial tracheitis, retropharyngeal abscess, and angioedema are other important conditions to consider. Particularly severe symptoms or presentation at a very young age should raise the possibility of an underlying problem such as subglottic stenosis. It is important to ensure that the diagnosis is correct, because several of these conditions require urgent and distinct forms of treatment.

Severity

Children who have stridor should be kept as calm as possible, and medical staff should avoid upsetting the child. Crying generates large negative intrathoracic pressures that exacerbate the collapse of the narrowed tracheal lumen and can provoke a vicious circle of increased distress caused by the increased difficulty breathing that leads to further crying and continued excessive airways narrowing. A number of croup scores have been devised, principally for the research setting. The most widely used is the one reported by Westley,[42] which has been used in a number of therapeutic trials. Although a number of emergency departments use these scores, evidence is lacking that the use of a scoring system improves treatment decisions or outcomes. It is argued consistently that clinical assessment of airways obstruction, which includes the patient's general appearance as well as the presence of stridor and recession, is critical, as is regular, repeated reassessment until the patient is clearly improving.[10,41,43] This approach can be viewed as a consensus position based on expertise rather than on objective studies. Pulse oximetry is widely used but is of limited significance, because values are normal or minimally affected in almost all infants. Low oxygen saturations caused by narrowing of the extrathoracic trachea, as seen in croup, is evidence of very severe narrowing. In distal airways obstruction, as seen in bronchiolitis, the huge number of airways within each generation means that hypoxia can be treated with supplemental oxygen without placing the patient at risk of catastrophic obstruction. In upper tracheal obstruction, however, the lumen narrows markedly before the child becomes hypoxic, and the patient then is at risk of catastrophic cardiorespiratory arrest. Therefore hypoxia caused by croup is an indication that the child should be transferred safely to an ICU or high-dependency unit. Conversely, patients who have mild disease may have evidence of mild hypoxia caused by concurrent involvement of the lower airways tract.

There is no evidence that any other investigation is helpful, and indeed investigations such as blood tests or radiographs, which may cause distress, can exacerbate the situation significantly, both in croup and in conditions that can mimic croup, such as epiglottitis.

Treatment

As noted earlier, the key change in the management of croup has been the widespread administration of corticosteroids, by a variety of routes, to patients who have moderate or severe croup (see **Table 1**). There is increasing evidence that a single dose of a corticosteroid may have benefits even in patients who have relatively mild symptoms, such as mild stridor and recession only when upset. It is widely believed that a single dose has no significant long-term effects, so the risk–benefit ratio favors the use of such agents. The Cochrane review addressing this issue[38] was updated most recently in 2004 and found significant benefits in a range of outcomes, including improvements in severity scores at 6 hours, reduced re-presentation and readmissions, shorter length of stay in those admitted to hospital, and a reduction in the use of epinephrine. The review was unable to show an effect on the need for intubation. When assessing the relative effectiveness of oral and inhaled therapy, the reviewers were unable to identify a clear benefit of one method of administration over the other, although there was a strong trend for inhaled fluticasone delivered via spacer to be less effective than dexamethasone or nebulized budesonide. The reviewers concluded, "In the absence of further evidence, a single oral dose of dexamethasone, probably 0.6 mg/kg, should be preferred because of its safety, efficacy, and cost-effectiveness. In a child who is vomiting, nebulized budesonide or intramuscular dexamethasone might be preferable." Studies to define optimal doses are on going, with a number of studies suggesting that lower doses are as effective as higher ones.[44,45]

The other pharmacologic agent shown to have a benefit is epinephrine. There is no meta-analysis, but a number of RTCs consistently have indicated that there are clinical benefits.[46–52] Although early studies reported using racemic adrenaline, this drug has not been shown to be superior to L-epinephrine.[46] Unlike corticosteroids, this form of therapy does not alter the natural history of the illness but does reduce the severity of symptoms transiently, probably through vasoconstriction leading to reduced hyperemia and edema. The onset is rapid (< 30 minutes), but the duration of efficacy is short (< 2 hours). The standard dose seems to be 0.5 mL/kg body weight nebulized up to a maximum of 5 mL (10 kgs or greater). Although there is good evidence that epinephrine can reduce symptom scores temporarily, there is no clear guidance as to when it should be used. It is used frequently to provide symptomatic relief in patients who have moderate to severe symptoms while waiting for corticosteroids to take effect. Tachycardia and pallor are relatively common; more serious side effects seem to be rare,[53] although a case of myocardial infarction has been reported following frequent administration in a young child who had severe obstruction.[54] Potentially, the most significant problem is that frequent use of epinephrine could mask a significant deterioration in the underlying obstruction.

Heliox (70/30 helium/oxygen mixture) also has been advocated as a therapeutic intervention in patients who have severe croup, on the basis that its lower density, as compared with air, improves gas flow. A small, double-blind, randomized trial comparing heliox with nebulized epinephrine in patients already receiving systemic steroids did not identify any benefit of heliox over epinephrine.[55] Unless further data support this form of therapy, it is unlikely that heliox can be recommended, given the increased complexity of its use.

A recent Cochrane review found no evidence to support the use of humidified air to treat children who have croup,[56] even though this practice has been widely advocated for many decades. The review identified only three small studies based in the emergency department and none in primary care. A subsequent study again found no benefit from humidification, and this practice cannot be recommended.[57]

Summary

Although there is little current controversy regarding the management of croup, assessment remains largely clinical. The natural history seems to be modified by a single dose of steroids. Although there is a benefit from oral, nebulized, or intramuscular treatment, oral dexamethasone seems to be the most acceptable method for most patients. Temporary benefit can be derived from the use of nebulized epinephrine, and studies indicate that patients can be discharged within 3 to 4 hours after the last dose, providing there is no deterioration after the effects of epinephrine have worn off and that the patient is continuing to improve.

REFERENCES

1. Elliott SP, Ray CG. Viral infections of the lower respiratory tract. In: Taussig L, Landau L, editors. Pediatric respiratory medicine. 2nd Edition. Philadelphia: Mosby Elsevier; 2008. p. 481–90.
2. Chonmaitree T, Revai K, Grady JJ, et al. Viral upper respiratory tract infection and otitis media complication in young children. Clin Infect Dis 2008;46:815–23.
3. Rihkanen H, Rönkkö E, Nieminen T, et al. Respiratory viruses in laryngeal croup of young children. J Pediatr 2008;152:661–5.
4. Brownlee JW, Turner RB. New developments in the epidemiology and clinical spectrum of rhinovirus infections. Curr Opin Pediatr 2008;20:67–71.
5. Sloots TP, Whiley DM, Lambert SB, et al. Emerging respiratory agents: new viruses for old diseases? J Clin Virol 2008;42(3):233–43.
6. Elphick HE, Ritson S, Rogers H, et al. When a 'wheeze' is not a wheeze—analysis of breath sounds in infancy. Eur Respir J 2000;16:593–7.
7. Elphick H, Everard ML. Noisy breathing in children. In: David T, editor. Recent advances in paediatrics. The Royal Society of Medicine. London; 2002.
8. Elphick H, Shirlock P, Foxall G, et al. Respiratory noises in early childhood—misuse of the term wheeze by parents and doctor. Arch Dis Child. 2001;84:35–9.
9. Cane RS, Ranganathan SC, McKenzie SA. What do parents of wheezy children understand by "wheeze"? Arch Dis Child 2000;82:327–32.
10. Asher MI, Grant CC. Infections of the upper respiratory tract. In: Taussig L, Landau L, editors. Pediatric respiratory medicine. 2nd Edition. Philadelphia: Mosby Elsevier; 2008. p. 453–80.
11. American Academy of Pediatrics Subcommittee on Diagnosis and Management of Bronchiolitis. Diagnosis and management of bronchiolitis. Pediatrics 2006;118: 1774–93.
12. SIGN. Bronchiolitis in children. Available at: http://www.sign.ac.uk. Accessed November 17, 2008.
13. Reynolds EOR, Cook CD. The treatment of bronchiolitis. J Pediatr 1963;63: 1205–7.

14. Blom D, Ermers M, Bont L, et al. Inhaled corticosteroids during acute bronchiolitis in the prevention of post-bronchiolitic wheezing. Cochrane Database Syst Rev 2007;(1):CD004881.
15. Gadomski AM, Bhasale AL. Bronchodilators for bronchiolitis. Cochrane Database Syst Rev 2006;(3):CD001266.
16. Spurling GK, Fonseka K, Doust J, et al. Antibiotics for bronchiolitis in children. Cochrane Database Syst Rev 2007;(1):CD005189.
17. Perrotta C, Ortiz Z, Roque M. Chest physiotherapy for acute bronchiolitis in paediatric patients between 0 and 24 months old. Cochrane Database Syst Rev 2005;(2):CD004873.
18. Patel H, Platt R, Lozano JM, et al. Glucocorticoids for acute viral bronchiolitis in infants and young children. Cochrane Database Syst Rev 2004;(3):CD004878.
19. Ventre K, Randolph A. Ribavirin for respiratory syncytial virus infection of the lower respiratory tract in infants and young children. Cochrane Database Syst Rev 2004;(4):CD000181.
20. Behrendt CE, Decker MD, Burch DM, et al. International variation in the management of infants hospitalized with respiratory syncytial virus. International RSV Study Group. Eur J Pediatr 1998;157:215–20.
21. Barben J, Hammer J. Current management of acute bronchiolitis in Switzerland. Swiss Med Wkly 2003;133:9–15.
22. Brand PL, Vaessen-Verberne AA. Differences in management of bronchiolitis between hospitals in The Netherlands. Dutch Paediatric Respiratory Society. Eur J Pediatr 2000;159:343–7.
23. Touzet S, Réfabert L, Letrilliart L, et al. Impact of consensus development conference guidelines on primary care of bronchiolitis: are national guidelines being followed? J Eval Clin Pract 2007;13:651–6.
24. Barben JU, Robertson CF, Robinson PJ. Implementation of evidence-based management of acute bronchiolitis. J Paediatr Child Health 2000;36:491–7.
25. Everard ML, Swarbrick A, Wrightham M, et al. Analysis of cells obtained by bronchial lavage of infants with respiratory syncytial virus infection. Arch Dis Child 1994;71:428–32.
26. Turner RB. The role of neutrophiles in the pathogenesis of rhinovirus infections. Pediatr Infect Dis J 1990;9:832–5.
27. Abu-Harb M, Bell F, Rao WH, et al. IL-8 and neutrophil inflammatory mediators in the upper respiratory tract of infants with RSV bronchiolitis. Eur Respir J 1999;14:150–4.
28. Evans GS, Jones A, Qui JM, et al. Neutrophil survival is prolonged in the airways of healthy infants and infants with RSV bronchiolitis. Eur Respir J 2002;20:651–7.
29. Martinez FD. Development of wheezing disorders and asthma in preschool children. Pediatrics 2002;109(2 Suppl):362–7.
30. Reddel H, Ware S, Marks G, et al. Differences between asthma exacerbations and poor asthma control. Lancet 1999;353:364–9.
31. Elphick H, Ritson S, Rigby AS, et al. Phenotype of acute respiratory syncytial virus lower respiratory tract illness in infancy and subsequent morbidity. Acta Paediatr 2007;96:1–3.
32. Pitrez PM, Brennan S, Sly PD. Inflammatory profile in nasal secretions of infants hospitalized with acute lower airway tract infections. Respirology 2005;10: 365–70.
33. BTS/SIGN. British guidelines on the management of asthma. Thorax 2003;58 (Suppl 1):1–96.
34. Bateman ED, Hurd SS, Barnes PJ, et al. Global strategy for asthma management and prevention: GINA executive summary. Eur Respir J 2008;31(1):43–78.

35. Bass JL, Gozal D. Oxygen therapy for bronchiolitis. Pediatr 2007;119:611.
36. Kairys SW, Olmstead EM, O'Connor GT. Steroid treatment of laryngotracheitis: a meta-analysis of the evidence from randomized trials. Pediatrics 1989;83:683–93.
37. Tibballs J, Shann FA, Landau LI. Placebo-controlled trial of prednisolone in children intubated for croup. Lancet 1992;340:745–8.
38. Russell K, Wiebe N, Saenz A, et al. Glucocorticoids for croup. Cochrane Database Syst Rev 2008;(Issue 2). John Wiley & Sons, Ltd.
39. Geelhoed G. Sixteen years of croup in a western Australian teaching hospital: effects of routine steroid treatment. Ann Emerg Med 1996;28:621–6.
40. Fisher JD. Out-of-hospital cardiopulmonary arrest in children with croup. Pediatr Emerg Care 2004;20:35–6.
41. Fitzgerald DA, Kilham HA. Croup: assessment and evidence-based management. Med J Aust 2003;179:372–7.
42. Westley CR, Cotton EK, Brooks JG. Nebulized racemic epinephrine by IPPB for the treatment of croup: a double-blind study. Am J Dis Child. 1978;132:484–7.
43. Bjornson CL, Johnson DW. Croup. Lancet 2008;371:329–39.
44. Geelhoed GC, Macdonald WB. Oral dexamethasone in the treatment of croup: 0.15 mg/kg versus 0.3 mg/kg versus 0.6 mg/kg. Pediatr Pulmonol 1995;20:362–8.
45. Chub-Uppakarn S, Sangsupawanich P. A randomized comparison of dexamethasone 0.15 mg/kg versus 0.6 mg/kg for the treatment of moderate to severe croup. Int J Pediatr Otorhinolaryngol 2007;71:473–7.
46. Waisman Y, Klein BL, Boenning DA, et al. Prospective randomized double-blind study comparing L-epinephrine and racemic epinephrine aerosols in the treatment of laryngotracheitis (croup). Pediatrics 1992;89:302–6.
47. Gardner H, Powell K, Roden V, et al. The evaluation of racemic epinephrine in the treatment of infectious croup. Pediatrics 1973;52:68–71.
48. Fogel J, Berg I, Gerber M, et al. Racemic epinephrine in the treatment of croup: nebulization alone versus nebulization with intermittent positive pressure breathing. J Pediatr 1982;101:1028–31.
49. Rizos J, DiGravio B, Sehl M, et al. The disposition of children with croup treated with racemic epinephrine and dexamethasone in the emergency department. J Emerg Med 1998;16:535–9.
50. Ledwith C, Shea L, Mauro RD. Safety and efficacy of nebulized racemic epinephrine in conjunction with oral dexamethasone and mist in the outpatient treatment of croup. Ann Emerg Med 1995;25:331–7.
51. Kunkel N, Baker M. Use of racemic epinephrine, dexamethasone, and mist in the outpatient management of croup. Pediatr Emerg Care 1996;12:156–9.
52. Prendergast M, Jones J, Hartman D. Racemic epinephrine in the treatment of laryngotracheitis: can we identify children for outpatient therapy? Am J Emerg Med 1994;12:613–6.
53. Zhang L, Sanguebsche L. The safety of nebulization with 3 to 5 ml of adrenaline (1:1000) in children: an evidence based review. J Pediatr (Rio J) 2005;81:193–7.
54. Butte M, Nguyen B, Hutchison T, et al. Pediatric myocardial infarction after racemic epinephrine administration. Pediatr 1999;104:e9.
55. Weber JE, Chudnofsky CR, Younger JG, et al. A randomized comparison of helium-oxygen mixture (Heliox) and racemic epinephrine for the treatment of moderate to severe croup. Pediatrics 2001;107:e96.
56. Moore M, Little P. Humidified air inhalation for treating croup. Cochrane Database Syst Rev 2006;(3):CD002870.
57. Scolnik D, Coates A, Stephens D, et al. Controlled delivery of high vs low humidity vs mist therapy for croup in emergency departments. JAMA 2006;295:1274–80.

Pneumonia and Other Respiratory Infections

Sarath C. Ranganathan, MBChB, PhD[a,b,c,*],
Samatha Sonnappa, MBBS, MD[d,e]

KEYWORDS

- Pneumonia • Tuberculosis • Respiratory infections
- Treatment of pneumonia
- Complications of community-acquired pneumonia

EPIDEMIOLOGY

Pneumonia is a leading killer of children, causing an estimated 1.9 million deaths worldwide in children under the age of 5 years (**Fig. 1**).[1,2] The true mortality caused by pneumonia probably is underestimated, because most deaths in developing nations occur at home without a true medical diagnosis. Ninety percent of the deaths are thought to occur in the developing world, with 50% of these occurring in Africa.[3] The incidence of pneumonia in North America and Europe is approximately 36 per 1000 per year.[4,5] Thus, although mortality is low, pneumonia causes significant morbidity even in developed countries.

DEFINITION

Pneumonia can be defined solely by clinical features[6] or with the addition of radiologic findings. In part because of the considerable overlap between the diagnosis of bronchiolitis and pneumonia in young children,[4] "lower respiratory illness" is a frequently used alternative term. Lower respiratory illness has been defined as fever, acute respiratory symptoms, and radiologic evidence of parenchymal infiltrates; the World Health Organization (WHO) guidelines use tachypnea as an important indicator of pneumonia when radiology facilities are unavailable.[6] Tachypnea is defined as a respiratory rate

[a] Department of Respiratory Medicine, Royal Children's Hospital Melbourne, Flemington Road, Parkville, Melbourne, VIC 3052, Australia
[b] Infection, Immunity & Environment Theme, Murdoch Children's Research Institute, Flemington Road, Parkville, Melbourne, VIC 3052, Australia
[c] Department of Paediatrics, University of Melbourne, Flemington Road, Parkville, Melbourne, VIC 3052, Australia
[d] Department of Respiratory Medicine, Great Ormond Street Hospital, Great Ormond Street, London WC1N 3JH, UK
[e] Portex Anaesthesia, Intensive Therapy and Respiratory Medicine Unit, Institute of Child Health, 30 Guilford Street, London WC1N 1EH, UK
* Corresponding author. Department of Respiratory Medicine, Royal Children's Hospital Melbourne, Flemington Road, Parkville, Melbourne, VIC 3052, Australia.
E-mail address: sarath.ranganathan@rch.org.au (S.C. Ranganathan).

Pediatr Clin N Am 56 (2009) 135–156
doi:10.1016/j.pcl.2008.10.005
0031-3955/08/$ – see front matter © 2009 Elsevier Inc. All rights reserved.
pediatric.theclinics.com

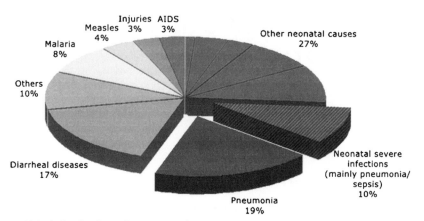

Fig. 1. Global distribution of cause-specific mortality among children under age 5 years in 2004. Pneumonia was the leading killer of children worldwide. (*From* UNICEF/WHO. Pneumonia: the forgotten killer of children. New York and Geneva: The United Nations Children's Fund (UNICEF)/World Health Organization (WHO); 2006; with permission.)

greater than 60 breaths per minute in infants younger than 2 months, greater than 50 breaths per minute in children 2 to 12 months, and greater than 40 breaths per minute in children over 1 year of age. In children who have been symptomatic for more than 3 days, tachypnea has a sensitivity of 74% and a specificity of 67% for radiologically diagnosed pneumonia.[7] In this study, sensitivity decreased when other clinical signs were included with tachypnea, but the addition of these other clinical signs increased specificity in relation to the reference standard of radiologically diagnosed pneumonia.

ETIOLOGY

Pneumonia usually begins as a colonization of the mucosa of the nasopharynx followed by spread into the lower respiratory tract. The infection can be community acquired or nosocomial. Bacteria, viruses, atypical organisms, and fungi are all known to cause pneumonia. In prospective research studies, a causative organism can be identified in nearly three quarters of cases of pneumonia. Respiratory viruses seem to be responsible for approximately 40% of cases of community-acquired pneumonia in children who are hospitalized, particularly in those under 2 years of age, whereas *Streptococcus pneumoniae* is responsible for 27% to 44% of the cases of community-acquired pneumonia.[8,9,10,11] Although infection with *Mycoplasma pneumoniae* and *Chlamydia pneumoniae* usually are considered to cause pneumonia in children of school age and in older patients, one study, in which preschool-aged children had as many episodes of atypical bacterial pneumonia episodes as older children, challenges this view.[9] In this study a bacterial cause was identified in 60% of cases of pneumonia, with *S. pneumoniae* causing 73% of the cases in which a bacterial cause was identified. Other bacterial causes such as *Staphylococcus aureus*, *Moraxhella catarrhalis*, group A Streptococci, *Streptococcus milleri*, and *Haemophilus* species (non–type b) were identified infrequently. *Mycoplasma pneumoniae* and *Chlamydia pneumoniae* were responsible for 14% and 9% of cases of pneumonia, respectively. The most severe disease occurred in patients who had infection with a typical bacterial organism or in the 23% in whom mixed bacterial (usually *S. pneumoniae*) and viral coinfection were identified.[9]

CLINICAL FEATURES

- Bacterial pneumonia is unlikely when wheeze is identified in young children (level of evidence: moderate).

Bacterial pneumonia should be considered in children if fever is higher than 38.5°C and is accompanied by tachypnea and recession.[12,13] Although auscultatory findings are not considered as reliable as other clinical signs in the diagnosis of pneumonia, crackles increase its likelihood. Wheeze in young children (preschool age and below) suggests a viral cause and in older subjects increases the possibility of infection by *M pneumoniae*. Fever, headache, and myalgia in older children are associated with *M pneumoniae*, whereas sticky eyes in a neonate are associated with *Chlamydia trachomatis* infection.[12,13]

MANAGEMENT OF A CHILD WHO HAS COMMUNITY-ACQUIRED PNEUMONIA AT PRESENTATION
Assess for Contributing Etiology

History is important in the evaluation of community-acquired pneumonia, and the physician should inquire about contacts, travel, immunization history, the possibility of foreign body aspiration or primary aspiration, stools consistent with malabsorption, sinusitis, asthma, and environmental exposure. The examination should evaluate general features such as growth, upper airway anatomy, dysmorphism suggesting syndrome, neuromuscular weakness, and swallowing and gag reflexes. The pulmonary examination should assess oxygen saturation, respiratory rate, accessory muscle use, wheezes, and other auscultatory findings such as crackles. Cardiovascular examination also is important to rule out signs of cardiac failure.

Assess for Severity of Pneumonia

In terms of severity, the WHO recommends that children who have chest indrawing be admitted to hospital.[13] The British Thoracic Society guidelines[12,14] regarding admission to hospital in the developed world are shown in **Box 1**.

Box 1
British Thoracic Society guidelines: factors indicating need for admission of a child who has pneumonia

- Oxygen saturations $\leq 92\%$
- Respiratory rate > 70 breaths per minute in infants or > 50 breaths per minute in older children
- Intermittent apnea, grunting
- Difficulty in breathing
- Infant not feeding or signs of dehydration in older children
- Family unable to provide appropriate observation or supervision

Data from British Thoracic Society. British Thoracic Society guidelines for the management of community acquired pneumonia in childhood. Thorax 2002;57(Suppl I):i1–24; and Kumar P, McKean MC. Evidence based paediatrics: review of BTS guidelines for the management of community acquired pneumonia in children. J Infect 2004;48(2):134–8.

AMBULATORY CARE OF A CHILD WHO HAS COMMUNITY-ACQUIRED PNEUMONIA

- Investigations are not indicated routinely in mild childhood pneumonia.
- The optimal duration of treatment is unknown, but most advocate treatment for 5 to 7 days (level of evidence: low).
- Numerous adjunctive therapies in addition to antibiotics are prescribed frequently for the treatment of pneumonia (**Table 1**).

INVESTIGATIONS OF A CHILD ADMITTED WITH PNEUMONIA

There are widespread variations in practice regarding the investigation of pneumonia in children who are admitted with this condition.

Chest Radiographs

- Chest radiographs should not be performed routinely in children suspected of having pneumonia (level of evidence: high).

Radiologic findings are accepted as the reference standard for defining pneumonia, but it is not clear to what extent chest radiographs alter the outcome of childhood pneumonia even though they frequently are used to confirm the presence, site, and extent of pulmonary infiltrates. In one study in children between 2 months and 5 years of age, recovery occurred at a median of 7 days, whether or not a chest radiograph

Table 1
Adjunct therapies used in the treatment of childhood community-acquired pneumonia

Medication/ Intervention	Recommendation	Grading of Recommendation (Based on Evidence of Benefit)	Quality of Supporting Evidence
Antipyretics	Pain, fever, and irritability; no benefit on duration or severity of pneumonia	Low	No randomized, controlled trials
Cough suppressants	Not recommended as adjunct to treat cough in pneumonia	Moderate	Systematic review concluded insufficient evidence[15]
Mucolytics	Not recommended in acute community-acquired pneumonia	Low	Systematic review concluded insufficient vidence[15]
Chest physical therapy	Not indicated in acute community-acquired pneumonia	High	Randomized, controlled trial[16]
Zinc supplementation	Zinc deficiency in high-mortality settings decreases prevalence and mortality of pneumonia	High	Meta-analysis of 17 randomized, controlled trials in children < 5 years[17]

had been performed, and there was no difference in subsequent health care use. Having a chest radiograph significantly increased the likelihood of being prescribed antibiotics, however. Routine use of chest radiography was not beneficial in ambulatory children over the age of 2 months who had acute lower respiratory tract infection.[18] The British Thoracic Society suggests that a chest radiograph be considered in a child younger than 5 years who has with a fever higher than 39°C of unknown origin and without features typical of bronchiolitis.[12] Although lobar infiltrates, effusions, abscesses, and cavities on a chest radiograph are likely to be a consequence of bacterial rather than viral pneumonia,[19] there are no other chest radiograph changes that are specific in differentiating bacterial from viral pneumonia and therefore indicating a need for treatment with antibiotics.

Blood Cultures

Blood cultures are positive in only 10% to 30% of children who have pneumonia and only in pneumonias where bacteremia occurs.[20] In a study in The Gambia, clinical signs that predicted a positive blood culture were high fever (>38°C), dehydration, nasal flaring, grunting, bronchial breath sounds, and diminished air entry.[21] Recent antibiotic use further reduces the chance of a positive blood culture, so in a developed country, where antibiotics are prescribed earlier in the course of lower respiratory illness, the clinical features that predict a positive blood culture are likely to be different. The British Thoracic Society guidelines recommend performing a blood culture in all children who are hospitalized and when bacterial pneumonia is suspected.[12]

Further Microbiology

- Lung aspirates should be considered when peripheral consolidation is proven by chest radiograph (level of evidence: moderate).
- Pleural aspiration is indicated when significant pleural effusion is identified (level of evidence: moderate).

Microbiologic investigations generally are not recommended for patients being managed in the community.[12] Within the hospital setting, older children may be able to provide a sputum sample, but younger children usually cannot. When pulmonary tuberculosis (TB) is suspected, consecutive early morning, preprandial, preambulatory gastric washings are indicated and are more sensitive than bronchoalveolar lavage. Induction of sputum using hypertonic saline may also be useful when TB is suspected, but this technique increases the chances of a typically noninfectious patient being rendered temporarily infectious during the procedure.[22] In hospitalized infants under 18 months of age a nasopharyngeal aspirate should be sent for viral antigen detection (such as immunofluorescence) with or without viral culture.[12] When significant pleural fluid is present, it should be aspirated and sent for microscopic aspiration and culture as early as possible during the course of disease, and a specimen should be saved for bacterial antigen detection.[12] If pleural fluid is associated with a complicated parapneumonic effusion, a sample of pleural fluid is likely to be obtained during the management of this complication, so in this circumstance an additional diagnostic pleural tap may not be in the best interest of the child. Lung aspirates are rarely performed, but the technique is safer than widely perceived and can provide a bacterial diagnosis in more than 50% of cases.[23] Lung aspirates therefore are more sensitive than blood cultures, but the organisms identified by this technique frequently are different from those identified by blood cultures taken in the same children.[24] The limitations of lung aspirates is that they are painful and result in a small (but usually clinically insignificant) pneumothorax, and the technique usually is limited to pneumonias associated with dense peripheral consolidations close to the chest wall. Lung aspiration in conjunction with use of nucleic amplification tests can potentially increase the yield further,[25] and therefore lung aspiration should be considered if the benefits of identifying the causative agent outweigh the modest risk of the procedure and equipment for and expertise in the management of the potential complication of a pneumothorax are available.

ORGANISMS CAUSING PNEUMONIA ACCORDING TO AGE
Neonates

Common organisms causing pneumonia in neonates are group B streptococci, gram-negative enteric bacteria, cytomegalovirus, Ureaplasma urealyticum, Listeria monocytogenes, and C trachomatis.

Less common organisms causing pneumonia in neonates are S pneumoniae, group D streptococcus, and anaerobes.

Infants

Common organisms causing pneumonia in infants are respiratory syncytial virus, parainfluenza viruses, influenza viruses, adenovirus, metapneumovirus, S pneumoniae, H influenzae, M pneumoniae, and Mycobacterium tuberculosis.

Less common organisms causing pneumonia in infants are Bordetella pertussis and Pneumocystis jiroveci.

Preschool Children

Common organisms causing pneumonia in preschool-age children are respiratory syncytial virus, parainfluenza viruses, influenza viruses, adenovirus, metapneumovirus, S pneumoniae, H influenzae, M pneumoniae, and M tuberculosis.

A less common organism causing pneumonia in preschool-age children is C pneumoniae

School-Age Children

Common organisms causing pneumonia in school-age children are M pneumoniae, C pneumoniae, S pneumonia, M tuberculosis, and respiratory viruses.

Organisms Rarely Causing Pneumonia

The following organisms rarely cause pneumonia:

Viruses: Coronavirus, Varicella-zoster, Epstein-Barr, Mumps
Atypical organisms: Chlamydia psittaci, Coxiella Burnetti
Bacteria: Klebsiella pneumoniae, Legionella, Streptococcus pyogenes, Brucella abortus
Fungi: Coccidioides immitis, Histoplasma capsulatum, Blastomyces dermatitidis

TREATMENT OF CHILDREN ADMITTED WITH PNEUMONIA
General

- Hypoxia (oxygen saturation $\leq 92\%$) should be treated with supplemental oxygen (level of evidence: moderate).

Initial management always should commence with an assessment of the airway, breathing, and circulation. Most children do not require admission to hospital. Children whose oxygen saturation is 92% or less in air should receive supplemental oxygen therapy.[12] In a Zambian study, the mortality from pneumonia was increased when hypoxemia was present, a finding that highlights the importance of oxygen in treatment.[26] Intravenous fluids rarely are indicated but may be required in the presence of severe dehydration, ongoing vomiting, severe electrolyte disturbances, or respiratory failure. In this context, inappropriate secretion of antidiuretic hormone may occur,[27] and intravenous fluids may need to be administered at 80% of full maintenance.

Antibiotics

- Children who have mild symptoms do not require treatment with antibiotics (level of evidence: moderate).
- Amoxicillin or co-amoxyclavulanic acid is the antibiotic of choice in preschool children (level of evidence: moderate).
- Children over 5 years of age also can be treated with amoxicillin or co-amoxyclavulanic acid or with a macrolide (or both) when atypical infection is suspected (level of evidence: moderate).
- Antibiotics administered orally are safe and effective for most children (level of evidence: high).
- The optimal duration of treatment for a child admitted with pneumonia is unknown, but most recommend 5 to 7 days of antibiotics (level of evidence: low).

When a decision has been made to treat with antibiotics, the oral route is the most appropriate for most children. Although co-trimoxazole is widely used as the first-choice antibiotic throughout the world, it is inferior to treatment with amoxicillin in severe pneumonia.[28,29] Amoxicillin is recommended as the first line of therapy for children under 5 years because it is relatively inexpensive, is well tolerated, and is effective against most of the pathogens in this age group. Co-amoxyclavulanic acid seems to be significantly more effective than oral amoxicillin alone but is more expensive.[29] In children older than 5 years, amoxicillin again is an appropriate first-line agent unless mycoplasma or chlamydia pneumonia is suspected, in which case a macrolide antibiotic, either alone or in addition, is appropriate. Erythromycin is equally as effective as[29] and is significantly cheaper than second-generation macrolides such as azithromycin, clarithromycin, or roxithromycin, but it has a shorter half-life and requires more frequent dosing. It also may be associated with more frequent adverse effects, especially involving the gastrointestinal tract.

There is no evidence that intravenous treatment is superior to oral treatment in community-acquired pneumonia. Intravenous antibiotics therefore are reserved for severe cases of pneumonia or for pneumonia in a child unable to tolerate oral antibiotics. Appropriate antibiotics to administer intravenously include benzyl penicillin, co-amoxyclavulanic acid, a second- or third-generation cephalosporin, and the addition of a macrolide if atypical infection is considered a possibility.

ANTIBIOTIC RESISTANCE

- Antibiotic resistance is common and increasing, partly in response to inappropriate antibiotic prescribing (level of evidence: moderate).

Principles of good antibiotic prescribing (eg, using the appropriate antibiotic with the narrowest spectrum, aiming for high tissue or plasma concentrations, a short-half life, and administered as a short, intensive course) are important and are less likely to induce antibiotic resistance.[30] Resistance to antibiotics usually is acquired through selective pressure on bacteria resulting from exposure to antibiotics and preferential survival of resistant organisms. Pneumococcal resistance has been documented in up to 40% of isolates,[31] and high rates have been reported in Spain, France, and the United States.[31,32] Mutations in genes coding for penicillin-binding proteins lead to decreased affinity for penicillin and consequently the failure of penicillin to inhibit the enzymes responsible for cell wall synthesis. Pneumococcal resistance to penicillin occurs when the mean inhibitory concentration is less than 2 μg/mL, but there is no evidence that treatment with high-dose penicillin or cephalosporins for pneumonia in which pneumococcal resistance is documented is associated with clinical failure.[33,34,35] Most, however, would consider using a third-generation cephalosporin or vancomycin if clinical resistance is suspected or when resistance is identified in a child who is immunosuppressed.

Up to 34% of isolates of *H influenzae* (including nontypeable strains) are resistant to ampicillin because of the production of ß-lactamases by the organism that inhibit the antibiotic.[36] Therefore, in areas of high endemic resistance, or when resistance is suspected clinically or is identified in an immunosuppressed individual, treatment with a third-generation cephalosporin is indicated.

Most strains of *S aureus* are penicillin resistant, because ß-lactamases are very prevalent. Methicillin/flucloxacillin resistance also is widespread now, particularly in hospital-acquired infection but also can be found in community-acquired infections.[37] Vancomycin or teicoplanin are the antibiotics of choice to treat such infections, at least when vancomycin resistance is not suspected. The outcome may be better when rifampicin is added to treatment with vancomycin,[38] but this benefit is not confirmed in community-acquired pneumonia. Apart from resistant *S aureus*, most other bacteria that cause hospital-acquired pneumonia are gram-negative organisms such as *Pseudomonas* species, Serratia species, *Escherichia coli*, and *Enterobacter* species. Multidrug resistance has been documented in each of these bacteria, so local guidelines are necessary for the appropriate selection of antibiotics.

PREVENTION
Vaccines

- Vaccines against *H influenzae* and *S pneumoniae* are effective (level of evidence: high).
- Vaccines are not currently available in populations where pneumonia has the highest mortality (level of evidence: high).

The recent development and introduction of conjugate vaccines for *H. influenzae* type b (Hib) and *S pneumoniae* has led to a degree of control of pneumonia caused by these two organisms in developed countries where they have been introduced into the immunization schedule. Hib vaccine was introduced in 1990. The first report from a bacterial pneumonia vaccine trial in the developing world was from The Gambia in 1997,[39] where Hib vaccination reduced clinical pneumonia by 4% and radiologic pneumonia by 20%. No lung aspirates were identified as culture positive for Hib in children who received the vaccine in this study. A further study in Chile also confirmed the clinical efficacy of Hib vaccine.[40] An Indonesian study, however, in which coverage with chest radiographs was much greater than in the other two studies, found no evidence for reduction of radiologic pneumonia as a result of the vaccine, even though a reduction in clinically diagnosed lower respiratory illness was confirmed.[41]

The first pneumococcal conjugate vaccine was introduced in 1990. Studies in the United States,[42] South Africa,[43] and The Gambia[44] have demonstrated its efficacy against development of clinically diagnosed pneumonia, severe pneumonia, radiologically defined pneumonia, and vaccine serotype–specific bacteremia or lung aspirate culture.[45] Newer vaccines that incorporate more serotypes than the nine included in the Gambian and South African studies are likely to offer improved efficacy when they are introduced. Because there are at least 90 pneumococcal serotypes, however, the risk is that serotype replacement eventually will result in diminished benefit from vaccination. The optimal schedule for administration of the seven-valent pneumococcal vaccine has not yet been determined.[46]

As antibiotics become less effective against common bacterial causes of childhood pneumonia, the role of primary vaccination will become increasingly important. Vaccination decreases the circulation of resistant organisms and, in the case of S pneumoniae, the current seven-valent vaccine is effective against the serotypes most commonly associated with antibiotic resistance.[47]

OTHER PREVENTION MEASURES

- Environmental, nutritional, and socioeconomic factors affect mortality in childhood pneumonia and are preventable (level of evidence: high).

Over the next decade, it is crucial that vaccines become available to children in the developing world, who are at greatest risk of dying from pneumonia. Failure to make these vaccines available would indicate that the motives behind vaccine development do not include a desire to affect significantly the global childhood mortality caused by pneumonia. Environmental, nutritional, and socioeconomic factors that affect equity of access are crucially important also.[48] A concerted effort to address these factors in many developed nations at the beginning of the last century resulted in the large reduction in mortality from pneumonia that occurred before the availability of antibiotics[49] and points out that mortality from pneumonia in childhood reflects socioeconomic disadvantage above all other factors.

COMMON RESPIRATORY ISSUES IN DEVELOPING COUNTRIES

The WHO estimates that nearly one fifth of childhood deaths are caused by pneumonia, which claims more than 2 million lives annually (see **Fig. 1**). Most of these deaths occur in Africa and Southeast Asia[2,50] and are caused either by community-acquired pneumonia or by infections secondary to measles, pertussis, or AIDS/HIV. Most of these deaths are preventable with available interventions.[51] Although few of these episodes result in death, they produce significant morbidity and short-term sequelae, which may have a detrimental effect on the child's nutritional status and also may influence the risk of other childhood diseases. Effective strategies to combat this problem include the WHO Integrated Management of Childhood Illness (IMCI) program, nutritional interventions, and immunization. The use of case management guidelines recommended by IMCI for childhood pneumonia has reduced overall and pneumonia-specific mortality in children significantly.[52,53,54]

INTEGRATED MANAGEMENT OF CHILDHOOD ILLNESS

The generic IMCI guidelines are meant to target the leading causes of mortality and severe morbidity in children below 5 years of age, who are a particularly vulnerable age group. The IMCI strategy incorporates assessment of feeding, updating immunization status, and provision of vitamin A prophylaxis. The three components of the IMCI program are improving the skills of health workers, improving the health system, and improving household and community practices. IMCI is considered to be among the most cost-effective interventions in both low- and middle-income countries and to be the program most likely to have the greatest impact on the global burden of disease. As of December 2000, more than 81 countries around the world had adopted IMCI guidelines.

MANAGEMENT OPTIONS FOR ACUTE RESPIRATORY INFECTION FOLLOWING THE INTEGRATED MANAGEMENT OF CHILDHOOD ILLNESS APPROACH

- Use oral co-trimoxazole rather than other oral/parenteral antibiotics in the treatment of nonsevere pneumonia (level of evidence: high).
- Use ambulatory short-course amoxicillin for treatment of severe pneumonia (level of evidence: high).
- Use parenteral chloramphenicol instead of ampicillin plus gentamicin for very severe pneumonia (level of evidence: high).

Community-based interventions to identify and treat pneumonia have a considerable effect on child mortality. The WHO guidelines for the case management of acute respiratory infections are based on simple signs such as fast breathing and indrawing of the chest and are designed for countries with an infant mortality rate higher than 40 per 1000 live births.[55] The WHO defines cases of suspected pneumonia as children reported to have an illness associated with a cough accompanied by fast and/or difficult breathing. It is recommended that children who have cough without fast breathing be treated as outpatients without antibiotics; those who have fast breathing (nonsevere pneumonia) be treated at home with oral co-trimoxazole or amoxicillin for 5 days; and those who have lower chest indrawing (severe pneumonia) and general danger signs (very severe disease) be referred to hospital and treated with parenteral ampicillin/penicillin.

A recent meta-analysis assessing the effect of the pneumonia case-management approach on mortality identified a 24% reduction in total mortality and a 36% reduction in pneumonia mortality in children under 5 years of age.[52] This analysis of nine studies[53,54,56–62] concluded that community-based interventions to identify and treat pneumonia have reduced child mortality considerably, with consistent results, despite the diversity of pneumonia interventions and developing-country settings in which these trials took place. A potential limitation of this analysis is that all the studies were undertaken more than a decade ago, and with the increasing prevalence of antimicrobial resistance their implications for public health programs are unclear.

In the last decade, and more recently, studies have looked at the efficacy of various antibiotic regimens in developing country settings.[28,63–68] All cases of suspected pneumonia in these settings should be treated with oral or parenteral antibiotics, depending on severity. The potential choice of antibiotics is wide but should be applicable for large-scale use in low-resource settings. Co-trimoxazole is a cheap and effective drug, and all the studies show that it compares favorably with other antibiotics for nonsevere pneumonia. A study comparing the efficacy of co-trimoxazole and that of amoxicillin for nonsevere pneumonia and examining the association with in vitro co-trimoxazole susceptibility found no difference in efficacy between co-trimoxazole and amoxicillin, despite high in vitro resistance to co-trimoxazole.[28] Another study comparing the clinical efficacy of twice-daily oral co-trimoxazole and twice-daily oral amoxicillin found that both were equally effective for the treatment of nonsevere pneumonia.[63] Three other studies comparing co-trimoxazole with chloramphenicol;[64] with procaine penicillin on day 1 followed by 5 days of oral ampicillin;[65] and with intramuscular procaine penicillin G or benzathine penicillin G in combination with procaine penicillin G[66] did not indicate any difference in efficacy with alternative antibiotic regimens. Another double-blind, randomized, controlled trial comparing a course of the standard dose (45 mg/kg/d) of oral amoxicillin for the treatment of nonsevere pneumonia versus a course of a double dose (80–90 mg/kg/d) found no difference between the two doses.[69] The only study assessing oral treatment for severe pneumonia concluded that home treatment with high-dose oral amoxicillin is equivalent to currently recommended hospitalization and parenteral ampicillin for treatment of severe pneumonia without underlying complications,[67] but a recent Cochrane review suggested that amoxicillin is better than co-trimoxazole for severe pneumonia.[29] Another study showed that the combination of parenteral ampicillin and gentamicin was more efficacious than parenteral chloramphenicol alone.[68] Based on these findings, the WHO has revised the guidelines for the management of severe pneumonia to include home treatment with high-dose oral amoxicillin or a combination of parenteral ampicillin and gentamicin for hospitalized patients.

TUBERCULOSIS IN CHILDREN AND ADOLESCENTS

The worsening TB pandemic remains a major threat to global health. TB kills nearly 2 million people every year (5000 per day).[70] Precise estimates for the burden of childhood TB are not readily available, primarily reflecting the difficulty in diagnosing TB accurately in children. Children represent an increasing proportion of the total number of cases in TB-endemic areas, however, with almost 500,000 children succumbing to the disease each year. Although the overwhelming burden of disease is in developing countries, several developed countries also have reported a recent increase in the number of TB cases in children.[71,72] Although in most children the initial infection occurs in the lungs, TB in children and adolescents should be considered, at least potentially, to be a systemic disease. The primary complex comprising the site of infection and the involved regional lymph nodes may heal, or complications may develop from enlargement or rupture of the regional lymph nodes or from the spread of tubercle bacilli into the bloodstream, giving rise to disseminated disease. The risk of dissemination is greatest in the first 5 years of life and within the first 12 to 24 months after infection and is seen more commonly in children than in adults.

Recently, the Tuberculosis Coalition for Technical Assistance and its partners have published international standards of care for the management of TB.[73] The reader is referred to this important document and its 17 standards relating to the diagnosis, treatment, and public health responsibilities of TB.

Diagnosis

Tuberculosis infection
Diagnosis of TB infection is based on tuberculin skin testing (TST) in the absence of signs or radiologic findings suggestive of TB disease. The interpretation of a positive test may be modified by the risk of infection, which is influenced by the contact history, duration of contact, medical history, and age of the individual and their Bacille Calmette-Guerin (BCG) vaccination status. The TST is an imperfect test. Its interpretation and subsequent clinical management depend on the prior probability of the test being positive and on the clinical circumstances of the individual or family.

Tuberculosis disease
Diagnosis of TB disease is based on clinical symptoms and signs, chest radiographs or other investigations, and smear and culture of infected body material. Although there are conflicting reports as to whether lateral chest radiographs increase the yield for detecting intrathoracic lymphadenopathy,[74,75] CT is considered an excellent tool for detecting mediastinal nodes. CT, however, requires a volumetric scanning protocol and should not be performed routinely because of the associated high radiation dose.

Even though the yield from cultures is low in children, microbiologic confirmation of TB should be sought. Treatment should be started as soon as samples have been obtained.

Microbiology

- In patients unable to produce sputum, gastric aspirates are the investigation of choice for pulmonary TB in children (level of evidence: moderate).

In younger children, when it is not possible to obtain sputum, gastric aspirates should be collected on 3 consecutive days. About 50 mL of gastric contents should be aspirated via a nasogastric tube early in the morning after the child has fasted for 8 to 10 hours, preferably while the child is still recumbent. Both a smear and culture should be performed on the aspirate.

If there is radiologic evidence of focal disease, such as lobar, segmental, or subsegmental collapse, or clinical evidence of bronchial obstruction, a flexible fiberoptic bronchoscopy may be indicated to identify and biopsy endobronchial lesions, ideally, with bronchoalveolar lavage performed in addition to gastric aspiration. Otherwise, bronchoscopy with bronchoalveolar lavage offers no advantages over gastric aspiration.[76]

Inhalation of nebulized sterile hypertonic saline (3% to 6%) via an ultrasonic nebulizer can be used to induce sputum in patients unable to expectorate sputum. The cough produced by this technique may be of sufficient force to aerosolize tubercle bacilli and infect health care workers, however. Ideally, sputum should be induced in areas with high-efficiency particulate air filters, and qualified personnel should wear appropriate respiratory protection.

ROLE OF INTERFERON-GAMMA RELEASE ASSAYS IN CHILDREN

The sensitivity of the currently available interferon-gamma release assays for the diagnosis of culture-confirmed TB disease in children is not high enough for these assays to be used alone to rule out TB.[77] In most studies interferon-gamma release assays and TST yield equivalent results for the detection of latent TB infection in children, once adjustment is made for interpretation of the TST based on differing cut-offs, and some evidence suggests these assays may be less sensitive than TST in children.[78] Limited data suggest that in situations in which the value of TST is greatly reduced (eg, in patients infected with HIV), interferon-gamma release assays may prove useful when used as an adjunct to TST to increase sensitivity. Other specific situations in which the interferon-gamma release assays might be indicated are

- To confirm infection in a child who has been vaccinated with BCG and the TST result is borderline positive/negative
- As a replacement for TST when repeat testing with TST is likely to result in a booster phenomenon
- If TST testing is considered likely to result in a blistering or a large painful response (eg, in a patient who has had a strong reaction to TST in the past)
- For a child who is unable or unlikely to return at 48 to 72 hours for reading of the TST

TREATMENT
Latent Tuberculosis Infection

Treatment of children who have latent TB infection and no evidence of TB disease is indicated for two reasons: first, to reduce the risk of the patient's developing disease in the years immediately after acquiring the infection, particularly in children under the age of 5 years, when extrapulmonary disease is more common, and second, to reduce the lifelong risk of developing TB disease as a consequence of infection. These goals can be achieved by the use of isoniazid therapy for a minimum of 6 months. Although a dose of isoniazid, 5 to10 mg/kg once daily, is recommended, a dose of 10 mg/kg is optimal: children eliminate isoniazid faster than adults, and therefore relatively larger doses are required to achieve comparable serum concentrations.[79]

Treatment of latent TB infection is particularly important in HIV—positive children, children in whom corticosteroid or immunosuppressive therapy is contemplated, and in those who have diabetes or other chronic diseases associated with malnutrition (eg, celiac disease).

Treatment of latent TB infection in children and adolescents has few side effects. The incidence of liver toxicity in children is extremely low, and routine monitoring of liver function is not recommended.

TREATMENT OF PULMONARY TUBERCULOSIS DISEASE

- A rifampicin-containing regime is the backbone of antituberculosis treatment for drug-susceptible *M tuberculosis* (level of evidence: high).
- At least 6 months' treatment is recommended using three or four drugs for 2 months with a further continuation phase of 4 months with isoniazid and rifampicin (level of evidence: high).

Children who have TB disease usually are treated with daily therapy with four drugs, isoniazid, rifampicin, pyrazinamide, and ethambutol, for 2 months, and then generally with two drugs, isoniazid and rifampicin, for a further 4 months. Normally these drugs are given daily, but supervised therapy given 3 days a week sometimes is necessary when adherence with daily therapy is considered to be poor.

Such short-course therapy (6 months) has been shown to be effective in children who have primary TB and complicated primary TB limited to the respiratory tract.

Infectivity

- Childhood TB is rarely contagious (level of evidence: high) because
- Children who have TB disease usually have a small bacterial load.
- Children are less able to generate the tussive forces needed to aerosolize bacilli.
- Children very rarely have cavitating disease.
- Young children swallow rather than expectorate sputum.
- Occasionally adolescents are seen with cavities caused by TB and then may be infectious.

Strategies to Improve Adherence

Adherence is a multidimensional phenomenon determined by the interplay of socio-economic, health system, disease-related, patient-related, and therapy-related factors.[73] A few pragmatic strategies to enhance treatment adherence include

- Emphasizing the importance of adherence at outset of treatment to child and family
- Assigning a key worker to each family with information on how to contact the worker
- Using professional interpreters to communicate if necessary, rather than family members
- Giving information about potential side effects to the child and the family
- Providing pill organizers for multidrug regimes
- Using combination antibiotic preparations when available and if tolerated
- Providing written information in appropriate languages

- Maintaining close liaison with the dispensing pharmacy regarding collection of scripts
- Having liquid preparations readily available for preschool children
- Providing easy access to follow-up

RESPIRATORY INFECTIONS IN HIV-INFECTED CHILDREN

- Parenteral benzyl penicillin or ampicillin should be used in combination with gentamicin (level of evidence: high).

The clinical expression of HIV disease in children is highly variable. HIV-related lower respiratory infections account for 30% to 40% of pediatric admissions and have a case fatality rate of up to 35%, much higher than the 10% for children not infected with HIV. In addition to *S pneumoniae* and *S aureus*, *P jiroveci*, gram-negative bacteria, and cytomegalovirus are important opportunistic infections in this group of children.[80] The WHO developed revised guidelines for presumptive treatment of pneumonia in young children in regions where the prevalence of HIV is high. It is recommended that children admitted with severe pneumonia in HIV-endemic areas receive benzyl penicillin or ampicillin in combination with gentamicin, irrespective of age, and that all infants receive high-dose co-trimoxazole because of the high prevalence of *P jiroveci*.[81] There are no reported studies assessing the efficacy of these treatment guidelines since publication. A study conducted before the publication of the guidelines used the same recommendations and concluded that in children older than 1 year the WHO guidelines were effective, irrespective of HIV status. For those aged younger than 1 year, however, the guidelines were found to be inadequate, because nearly half of the infants did not respond to therapy. This failure was attributed to polymicrobial disease.[82]

COMMON TROPICAL RESPIRATORY INFECTIONS
Pulmonary Hydatid Cyst (Echinococcosis)

- Surgical excision of the cyst in conjunction with benzimidazoles is recommended (level of evidence: moderate).
- Exclusive medical therapy is reserved for patients who are poor candidates for surgery (level of evidence: moderate).

Echinococcosis or hydatid disease is caused by the cystic larval stage of the tapeworm *Echinococcus*. The liver is the most common site of cyst formation, followed by the lung in 10% to 30% of cases. Pulmonary disease seems to be more common in children and younger individuals. Although most patients are asymptomatic, some may expectorate the contents of the cyst or develop symptoms related to compression of the surrounding structures. Surgical excision of the cyst is the treatment of choice whenever feasible, because the parasite can be removed completely and the patient cured.[83] The surgical options for lung cysts include lobectomy, wedge resection, pericystectomy, intact endocystectomy, and capitonnage. Medical therapy with benzimidazoles is valuable in disseminated disease, including secondary lung or pleural hydatidosis, in patients who are poor surgical risks, and when there is intraoperative spillage of hydatid fluid.[84]

PULMONARY AMEBIASIS

- Tissue amebicides are effective treatment (level of evidence: moderate).
- Surgical management is reserved for patients who have advanced disease (level of evidence: moderate).

Amebiasis caused by *Entameba histolytica* is endemic in the tropical countries. The lungs are the second most common extraintestinal site after amebic liver abscess. Pleuropulmonary amebiasis most often is a consequence of the direct extension of an amebic liver abscess manifested by consolidation, lung abscess, pleural effusion/empyema or hepato-bronchial fistula. Tissue amebicides such as metronidazole, chloroquine, and dehydroemetine are effective in most patients who have pulmonary disease.[85,86] Percutaneous pleural drainage and surgical decortication have a role in patients who have advanced disease.[87,88]

TROPICAL EOSINOPHILIA

- A 3-week course of diethylcarbamazine is recommended (level of evidence: moderate).

Tropical eosinophilia is a syndrome characterized by a generalized tissue reaction in which pulmonary manifestations predominate. An underlying hypersensitivity reaction to the filarial parasites *Wuchereria bancrofti* or *Brugia malayi* results in cough, breathlessness, wheeze, marked increase in peripheral eosinophilia, and eosinophilic pulmonary infiltrates.[89,90] Treatment is with a 3-week course of diethylcarbamazine.[91,92]

MANAGEMENT OF COMPLICATIONS OF RESPIRATORY INFECTIONS
Empyema

- Use a chest drain with intrapleural fibrinolytics (level of evidence: high).
- Use video-assisted thoracoscopic surgery (level of evidence: high).

A number of treatment options currently are available for empyema, including systemic antibiotics alone or in combination with thoracocentesis; chest drain insertion, with or without intrapleural fibrinolytics; and surgical techniques such as video-assisted thoracoscopic surgery (VATS), mini-thoracotomy, and standard thoracotomy with decortication. All these treatment options are safe and effective. Chest drain with intrapleural fibrinolytics, particularly urokinase,[93,94] and VATS[94,95] have been shown to be effective primary approaches in the treatment of empyema, with a shorter duration of hospital stay, which is used consistently as an outcome measure. The failure rates are similar with both modalities of treatment. The cost of treatment with intrapleural urokinase is around 25% cheaper than VATS, and, because the expertise to perform VATS may not be universally available, intrapleural urokinase is advocated as first-line management.[94]

A meta-analysis comparing the results of nonoperative and primary operative therapy for the treatment of pediatric empyema reviewed 67 studies.[96] Data were aggregated from reports of children treated nonoperatively (3418 cases from 54 studies) and from children treated with a primary operative approach (363 cases from 25 studies). Data analysis showed that primary operative therapy was associated with a lower mortality rate, lower re-intervention rate, shorter length of hospitalization, decreased time with a thoracostomy tube, and shorter course of antibiotic therapy, compared with nonoperative therapy. The limitations of this analysis are that most of the studies included were observational or retrospective case note reviews. The observational data from the analysis show that the length of stay is similar for primary fibrinolytic therapy (10.7 days), thoracotomy (10.6 days), and VATS (11.2 days). The analysis also suggests that current surgical options for childhood empyema seem safe, with no reported mortality and little morbidity, and that there is complete resolution of the disease, whatever the treatment.

Pneumatoceles

- Pneumatoceles resolve without treatment (level of evidence: moderate).
- Refractory cases require surgery (level of evidence: moderate).

Pneumatoceles are associated most frequently with staphylococcal pneumonia but also are seen in pneumonias caused by *S pneumoniae, H influenzae, E coli*, and *Klebsiella*. They usually do not produce any additional symptoms to the underlying infective process and regress spontaneously.[97,98] Surgical management, including drainage, resection, or decortication, is required only in refractory cases or those that are symptomatic.[98]

Lung Abscess

- Lung abscess resolves with a prolonged course of antibiotics (level of evidence: moderate).
- Abscess drainage hastens recovery (level of evidence: moderate).

Lung abscesses coexisting with necrotizing pneumonia or empyema usually do not require surgical drainage and resolve with a prolonged course of antibiotics administered for the pneumonic process.[99] In the last decade, however, there has been increasing interest in the early use of interventional radiology for the aspiration of lung abscesses, with or without placement of an external drain, as a way of hastening recovery and decreasing hospital stay. Surgical resection of the affected lobe is associated with significant morbidity and is very rarely advocated.[100,101,102]

Bronchopleural Fistulae and Pyopneumothorax

- Bronchopleural fistula resolves with continued drainage (level of evidence: moderate).
- Surgical management is useful in protracted cases (level of evidence: moderate).

Bronchopleural fistulae associated with necrotizing pneumonias and empyema usually are peripheral and resolve with continued chest drainage.[103] Sometimes, however, they are slow to resolve, and surgical management must be considered. Talc pleurodesis and limited decortication with muscle flap around the bronchopleural fistula have been used successfully in protracted cases.[104,105]

REFERENCES

1. Wardlaw T, Salama P, Johansson EW, et al. Pneumonia: the leading killer of children. Lancet 2006;368(9541):1048–50.
2. Williams BG, Gouws E, Boschi-Pinto C, et al. Estimates of world-wide distribution of child deaths from acute respiratory infections. Lancet Infect Dis 2002;2(1): 25–32.
3. World Health Organization. The World Health Organization report 2005. Available at: http://www.who.int/whr/en. 2005. Accessed July 2008.
4. Jokinen C, Heiskanen L, Juvonen H, et al. Incidence of community-acquired pneumonia in the population of four municipalities in eastern Finland. Am J Epidemiol 1993;137(9):977–88.
5. McCracken GH Jr. Etiology and treatment of pneumonia. Pediatr Infect Dis J 2000;19(4):373–7.
6. World Health Organisation. The management of acute respiratory infections in children. practical guidelines for outpatient care. Geneva: WHO; 1995.

7. Palafox M, Guiscafre H, Reyes H, et al. Diagnostic value of tachypnoea in pneumonia defined radiologically. Arch Dis Child 2000;82(1):41–5.
8. Heiskanen-Kosma T, Korppi M, Jokinen C, et al. Etiology of childhood pneumonia: serologic results of a prospective, population-based study. Pediatr Infect Dis J 1998;17(11):986–91.
9. Michelow IC, Olsen K, Lozano J, et al. Epidemiology and clinical characteristics of community-acquired pneumonia in hospitalized children. Pediatrics 2004; 113(4):701–7.
10. Wubbel L, Muniz L, Ahmed A, et al. Etiology and treatment of community-acquired pneumonia in ambulatory children. Pediatr Infect Dis J 1999;18(2): 98–104.
11. Juven T, Mertsola J, Waris M, et al. Etiology of community-acquired pneumonia in 254 hospitalized children. Pediatr Infect Dis J 2000;19(4):293–8.
12. British Thoracic Society. British Thoracic Society guidelines for the management of community acquired pneumonia in childhood. Thorax 2002;57(Suppl I):i1–24.
13. Pio A. Standard case management of pneumonia in children in developing countries: the cornerstone of the Acute Respiratory Infection Programme. Bull World Health Organ 2003;81(4):298–300.
14. Kumar P, McKean MC. Evidence based paediatrics: review of BTS guidelines for the management of community acquired pneumonia in children. J Infect 2004; 48(2):134–8.
15. Chang CC, Cheng AC, Chang AB. Over-the-counter (OTC) medications to reduce cough as an adjunct to antibiotics for acute pneumonia in children and adults. Cochrane Database Syst Rev 2007;(4):CD006088.
16. Paludo C, Zhang L, Lincho CS, et al. Chest physical therapy for children hospitalized with acute pneumonia: a randomized controlled trial. Thorax 2008;63(9): 791–4.
17. Aggarwal R, Sentz J, Miller MA. Role of zinc administration in prevention of childhood diarrhea and respiratory illnesses: a meta-analysis. Pediatrics 2007; 119(6):1120–30.
18. Swingler GH, Hussey GD, Zwarenstein M. Randomised controlled trial of clinical outcome after chest radiograph in ambulatory acute lower-respiratory infection in children. Lancet 1998;351(9100):404–8.
19. Davies HD, Wang EE, Manson D, et al. Reliability of the chest radiograph in the diagnosis of lower respiratory infections in young children. Pediatr Infect Dis J 1996;15(7):600–4.
20. Anonymous. Pneumonia in childhood. Lancet 1988;1(8588):741–3.
21. Banya WA, O'Dempsey TJ, McArdle T, et al. Predictors for a positive blood culture in African children with pneumonia. Pediatr Infect Dis J 1996;15(4):292–7.
22. Zar HJ, Hanslo D, Apolles P, et al. Induced sputum versus gastric lavage for microbiological confirmation of pulmonary tuberculosis in infants and young children: a prospective study. Lancet 2005;365(9454):130–4.
23. Vuori-Holopainen E, Peltola H. Reappraisal of lung tap: review of an old method for better etiologic diagnosis of childhood pneumonia. Clin Infect Dis 2001;32(5): 715–26.
24. Falade AG, Mulholland EK, Adegbola RA, et al. Bacterial isolates from blood and lung aspirate cultures in Gambian children with lobar pneumonia. Ann Trop Paediatr 1997;17(4):315–9.
25. Vuori-Holopainen E, Salo E, Saxen H, et al. Etiological diagnosis of childhood pneumonia by use of transthoracic needle aspiration and modern microbiological methods. Clin Infect Dis 2002;34(5):583–90.

26. Smyth A, Carty H, Hart CA. Clinical predictors of hypoxaemia in children with pneumonia. Ann Trop Paediatr 1998;18(1):31–40.

27. Dhawan A, Narang A, Singhi S. Hyponatraemia and the inappropriate ADH syndrome in pneumonia. Ann Trop Paediatr 1992;12(4):455–62.

28. Straus WL, Qazi SA, Kundi Z, et al. Antimicrobial resistance and clinical effectiveness of co-trimoxazole versus amoxycillin for pneumonia among children in Pakistan: randomised controlled trial. Pakistan Co-trimoxazole Study Group. Lancet 1998;352(9124):270–4.

29. Kabra SK, Lodha R, Pandey RM. Antibiotics for community acquired pneumonia in children. Cochrane Database Syst Rev 2006;3:CD004874.

30. Schrag SJ, McGee L, Whitney CG, et al. Emergence of Streptococcus pneumoniae with very-high-level resistance to penicillin. Antimicrobial Agents Chemother 2004;48(8):3016–23.

31. Low DE, Pichichero ME, Schaad UB. Optimizing antibacterial therapy for community-acquired respiratory tract infections in children in an era of bacterial resistance. Clin Pediatr (Phila) 2004;43(2):135–51.

32. Whitney CG, Farley MM, Hadler J, et al. Increasing prevalence of multidrug-resistant Streptococcus pneumoniae in the United States. N Engl J Med 2000; 343(26):1917–24.

33. Deeks SL, Palacio R, Ruvinsky R, et al. Risk factors and course of illness among children with invasive penicillin-resistant Streptococcus pneumoniae. The Streptococcus pneumoniae Working Group. Pediatrics 1999;103(2):409–13.

34. Friedland IR. Comparison of the response to antimicrobial therapy of penicillin-resistant and penicillin-susceptible pneumococcal disease. Pediatr Infect Dis J 1995;14(10):885–90.

35. Tan TQ, Mason EO Jr, Barson WJ, et al. Clinical characteristics and outcome of children with pneumonia attributable to penicillin-susceptible and penicillin-non-susceptible Streptococcus pneumoniae. Pediatrics 1998;102(6):1369–75.

36. Doern GV, Jones RN, Pfaller MA, et al. Haemophilus influenzae and Moraxella catarrhalis from patients with community-acquired respiratory tract infections: antimicrobial susceptibility patterns from the SENTRY Antimicrobial Surveillance Program (United States and Canada, 1997). Antimicrob Agents Chemother 1999;43(2):385–9.

37. Gorak EJ, Yamada SM, Brown JD. Community-acquired methicillin-resistant Staphylococcus aureus in hospitalized adults and children without known risk factors. Clin Infect Dis 1999;29(4):797–800.

38. Gang RK, Sanyal SC, Mokaddas E, et al. Rifampicin as an adjunct to vancomycin therapy in MRSA septicaemia in burns. Bur 1999;25(7):640–4.

39. Mulholland K, Hilton S, Adegbola R, et al. Randomised trial of Haemophilus influenzae type-b tetanus protein conjugate vaccine [corrected] for prevention of pneumonia and meningitis in Gambian infants. Lancet 1997; 349(9060):1191–7.

40. Levine OS, Lagos R, Munoz A, et al. Defining the burden of pneumonia in children preventable by vaccination against Haemophilus influenzae type b. Pediatr Infect Dis J 1999;18(12):1060–4.

41. Gessner BD, Sutanto A, Linehan M, et al. Incidences of vaccine-preventable Haemophilus influenzae type b pneumonia and meningitis in Indonesian children: hamlet-randomised vaccine-probe trial. Lancet 2005;365(9453):43–52.

42. Black S, Shinefield H, Fireman B, et al. Efficacy, safety and immunogenicity of heptavalent pneumococcal conjugate vaccine in children. Northern California

Kaiser Permanente Vaccine Study Center Group. Pediatr Infect Dis J 2000;19(3): 187–95.

43. Klugman KP, Madhi SA, Huebner RE, et al. A trial of a 9-valent pneumococcal conjugate vaccine in children with and those without HIV infection. N Engl J Med 2003;349(14):1341–8.

44. Cutts FT, Zaman SM, Enwere G, et al. Efficacy of nine-valent pneumococcal conjugate vaccine against pneumonia and invasive pneumococcal disease in The Gambia: randomised, double-blind, placebo-controlled trial. Lancet 2005; 365(9465):1139–46.

45. Obaro SK, Madhi SA. Bacterial pneumonia vaccines and childhood pneumonia: are we winning, refining, or redefining? Lancet Infect Dis 2006;6(3):150–61.

46. Whitney CG, Pilishvili T, Farley MM, et al. Effectiveness of seven-valent pneumococcal conjugate vaccine against invasive pneumococcal disease: a matched case-control study. Lancet 2006;368(9546):1495–502.

47. Cohen R, Levy C, de La RF, et al. Impact of pneumococcal conjugate vaccine and of reduction of antibiotic use on nasopharyngeal carriage of nonsusceptible pneumococci in children with acute otitis media. Pediatr Infect Dis J 2006; 25(11):1001–7.

48. Mulholland K. Childhood pneumonia mortality—a permanent global emergency. Lancet 2007;370(9583):285–9.

49. Grove RD, Hetzel AM. Vital statistics rates in the United States 1940–1960. Washington DC: US National Center for Health Statistics; 1968. 2008.

50. Bryce J, Boschi-Pinto C, Shibuya K, et al. WHO estimates of the causes of death in children. Lancet 2005;365(9465):1147–52.

51. Jones G, Steketee RW, Black RE, et al. How many child deaths can we prevent this year? Lancet 2003;362(9377):65–71.

52. Sazawal S, Black RE. Effect of pneumonia case management on mortality in neonates, infants, and preschool children: a meta-analysis of community-based trials. Lancet Infect Dis 2003;3(9):547–56.

53. Pandey MR, Sharma PR, Gubhaju BB, et al. Impact of a pilot acute respiratory infection (ARI) control programme in a rural community of the hill region of Nepal. Ann Trop Paediatr 1989;9(4):212–20.

54. Pandey MR, Daulaire NM, Starbuck ES, et al. Reduction in total under-five mortality in western Nepal through community-based antimicrobial treatment of pneumonia. Lancet 1991;338(8773):993–7.

55. WHO. Programme for the control of acute respiratory infections. Technical basis for the WHO recommendations on the management of pneumonia in children at first level health facilities. Geneva, Switzerland: World Health Organization; 1991.

56. Kielmann AA, Taylor CE, DeSweemer C, et al. The Narangwal experiment on interactions of nutrition and infections: II. Morbidity and mortality effects. Indian J Med Res 1978;68(Suppl):21–41.

57. Mtango FD, Neuvians D. Acute respiratory infections in children under five years. Control project in Bagamoyo District, Tanzania. Trans R Soc Trop Med Hyg 1986;80(6):851–8.

58. Khan AJ, Khan JA, Akbar M, et al. Acute respiratory infections in children: a case management intervention in Abbottabad District, Pakistan. Bull World Health Organ 1990;68(5):577–85.

59. World Health Organization. Case management of acute respiratory infections in children: intervention studies. WHO/ARI/88 2. Geneva: WHO; 1998.

60. Bang AT, Bang RA, Tale O, et al. Reduction in pneumonia mortality and total childhood mortality by means of community-based intervention trial in Gadchiroli, India. Lancet 1990;336(8709):201–6.
61. Fauveau V, Stewart MK, Chakraborty J, et al. Impact on mortality of a community-based programme to control acute lower respiratory tract infections. Bull World Health Organ 1992;70(1):109–16.
62. Roesin R, Sutanto A, Sastra K. ARI intervention study in Kediri, Indonesia (a summary of study results). Bull Int Union Tuberc Lung Dis 1990;65(4):23.
63. CATCHUP study group. Clinical efficacy of co-trimoxazole versus amoxicillin twice daily for treatment of pneumonia: a randomised controlled clinical trial in Pakistan. Arch Dis Child 2002;86(2):113–8.
64. Mulholland EK, Falade AG, Corrah PT, et al. A randomized trial of chloramphenicol vs. trimethoprim-sulfamethoxazole for the treatment of malnourished children with community-acquired pneumonia. Pediatr Infect Dis J 1995;14(11):959–65.
65. Campbell H, Byass P, Forgie IM, et al. Trial of co-trimoxazole versus procaine penicillin with ampicillin in treatment of community-acquired pneumonia in young Gambian children. Lancet 1988;2(8621):1182–4.
66. Sidal M, Oguz F, Unuvar A, et al. Trial of co-trimoxazole versus procaine penicillin G and benzathin penicillin + procaine penicillin G in the treatment of childhood pneumonia. J Trop Pediatr 1994;40(5):301–4.
67. Hazir T, Fox LM, Nisar YB, et al. Ambulatory short-course high-dose oral amoxicillin for treatment of severe pneumonia in children: a randomised equivalency trial. Lancet 2008;371(9606):49–56.
68. Asghar R, Banajeh S, Egas J, et al. Chloramphenicol versus ampicillin plus gentamicin for community acquired very severe pneumonia among children aged 2–59 months in low resource settings: multicentre randomised controlled trial (SPEAR study). BMJ 2008;336(7635):80–4.
69. Hazir T, Qazi SA, Bin NY, et al. Comparison of standard versus double dose of amoxicillin in the treatment of non-severe pneumonia in children aged 2–59 months: a multi-centre, double blind, randomised controlled trial in Pakistan. Arch Dis Child 2007;92(4):291–7.
70. Maher D, Raviglione M. Global epidemiology of tuberculosis. Clin Chest Med 2005;26(2):167–82.
71. Atkinson P, Taylor H, Sharland M, et al. Resurgence of paediatric tuberculosis in London. Arch Dis Child 2002;86(4):264–5.
72. Shah NS, Harrington T, Huber M, et al. Increased reported cases of tuberculosis among children younger than 5 years of age, Maricopa County, Arizona, 2002–2003. Pediatr Infect Dis J 2006;25(2):151–5.
73. Tuberculosis Coalition for Technical Assistance. International standards for tuberculosis care. 2008. Available at: www.istcweb.org/materials.html. Accessed July 2008.
74. Smuts NA, Beyers N, Gie RP, et al. Value of the lateral chest radiograph in tuberculosis in children. Pediatr Radiol 1994;24(7):478–80.
75. Swingler GH, du TG, Andronikou S, et al. Diagnostic accuracy of chest radiography in detecting mediastinal lymphadenopathy in suspected pulmonary tuberculosis. Arch Dis Child 2005;90(11):1153–6.
76. Abadco DL, Steiner P. Gastric lavage is better than bronchoalveolar lavage for isolation of Mycobacterium tuberculosis in childhood pulmonary tuberculosis. Pediatr Infect Dis J 1992;11(9):735–8.
77. Ranganathan S, Connell T, Curtis N. Interferon-gamma release assays in children—no better than tuberculin skin testing? J Infect 2007;54(4):412–3.

78. Connell TG, Curtis N, Ranganathan SC, et al. Performance of a whole blood interferon gamma assay for detecting latent infection with Mycobacterium tuberculosis in children. Thorax 2006;61(7):616–20.

79. Schaaf HS, Parkin DP, Seifart HI, et al. Isoniazid pharmacokinetics in children treated for respiratory tuberculosis. Arch Dis Child 2005;90(6):614–8.

80. Simoes EA, Cherian T, Chow J, et al. Acute respiratory infections in children. In: Jamieson DT, Breman JG, Measham AR, et al, editors. Disease control priorities in developing countries. New York: Oxford University Press; 2006. p. 483–98.

81. Management of children with pneumonia and HIV in low-resource settings. Report of a consultative meeting. Harare, Zimbabwe, 2003. Geneva: World Health Organization; 2004.

82. McNally LM, Jeena PM, Gajee K, et al. Effect of age, polymicrobial disease, and maternal HIV status on treatment response and cause of severe pneumonia in South African children: a prospective descriptive study. Lancet 2007; 369(9571):1440–51.

83. Qian ZX. Thoracic hydatid cysts: a report of 842 cases treated over a thirty-year period. Ann Thorac Surg 1988;46(3):342–6.

84. Kilani T, El HS. Pulmonary hydatid and other lung parasitic infections. Curr Opin Pulm Med 2002;8(3):218–23.

85. Cohen HG, Reynolds TB. Comparison of metronidazole and chloroquine for the treatment of amoebic liver abscess. A controlled trial. Gastroenterology 1975; 69(1):35–41.

86. Cameron EW. The treatment of pleuropulmonary amebiasis with metronidazole. Chest 1978;73(5):647–50.

87. Ibarra-Perez C, Selman-Lama M. Diagnosis and treatment of amebic "empyema": report of eighty-eight cases. Am J Surg 1977;134(2):283–7.

88. Ibarra-Perez C. Thoracic complications of amebic abscess of the liver: report of 501 cases. Chest 1981;79(6):672–7.

89. Parab PB, Samuel AM, Udwadia FE, et al. Hypersensitivity reaction in tropical eosinophilia. Indian J Med Res 1979;69:122–7.

90. Ottesen EA, Nutman TB. Tropical pulmonary eosinophilia. Annu Rev Med 1992; 43:417–24.

91. Ganatra RD, Sheth UK, Lewis RA. Diethylcarbamazine (Hetrazan) in tropical eosinophilia. Indian J Med Res 1958;46(2):205–22.

92. Pinkston P, Vijayan VK, Nutman TB, et al. Acute tropical pulmonary eosinophilia. Characterization of the lower respiratory tract inflammation and its response to therapy. J Clin Invest 1987;80(1):216–25.

93. Thomson AH, Hull J, Kumar MR, et al. Randomised trial of intrapleural urokinase in the treatment of childhood empyema. Thorax 2002;57(4):343–7.

94. Sonnappa S, Cohen G, Owens CM, et al. Comparison of urokinase and video-assisted thoracoscopic surgery for treatment of childhood empyema. Am J Respir Crit Care Med 2006;174(2):221–7.

95. Kurt BA, Winterhalter KM, Connors RH, et al. Therapy of parapneumonic effusions in children: video-assisted thoracoscopic surgery versus conventional thoracostomy drainage. Pediatrics 2006;118(3):e547–53 [Epub 2006 Aug 14].

96. Avansino JR, Goldman B, Sawin RS, et al. Primary operative versus nonoperative therapy for pediatric empyema: a meta-analysis. Pediatrics 2005;115(6): 1652–9.

97. Victoria MS, Steiner P, Rao M. Persistent postpneumonic pneumatoceles in children. Chest 1981;79(3):359–61.

98. Imamoglu M, Cay A, Kosucu P, et al. Pneumatoceles in postpneumonic empyema: an algorithmic approach. J Pediatr Surg 2005;40(7):1111–7.

99. Asher MI, Spier S, Beland M, et al. Primary lung abscess in childhood: the long-term outcome of conservative management. Am J Dis Child 1982;136(6):491–4.

100. van Sonnenberg E, D'Agostino HB, Casola G, et al. Lung abscess: CT-guided drainage. Radiology 1991;178(2):347–51.

101. Yen CC, Tang RB, Chen SJ, et al. Pediatric lung abscess: a retrospective review of 23 cases. J Microbiol Immunol Infect 2004;37(1):45–9.

102. Chan PC, Huang LM, Wu PS, et al. Clinical management and outcome of childhood lung abscess: a 16-year experience. J Microbiol Immunol Infect 2005;38(3):183–8.

103. Balfour-Lynn IM, Abrahamson E, Cohen G, et al. BTS guidelines for the management of pleural infection in children. Thorax 2005;60(Suppl 1):i1–21.

104. Puskas JD, Mathisen DJ, Grillo HC, et al. Treatment strategies for bronchopleural fistula. J Thorac Cardiovasc Surg 1995;109(5):989–95.

105. Hallows MR, Parikh DH. Surgical management of children with pyopneumothorax: serratus anterior digitation flap. J Pediatr Surg 2004;39(7):1122–4.

Bronchiectasis in Children

Gregory J. Redding, MD[a,b,*]

KEYWORDS

- Cystic fibrosis • Bronchiectasis • Children • Lung treatments

Bronchiectasis is a chronic disease of the conducting airways that produces persistent productive cough, recurrent respiratory infectious exacerbations, and obstructive lung disease in children and adults. The hallmarks of bronchiectasis are stasis of infected airway secretions; reduced airway mucus clearance; and regional or diffuse airway wall dilation, thickening, and destruction with loss of airway structural integrity. Bronchiectasis is associated with a prolonged neutrophilic inflammatory and secretory response within the airways, producing a "wet" sounding cough in infants and young children and mucopurulent sputum expectoration in older children. Bronchiectasis is diagnosed by characteristic images of airways obtained with high-resolution computerized tomographic scans of the chest.[1]

Bronchiectasis is most commonly associated with cystic fibrosis (CF) in industrialized countries, although there are many etiologies for bronchiectasis unrelated to CF. The pathogenic mechanisms that predispose to bronchiectasis range from narrowing of proximal airways (eg, airway compression, intraluminal obstruction) to injury of conducting airways after viral, bacterial, and some fungal infections. Underlying conditions that affect pulmonary host defenses, such as CF, primary ciliary dyskinesia, and primary and acquired immunodeficiencies, also lead to bronchiectasis. Clinical evaluation includes identifying an underlying condition that can be treated with specific and supportive care and disorders that affect not only the lungs but other organs as well. Conditions and diseases that predispose to bronchiectasis are listed in **Box 1**.

This article focuses on the grading and recommendations for chronic therapies of bronchiectasis caused by CF- and non–CF-related conditions. Chronic therapies do not necessarily mean daily therapies. For example, aerosol tobramycin is administered to children who have CF every other 28-day period but on a regular basis long

Funding was provided in part by the Maternal Child Health Bureau (grant T72MC000007). There are no financial conflicts of interest pertaining to this article.

[a] Department of Pediatrics, University of Washington School of Medicine, Health Sciences, RR 314, Box 356320, 1959 NE Pacific Street Seattle, WA 98195-6320, USA
[b] Pulmonary Division, Seattle Children's Hospital, Room A-5937, 4800 Sand Point Way NE, Health Sciences, RR 314, Box 356320, 1959 NE Pacific Street Seattle, WA, USA
* Pulmonary Division, Seattle Children's Hospital, Room A-5937, 4800 Sand Point Way NE, Seattle, WA, USA.
E-mail address: gredding@u.washington.edu

Pediatr Clin N Am 56 (2009) 157–171
doi:10.1016/j.pcl.2008.10.014
0031-3955/08/$ – see front matter © 2009 Published by Elsevier Inc.

Box 1
Conditions that predispose to bronchiectasis in children

Proximal airway narrowing

    Airway wall compression (ie, vascular ring, adenopathy impinging on airways)

    Airway intraluminal obstruction (eg, inhaled foreign body, granulation tissue)

    Airway stenosis and malacia

Airway injury

    Bronchiolitis obliterans (eg, postviral, after lung transplantation)

    Recurrent pneumonitis or pneumonia (eg, pneumococcal pneumonia, aspiration pneumonia)

Altered pulmonary host defenses

    CF

    Ciliary dyskinesia

    Impaired cough (eg, neuromuscular weakness conditions)

Altered immune states

    Primary abnormalities (eg, hypogammaglobulinemia)

    Secondary abnormalities (eg, HIV infection, immunosuppressive agents)

Other

    Allergic bronchopulmonary aspergillosis

    Plastic bronchitis

---

term.[2] Chronic therapy even might include regular hospitalization for inpatient treatment, but the scope of this article is to focus on outpatient treatment and not include as-needed treatment for mild or severe pulmonary exacerbations associated with bronchiectasis. The grading process, as described by the Grade Working Group,[3] includes quality of evidence, pertinent outcomes of treatment that are disease specific and relevant to children, and their benefits relative to potential risks. Quality of evidence depends on study design and quality, direct relevance of evidence to the clinical problem, and consistency of findings among studies. Readers are directed to the Cochrane Collaboration's database of systematic reviews.[4] These reviews address clinical treatments for specific conditions, search the literature for large and small clinical randomized controlled trials (RCTs), and render decisions as to whether publications are numerous and rigorous enough to make recommendations about treatment practices. Chronic therapies for bronchiectasis that have Cochrane reviews completed are listed in **Table 1**.

Bronchiectasis unrelated to CF has been considered an "orphan disease" based on a low prevalence compared with CF in developed countries.[5] Much more research about treatments has been conducted among patients who have CF than for bronchiectasis attributable to other etiologies. As a result, most research evaluating therapies for idiopathic bronchiectasis has been conducted in adults rather than in children and it is debatable whether this information can be extrapolated to younger patients. Idiopathic bronchiectasis is more prevalent than CF-related disease in certain high-risk groups, such as indigenous populations, and in developing countries.[6–8] There are no treatment RCTs in children belonging to these high-risk groups.

Table 1
Chronic pulmonary therapies for bronchiectasis related and unrelated to cystic fibrosis

Treatment Category	Cystic Fibrosis	Non–Cystic Fibrosis–Related Bronchiectasis
Long-term antibiotics		
Aerosol	2003	
Oral	2004, 2006	2007
Airway hydration		
Hypertonic saline	2005	2006
Mannitol		2002
Mucoactive drugs		
DNase	2003	2001
N-acetylcysteine		
Anti-inflammatory drugs		
Oral corticosteroids	2000	2001
Inhaled corticosteroids	2000	
Nonsteroidal agents	2007	2007
Chest physiotherapy	2005	1998
Vaccine		
Influenza	2000	2007
Pneumococcal		2007
Bronchodilator	2005	
Adrenergics		2005
Anticholinergic		2001
Leukotriene antagonists		2000
Oxygen	2008	2000
Surgical resection		

Date of Cochrane review.

Bronchiectasis in this article refers to CF-related and non–CF-related disease based on the relatively unique pathophysiology of CF and the amount of research published on therapies for this condition. This is an oversimplified designation, however. Treatment for different etiologies of non–CF-related bronchiectasis needs to be individualized based on the etiology of the disease. This is particularly true for underlying conditions, such as immunodeficiencies. For example, there are differences between postinfectious bronchiectasis, in which distribution of initial airway injury dictates distribution of bronchiectasis, and primary ciliary dyskinesia, in which the defect in ciliary function is distributed evenly throughout the conducting airways. The endobronchial pathogens related to bronchiectasis resulting from chronic aspiration differ from those in children who have bronchiectasis associated with primary hypogammaglobulinemia.[9,10] The most substantial differences may exist between idiopathic or postinfectious bronchiectasis and bronchiectasis attributable to CF. These include differences in airway pathogens and the age at which they are acquired, sputum rheologic and transport properties, airway hydration, distribution of disease, sputum DNA content, extrapulmonary contributors to disease (eg, pancreatic insufficiency), and overall progressive nature of the disease.[11–13] These differences may result in different efficacies for some of the chronic therapies directed toward bronchiectasis.

CLINICAL COURSE OF BRONCHIECTASIS AND EFFECT OF MANAGEMENT PROGRAMS

The natural course of bronchiectasis is dictated by the underlying etiology, severity at the time of diagnosis, and impact of proactive management programs in specialized centers of expertise. National guidelines for care have been developed by the Cystic Fibrosis Foundation addressing all aspects of the disease management on a quarterly basis to diagnose new infections, nutritional depletion, psychosocial aspects of chronic progressive disease, adherence to treatment plans, and associated CF-related conditions, (eg, diabetes mellitus) that may arise at different ages.[14] In patients who have CF, the median age of survival has significantly increased over time **(Fig. 1)**.[15] Similar programs have been developed for primary ciliary dyskinesia in pediatric pulmonary referral centers. In children who have ciliary dyskinesia, a proactive management regimen that included medical evaluations every 3 months led to stabilizing the progressive decline in lung functions over a median interval of 7 years.[16] The relative contribution of each treatment to the overall improvement in outcomes is difficult to assess, but longitudinal studies demonstrate that comprehensive proactive management programs improve pulmonary outcomes of children and adults with these diagnoses.

In children who have idiopathic bronchiectasis, there is a spectrum of airway disease and injury at the time of diagnosis. Differentiation between radiographic features of "cylindric" and "saccular" bronchiectasis is made assuming that the former might be reversible and that the latter, even with medical therapy, is not. Several published series have cited complete resolution of symptoms related to idiopathic bronchiectasis over time.[8,17] Radiographic resolution of bronchiectasis can occur shortly after pneumococcal pneumonia and after chronic foreign body removal.[18] In contrast, idiopathic bronchiectasis in childhood can also progress by extension to new areas and by evolving into irreversible saccular changes in previously involved lung regions.[19,20] The presence, extension, and progression of airway obstruction in children who have idiopathic

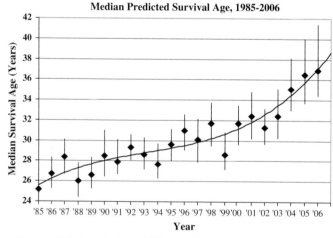

Fig. 1. The median predicted survival was 36.9 years for 2006. The data are based on the ages of patients who have CF in the Cystic Fibrosis Foundation Registry and the mortality distribution of the deaths in 2006. The 95% confidence indicators are noted for each year. In 2006, the median predicted survival was between 34.4 and 41.4 years. (*Adapted from* Cystic Fibrosis Foundation. Cystic fibrosis foundation patient registry. 2006 annual data report to the center directors. Bethesda (MD): Cystic Fibrosis Foundation; 2007; with permission.)

bronchiectasis vary with extent and distribution of disease but progress more slowly than in children who have CF. This is illustrated in **Fig. 2** based on longitudinal trends in best lung function (forced expiratory volume in 1 second [FEV$_1$]) assessed annually among children with CF- and non–CF-related bronchiectasis.[11] Comprehensive management programs have been recommended for idiopathic bronchiectasis of childhood similar to those for CF and ciliary dyskenesia.[6] Long-term results of such programs for idiopathic bronchiectasis have not been evaluated, however.

SPECIFIC THERAPIES

Individual treatments for bronchiectasis fall into several larger categories as depicted in **Table 1**. Those that have been addressed by the Cochrane database and the date of the report are also noted in **Table 1**. These include prevention and reduction of infection, enhanced mucus clearance, improvements in sputum rheology, treatment of reversible airway obstruction if present, improved respiratory muscle strength and endurance, and reductions in airway inflammation. For severe disease, lung transplantation is an option for patients who have CF.[21] Surgical resection of localized bronchiectatic regions also is a treatment option.

A recent report by the Pulmonary Therapies Committee of the Cystic Fibrosis Foundation graded the quality of evidence in the literature pertaining to chronic treatments for CF-related lung disease.[22] As part of that evidence-based process, the committee assessed treatment effects based on whether patients had mild or severe lung disease at the onset of treatment. This valuable distinction has not been made for other etiologies of bronchiectasis. The reader is directed to that publication to review how efficacies of different therapies differ between mild and severe bronchiectasis attributable to CF. In addition, published studies use various short- and long-term outcome measures to assess the utility of different treatments. For purposes of this article, a long-term outcome has been chosen arbitrarily is one measured over at least a 6-month interval. Lung-related and extrapulmonary outcome measures described for the treatment of chronic bronchiectasis are listed in **Box 2**.

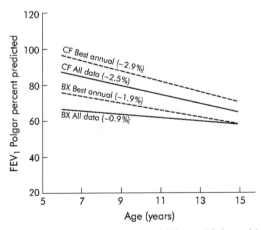

Fig. 2. Linear mixed-model estimated FEV$_1$ among children with bronchiectasis and children with CF using best FEV$_1$ data (*dotted line*) and all annual data (*solid line*) using FEV$_1$ as a percent predicted value obtained longitudinally. (*From* Twiss J, Stewart AW, Byrnes CA. Longitudinal pulmonary function of childhood bronchiectasis and comparison with cystic fibrosis. Thorax 2006;61:417; with permission.)

Box 2
Outcome variables for treatment of bronchiectasis

Lung-related

    Spirometry: forced vital capacity

    FEV_1

    Rate of decline in FEV_1

    Time to first acute exacerbation after onset of therapy

    Exacerbation frequency per time interval

    Number of antibiotic courses

    Days of hospital treatment of pulmonary status

    Sputum volume

    Sputum viscoelasticity

    Airway reactivity (methacholine responsiveness)

    Sputum neutrophils and cytokine levels

Extrapulmonary

    Weight velocity

    Bacterial density in sputum

    C-reactive protein

    Days of lost work

    Quality of life assessment

Antimicrobial Therapy

Chronic antibiotic therapy directed toward endobronchial pathogens producing infection, inflammation, and secretion production in patients who have bronchiectasis have been studied in CF- and non–CF-related bronchiectasis.[3,23–30] The treatments have been targeted toward specific pathogens, such as *Pseudomonas* and *Staphylococcus*, and for idiopathic bronchiectasis, *Haemophilus influenzae* non-type B. Aerosol treatment with tobramycin for *Pseudomonas* endobronchial infection in children who have CF, reported in seven RCTs, has led to short- and long-term benefits, including improvement in lung functions, reduction in acute exacerbations and days of hospitalization, and reduced rate of decline in lung functions for longer than 32 months.[3,28,29,31–33] The risk for producing resistant strains of *Pseudomonas* exists for up to 30% of patients, compared with 17% of patients in the control group, but occurs infrequently enough that benefits outweigh the risks.[29] Aerosol tobramycin is recommended as a chronic therapy for mild to severe lung disease related to CF in children with documented *Pseudomonas* endobronchial infection.[22]

Use of inhaled colistin has been less well studied, and its role is based on two RCTs of short duration (48–90 days).[34,35] In a randomized trial, colistin administered by inhalation initially over 4 weeks and subsequently over 5 months did not improve FEV_1, in contrast to a mean 7% improvement with aerosolized tobramycin over the same duration in children with CF.[35] Additional aerosolized antibiotics directed toward *Pseudomonas*, such as aztreonam, are currently in clinical trials in patients who have CF.[36] A systematic review of five RCTs using antistaphycoccal treatment for existing bronchiectasis with staphylococcal infection in patients who have CF found that no outcome was consistently improved.[37] Eradication of *Staphylococcus* from sputum was most commonly described, but reductions in cough frequency, respiratory exacerbations, and antibiotic courses were not consistently demonstrated across studies. Use of continuous (>200 days per year) antistaphylococcal antibiotics was associated with a significantly higher rate of new-onset *Pseudomonas* airway colonization than was intermittent antistaphylococcal therapy in young children who had CF.[38] The latter antibiotic has not been recommended for use on a chronic basis in children who have CF based on this risk compared with the modest reported benefits.[22]

Oral macrolide therapy has been studied with the rationale that this class of antibiotics has anti-inflammatory and antisecretogogue properties in addition to antimicrobial properties and that the former may be a more important mechanism of efficacy.[39] Three RCTs involving adults and children who had CF have reported a consistent and modest improvement in FEV$_1$ values (average of 5.8%) when oral macrolides are administered daily to three times per week over a 3- to 6-month period.[27,30,40,41] The study by Wolter and colleagues[30] also reported a reduction in hospital days and serum C-reactive protein levels and a reduced rate of decline in lung functions over a 3-month interval among adults with CF. Azithromycin administered two times per week over 6 months reduced use of oral antibiotics for acute exacerbations and improved quality-of-life survey results but did not affect lung functions among adults who had non–CF-related bronchiectasis.[26] Two small, short-term, randomized studies in children with non–CF-related bronchiectasis found no changes in lung function but reduced airway hyperreactivity and reduced proinflammatory cytokine levels in bronchoalveolar lavage after 3 months of roxithromycin and clarithromycin, respectively.[42,43]

Among children with non–CF-related bronchiectasis, there have been no long-term RCTs using antibiotics by any route on a chronic basis. Antipseudomonal treatment in non–CF-related bronchiectasis is limited to adults and some older children with non–CF-related bronchiectasis because the age acquisition of *Pseudomonas* is later than among children who have CF.[44,45] In these older age groups, *Pseudomonas* eradication can occur with 4-week courses of aerosolized tobramycin.[46] Short-term (weeks) of therapy with amoxicillin reduced sputum volume and improved lung function in children with non–CF-related bronchiectasis.[24] Daily amoxicillin over 32 weeks reduced time away from work and daily expectorated sputum volume but did not influence exacerbation rates in adults with non–CF-related bronchiectasis.[25]

Airway Hydration, Mucolytic Treatment, and Chest Physiotherapy

Reduced periciliary airway lining fluid is considered a primary pathogenic mechanism in CF that impairs mucus clearance by reducing the function of airway cilia.[12] In addition, rheologic and transport properties of mucus are abnormal in patients who have CF and patients who have ciliary dyskinesia, more so than among children who have idiopathic bronchiectasis.[47] Therapies that hydrate the airway and airway mucus and those that modify mucus rheology in a way that improves mucus transport have been studied in CF- and non–CF-related bronchiectasis.

Airway hydration has been accomplished with inhalation of hypertonic (6%–7% saline), which draws water from cells and tissues into the airway lumen as a result of its hyperosmolality. Use of 7% saline daily for 48 weeks in an RCT involving adults and children who had CF led to a reduction in exacerbations and improvement in FEV$_1$ but no change in the rate of decline in FEV$_1$ compared with controls.[48] Short-term use of 6% inhaled saline over a 2-week period in patients who had CF improved

FEV_1, suggesting that the effect is rapid in onset.[49] The risk for bronchospasm, which can occur with inhalation of hyperosmolar agents, is substantially reduced with pre-treatment with albuterol.[50] Inhaled dry powder mannitol is an alternative hydrating agent that improves secretion clearance in a dose-dependent manner (160–480 mg per inhalation) acutely among adults who have non–CF-related bronchiectasis.[51] In several short-term (2-week) studies, inhaled mannitol increased FEV_1 by 7% in adults who had CF and improved quality of life in surveys among adult patients who had non–CF-related bronchiectasis.[52,53] Long-term studies using RCT designs are needed to see if this mannitol proves as useful as hypertonic saline to improve secretion clearance in CF- and non–CF-related bronchiectasis.[54]

Mucolytic agents directly alter physical viscoelastic and transport properties of mucus, which are abnormal among children and adults who have CF and primary ciliary dyskinesia.[47] The most studied agent is dornase-α or recombinant human DNase, which degrades extracellular polymers of DNA derived from inflammatory cell breakdown and debris. Used for periods of 6 days to 96 weeks, inhaled DNase once or twice per day increases FEV_1, reduces hospitalizations, improves quality of life, and reduces the decline in lung functions associated with bronchiectasis attributable to CF.[32,55–60] Nine long-term RCTs have demonstrated the consistency of this finding in patients who had mild and severe lung disease attributable to CF, and the daily use of DNase to improve mucus clearance is recommended for both groups of patients who have CF.[22]

In contrast to these findings, the use of DNase among adults with non–CF-related bronchiectasis has not provided any benefit. O'Donnell[61] reported the one RCT of twice-daily DNase, compared with placebo, for 24 weeks among adults who had idiopathic bronchiectasis. Patients receiving DNase had significantly more protocol-defined exacerbations, a greater annual rate of decline in FEV_1, and more days of antibiotic use compared with patients receiving placebo. The reasons for these findings are not clear, although in vitro sputum transportability is worsened by DNase when sputum samples from adults who had idiopathic bronchiectasis were tested.[62] These results underscore the need for clinical trials in non–CF-related bronchiectasis without extrapolation of results from patients who have CF.

N-acetylcysteine disrupts sulfide bonds and thereby reduces the viscosity of purulent mucus sampled from children who have CF. It has been studied in a small number of children who have CF over short periods. Although modest improvements were noted compared with placebo-treated patients over 12 weeks, the changes in lung function were small.[63,64] Given the impact of DNase for patients who have CF, N-acetylcysteine is not a long-term treatment of choice as a mucolytic agent.

Chest physiotherapy (CPT) includes multiple techniques to improve mucus clearance in conjunction with spontaneous or directed cough. Short-term studies have been reported comparing CPT with no CPT, often in a hospital setting, and also comparing different CPT techniques with one another among patients who have CF and adults who have idiopathic bronchiectasis. Short-term outcomes of benefit include volume, weight, and viscoelasticity of sputum, but long-term studies have not consistently demonstrated the benefit of this therapy in patients who have CF.[65] CPT using positive expiratory devices has recently been reviewed by the Cochrane collaboration separately.[66] Those studies of sufficient quality were conducted over 3 months and failed to show an improvement in FEV_1 values. Of note, patients who had CF preferred these devices and also self-directed therapies more than conventional CPT techniques.[67] Among adults who have chronic obstructive lung disease and bronchiectasis, there have not been enough or sufficient quality studies to assess the impact of CPT techniques on long-term outcomes.[68]

ANTI-INFLAMMATORY AGENTS

Therapies for bronchiectasis have been designed to reduce chronic neutrophilic inflammation in addition to eradicating infection. Corticosteroids and nonsteroidal anti-inflammatory treatment have been studied. The use of long-term oral corticosteroids (1–2 mg/kg every other day) consistently increased FEV_1 and reduced the rate of decline in lung function over 4 years in children who had CF.[69–71] The largest of these RCTs also reported adverse side effects, however, which included abnormalities in glucose metabolism, reduced height velocity, and cataracts.[70] Risks therefore outweighed the reported benefits, and long-term corticosteroids are thus not recommended to treat CF-related bronchiectasis. Inhaled corticosteroids have also been studied in hopes of reducing systemic side effects associated with oral corticosteroids. Seven RCTs with a duration of up to 6 months involving children and adults who had CF have been reported using different compounds at various doses.[72] No improvements in lung functions, time to exacerbations, or decline in lung functions over time occurred in any of the studies.

Use of nonsteroidal anti-inflammatory agents also has potential to reduce neutrophilic airway inflammation without the side effects of oral corticosteroid therapy. Konstan and colleagues[73] reported a reduction in the rate of lung function decline and improved weight gain but no change in the frequency of pulmonary exacerbations when high doses of ibuprofen given twice daily were used for 4 years in children who had CF. Change in the rate of decline in FEV_1 produced by ibuprofen is illustrated in **Fig. 3.** An additional trial has reported similar findings.[74] Severe gastrointestinal bleeding in less than 1% of patients receiving drug was considered an acceptable risk compared with the benefits of long-term use among patients who have mild pulmonary disease.[75]

Long-term oral steroid therapy has not been studied in idiopathic bronchiectasis. Steroids are indicated in the treatment of allergic bronchopulmonary aspergillosis, whether bronchiectasis is present or absent. Steroid therapy for bronchiectasis in children is therefore etiology specific. Among children who have idiopathic

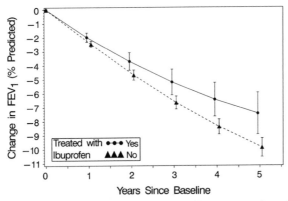

Fig. 3. Estimated average change from baseline FEV_1 as percentage of predicted value over 5 years between patients who had CF and were treated or not treated with high-dose ibuprofen, based on Cystic Fibrosis Foundation Registry data from 1996 through 2002. (*From* Konstan MW, Schluchter MD, Xue W, et al. Clinical use of ibuprofen is associated with slower FEV_1 decline in childre with cystic fibrosis. Am J Respir Crit Care Med 2007;176(11):1084–9; with permission. Copyright © 2007, American Thoracic Society.)

Box 3
Summary of long-term treatment recommendations for childhood

1. Comprehensive interdisciplinary chronic disease management programs should treat children with bronchiectasis (CF- and non–CF-related bronchiectasis).

   Grade: low evidence; evidence: cohort studies

2. Pathogen-directed aerosolized tobramycin treatment should be used long term on a regular basis to improve the course of CF-related bronchiectasis.

   Grade: high; evidence: Cochrane reviews, RCTs

3. Oral macrolide antibiotic use short term (up to 6 months) improves lung function among children with CF-related bronchiectasis.

   Grade: moderate; evidence: Cochrane reviews, few RCTs

4. Long-term antibiotic use (oral or aerosolized) in children with non–CF-related bronchiectasis has not been studied enough to warrant routine use.

   Grade: extremely low; evidence: no RCTs or cohort studies

5. Hypertonic saline administered by inhalation used long term (48 weeks) improves lung function and is safer when used with pretreatment bronchodilator therapy among children who have CF.

   Grade: moderate; evidence: Cochrane review, few RCTs

6. Nebulized dornase-α improves multiple pulmonary outcomes of children who have CF and is indicated for long-term use.

   Grade: high; evidence: Cochrane review, RCTs

7. The risks for long-term oral corticosteroid use outweigh pulmonary benefits in the treatment of CF-related bronchiectasis.

   Grade: moderate; evidence: RCTs

8. High-dose ibuprofen therapy reduces the rate of decline among children with mild CF-related bronchiectasis and is indicated for long-term use.

   Grade: moderate; evidence: Cochrane reviews, few RCTs

9. Mucolytic agents, airway hydrating treatments, anti-inflammatory therapy, CPT, and bronchodilator therapy have not been studied sufficiently long term in children with non–CF-related bronchiectasis to merit their routine use.

   Grade: low; evidence: no RCTs

---

bronchiectasis, no long-term RCTs have been conducted to assess the effects of inhaled corticosteroids or oral ibuprofen.[76]

OTHER THERAPIES

Remarkably, there are insufficient RCTs to grade the evidence for many pulmonary therapies for bronchiectasis in children who do not have CF. These therapies include short- and long-acting β-adrenergic agonists, nonsteroidal anti-inflammatory agents, leukotriene receptor antagonists, pneumococcal vaccines, and annual influenza vaccines.[77–81] Among adults who have bronchiectasis, only subpopulations of patients with bronchial hyperreactivity respond to chronic bronchodilator treatment.[78] Although far more patients who have bronchiectasis are treated medically than in the past, there are no randomized trials to compare medical therapy versus surgical removal of bronchiectatic regions.[82] Surgery remains a consideration when bronchiectasis is localized to one lobe.

The chronic therapy for bronchiectasis for children who have CF and those who do not have CF has been additive as new modalities are studied. The sequence of albuterol, hypertonic saline, DNAase, and aerosol antibiotic treatments two to three times per day constitutes an increasing burden of care for patients and families. The additivity or synergy of these different therapies has not been demonstrated, nor has the importance of each therapy relative to the others been studied. Data addressing efficacy of different combinations of therapies for non–CF-related bronchiectasis in children are nonexistent. Although it has become customary for patients who have CF to use multiple therapies for bronchiectasis determined at referral CF centers, the same is not true for non–CF-related bronchiectasis. A similar network for children with non–CF-related bronchiectasis is necessary if treatments for this group of children are to be studied and recommendations for treatment are to be derived.

SUMMARY

A summary of the recommendations and graded evidence for long-term treatment of CF- and non–CF-related bronchiectasis is provided in **Box 3**. Bronchiectasis is a chronic airway condition that responds to multiple modalities of chronic treatment directed toward airway infection, inflammation, hydration, and mucus stasis. Rigorous studies addressing treatment of bronchiectasis in children who have CF have led to standards of care that are widely practiced. Similar data for children who have bronchiectasis unrelated to CF is lacking. Although approaches to chronic treatment are extrapolated from studies pertaining to CF in children and non–CF-related bronchiectasis in adults, treatments may not produce the same responses or benefits for children with non–CF-related bronchiectasis. Studies directed toward this condition have an impact, particularly in the developing world and among children with other underlying conditions in industrialized countries.

ACKNOWLEDGMENTS

The author thanks Holly Kaopuiki for her assistance in preparing the manuscript and figures for publication.

REFERENCES

1. Westcott JL. Bronchiectasis. Radiol Clin North Am 1991;29:1031–42.
2. Murphy TD, Anbar RD, Lester LA, et al. Treatment with tobramycin solution for inhalation reduces hospitalizations in young CF subjects with mild lung disease. Pediatr Pulmonol 2004;38:314–20.
3. Grade Working Group. Education and debate—grading quality of evidence and strength of recommendations. BMJ 2007;328:1–8.
4. Available at: http://www.cochrane.org/reviews.
5. Callahan CW, Redding GJ. Bronchiectasis in children: orphan disease or persistent problem? Pediatr Pulmonol 2002;33:492–6.
6. Chang AB, Grimwood K, Mulholland EK, et al. Bronchiectasis in indigenous children in remote Australian communities. Med J Aust 2002;177:200–4.

7. Edwards EA, Asher MI, Byrnes CA. Paediatric bronchiectasis in the twenty-first century: experience of a tertiary children's hospital in New Zealand. J Paediatr Child Health 2003;39:111–7.

8. Singleton R, Morris A, Redding G, et al. Bronchiectasis in Alaska Native children: causes and clinical courses. Pediatr Pulmonol 2000;29:182–7.

9. Brook I, Finegold SM. Bacteriology of aspiration pneumonia in children. Pediatrics 1980;65:1115–20.

10. Lischner HW, Huang NN. Respiratory complications of primary hypogammaglobulinemia. Pediatr Ann 1977;6:514–25.

11. Twiss J, Stewart AW, Byrnes CA. Longitudinal pulmonary function of childhood bronchiectasis and comparison with cystic fibrosis. Thorax 2006;61:414–8.

12. Gibson RL, Burns JL, Ramsey BW. Pathophysiology and management of pulmonary infections in cystic fibrosis. Am J Respir Crit Care Med 2003;168:918–51.

13. Chang AB, Redding GJ, Bronchiectasis. In: Chernick V, Boat TF, Wilmott RW, et al, editors. Disorders of the respiratory tract in children, vol 7. Philadelphia: Elsevier Inc., 2006. p. 463–77.

14. Aitken ML, Bergman D, Bolek J, et al. Clinical practice guidelines for cystic fibrosis. Bethesda (MD): Cystic Fibrosis Foundation; 1997.

15. Cystic Fibrosis Foundation, Cystic Fibrosis Foundation patient registry. 2006 annual data report to the center directors, Bethesda (MD), 2007.

16. Ellerman A, Bisgaard H. Longitudinal study of lung function in a cohort of primary ciliary dyskinesia. Eur Respir J 1997;10:2376–9.

17. Landau LI, Phelan PD, Williams HE. Ventilatory mechanics in patients with bronchiectasis starting in childhood. Thorax 1974;29:304–12.

18. Gaillard EA, Carty H, Heaf D, et al. Reversible bronchial dilatation in children. Comparison of serial high-resolution computed tomography scans of the lungs. Eur J Radiol 2003;47:215–20.

19. Clark NS. Bronchiectasis in childhood. BMJ 1963;1:80–8.

20. Wilson JF, Decker AM. The surgical management of childhood bronchiectasis. Ann Surg 1982;195:354–63.

21. Orens JB, Estenne M, Arcasoy S, et al. International guidelines for the selection of lung transplant candidates: 2006 update—a consensus report from the Pulmonary Scientific Council of the International Society for Heart and Lung Transplantation. J Heart Lung Transplant 2006;25:745–55.

22. Flume PA, O'Sullivan BP, Robinson KA, et al. Cystic fibrosis pulmonary guidelines: chronic medications for maintenance of lung health. Am J Respir Crit Care Med 2007;176:957–69.

23. Chang AB, Redding GJ, Everard ML. Chronic wet cough: protracted bronchitis, chronic suppurative lung disease and bronchiectasis. Pediatr Pulmonol 2008;43:519–31.

24. Cole PJ, Roberts DE, Davies SF, et al. A simple oral antimicrobial regimen effective in severe chronic bronchial suppuration associated with culturable *Haemophilus influenzae*. J Antimicrob Chemother 1983;11:109–13.

25. Currie DC, Garbett ND, Chan KL, et al. Double-blind randomized study of prolonged higher-dose oral amoxicillin in purulent bronchiectasis. QJM 1990;76:799–816.

26. Cymbala AA, Edmonds LC, Bauer MA, et al. The disease-modifying effeccts of twice-weekly oral azithromycin in patients with bronchiectasis. Treat Respir Med 2005;4:117–22.

27. Equi A, Balfour-Lynn IM, Bush A, et al. Long term azithromycin in children with cystic fibrosis: a randomised, placebo-controlled crossover trial. Lancet 2002; 360:978–84.

28. MacLusky IB, Gold R, Corey M, et al. Long-term effects of inhaled tobramycin in patients with cystic fibrosis colonized with *Pseudomonas aeruginosa.* Pediatr Pulmonol 1989;7:42–8.

29. Ramsey BW, Pepe MS, Quan M, et al. Cystic Fibrosis Inhaled Study Group. Intermittent administration of inhaled tobramycin in patients with cystic fibrosis. N Engl J Med 1999;340:23–30.

30. Wolter J, Seeney S, Bell S, et al. Effect of long term treatment with azithromycin on disease parameters in cystic fibrosis: a randomised trial. Thorax 2002; 57:212–6.

31. Ramsey BW, Astley SJ, Aitken ML, et al. Efficacy and safety of short-term administration of aerosolised recombinant human deoxyribonuclease in patients with cystic fibrosis. Am Rev Respir Dis 1993;148:145–51.

32. Ramsey BW, Dorkin HL, Eisenberg JD, et al. Efficacy of aerosolized tobramycin in patients with cystic fibrosis. N Engl J Med 1993;328:1740–6.

33. Wiesemann HG, Steinkamp G, Ratjen F, et al. Placebo-controlled, double-blind, randomized study of aerosolized tobramycin for early treatment of *Pseudomonas aeruginosa* colonization in cystic fibrosis. Pediatr Pulmonol 1998;25:88–92.

34. Adeboyeku D, Scott S, Hodson ME. Open follow-up study of tobramycin nebuliser solution and colistin patients with cystic fibrosis. J Cyst Fibros 2006;5:261–3.

35. Hodson ME, Gallagher CG, Govan JRW. A randomised clinical trial of nebulilsed tobramycin or colistin in cystic fibrosis. Eur Respir J 2002;20:658–64.

36. Gibson RL, Retsch-Bogart GZ, Oermann C, et al. Microbiology, safety, and pharmacokinetics of aztreonam lysinate for inhalation in patients with cystic fibrosis. Pediatr Pulmonol 2006;41:656–65.

37. McCaffery K, Olver RE, Franklin M, et al. Systematic review of antistaphylococcal antibiotic therapy in cystic fibrosis. Thorax 1999;54:380–3.

38. Ratjen F, Comes G, Paul K, et al. Effect of continuous antistaphylococcal therapy on the rate of *P. aeruginosa* acquisition in patients with cystic fibrosis. Pediatr Pulmonol 2001;31:13–6.

39. Bush A, Rubin BK. Macrolides as biological response modifiers in cystic fibrosis and bronchiectasis. Semin Respir Crit Care Med 2003;24:737–47.

40. Saiman L, Marshall BC, Mayer-Hamblett N, et al. Azithromycin in patients with cystic fibrosis chronically infected with *Pseudomonas aeruginosa*: a randomized controlled trial. JAMA 2003;290:1749–56.

41. Southern KW, Barker PM, Solis A. Macrolide antibiotics for cystic fibrosis. Cochrane Database Syst Rev 2004;(2):CD002203.

42. Koh YY, Lee MH, Sun YH, et al. Effect of roxithromycin on airway responsiveness in children with bronchiectasis: a double-blind, placebo-controlled study. Eur Respir J 1997;10:994–9.

43. Yalcin E, Kiper N, Ozcelik U, et al. Effects of clarithromycin on inflammatory parameters and clinical conditions in children with bronchiectasis. J Clin Pharm Ther 2006;31:49–55.

44. Noone PG, Leigh MW, Sannuti A, et al. Primary ciliary dyskinesia—diagnostic and phenotypic features. Am J Respir Crit Care Med 2004;169:459–67.

45. Rosenfeld M, Gibson RL, McNamara S, et al. Early pulmonary infection, inflammation, and clinical outcomes in infants with cystic fibrosis. Pediatr Pulmonol 2001;32:356–66.

46. Barker AJ, Couch L, Fiel SB, et al. Tobramycin solution for inhalation reduces sputum *Pseudomonas aeruginosa* density in bronchiectasis. Am J Respir Crit Care Med 2000;162:481–5.

47. Bush A, Payne D, Pike S, et al. Mucus properties in children with primary ciliary dyskinesia: comparison with cystic fibrosis. Chest 2006;129:118–23.

48. Elkins MR, Robinson M, Rose BR, et al. A controlled trial of long-term inhaled hypertonic saline in patients with cystic fibrosis. N Engl J Med 2006;354: 229–40.

49. Eng PA, Morton J, Douglass JA, et al. Short-term efficacy of ultrasonically nebulized hypertonic saline in cystic fibrosis. Pediatr Pulmonol 1996;21:77–83.

50. Delvaux M, Henket M, Lau L, et al. Nebulised salbutamol administered during sputum induction improves bronchoprotection in patients with asthma. Thorax 2004;59:111–5.

51. Daviskas E, Anderson SD, Eberl S, et al. Effect of increasing doses of mannitol on mucus clearance in patients with bronchiectasis. Eur Respir J 2008;31:765–72.

52. Daviskas E, Anderson SD, Gomes K, et al. Inhaled mannitol for the treatment of mucociliary dysfunction in patients with bronchiectasis: effect on lung function, health status and sputum. Respirology 2005;10:46–56.

53. Jaques A, Daviskas E, Turton JA, et al. Inhaled mannitol improves lung function in cystic fibrosis. Chest 2008;133:1388–96.

54. Wills PJ, Greenstone M. Inhaled hyperosmolar agents for bronchiectasis. Cochrane Database Syst Rev 2006;(2):CD002996.

55. Fuchs HJ, Borowitz DS, Christiansen DH, et al. Pulmozyme Study Group. Effect of aerosolized recombinant human DNase on exacerbations of respiratory symptoms and on pulmonary function in patients with cystic fibrosis. N Engl J Med 1994;331:637–42.

56. Furuya MEY, Lezana-Fernandez JL, Vargas MH, et al. Efficacy of human recombinant DNase in pediatric patients with cystic fibrosis. Arch Med Res 2001;32:30–4.

57. Laube BL, Auci RM, Shields DE, et al. Effect of rhDNase on airflow obstruction and mucociliary clearance in cystic fibrosis. Am J Respir Crit Care Med 1996; 153:752–60.

58. Quan JM, Tiddens HAWM, Sy JP, et al. A two-year randomized placebo-controlled trial of dornase alfa in young patients with cystic fibrosis with mild lung function abnormalities. J Pediatr 2001;139:813–20.

59. Ranasinha C, Assoufi B, Shak S, et al. Efficacy and safety of short-term administration of aerosolised recombinant human DNase I in adults with stable stage cystic fibrosis. Lancet 1993;342:199–202.

60. Shah PL, Scott SF, Knight RA, et al. *In vivo* effects of recombinant human DNase I on sputum in patients with cystic fibrosis. Thorax 1996;51:119–25.

61. O'Donnell AE, Barker AF, Ilowite JS, et al. Treatment of idiopathic bronchiectasis with aerosolized recombinant human DNase I. rhDNase Study Group. Chest 1998;113:1329–34.

62. Wills PJ, Wodehouse T, Corkery K, et al. Short-term recombinant human DNase in bronchiectasis. Effect on clinical state and in vitro sputum transportability. Am J Respir Crit Care Med 1996;154:413–7.

63. Ratjen F, Wonne R, Posselt HG, et al. A double-blind placebo controlled trial with oral ambroxol and *N*-acetylcysteine for mucolytic treatment in cystic fibrosis. Eur J Pediatr 1985;144:374–8.

64. Stafanger G, Garne S, Howitz P, et al. The clinical effect and the effect on the ciliary motility of oral N-acetylcysteine in patients with cystic fibrosis and primary ciliary dyskinesia. Eur Respir J 1988;1:161–7.

65. Jones AP, Rowe BH. Bronchopulmonary hygiene physical therapy for chronic obstructive pulmonary disease and bronchiectasis. Cochrane Database Syst Rev 2000;(2):CD000045.

66. Elkins MR, Jones A, Van der Schans C. Positive expiratory pressure physiotherapy for airway clearance in people with cystic fibrosis. Cochrane Database Syst Rev 2006;(2):CD003147.

67. Main E, Prasad A, Schans C. Conventional chest physiotherapy compared to other airway clearance techniques for cystic fibrosis. Cochrane Database Syst Rev 2005;(1):CD002011.

68. McCool FD, Rosen MJ. Nonpharmacologic airway clearance therapies. Chest 2006;129:250S–9S.

69. Auerbach HS, Williams M, Kirkpatrick JA, et al. Alternate-day prednisone reduces morbidity and improves pulmonary function in cystic fibrosis. Lancet 1985;2: 686–8.

70. Eigen H, Rosenstein BJ, FitzSimmons S, et al. A multicenter study of alternate-day prednisone therapy in patients with cystic fibrosis. Cystic Fibrosis Foundation Prednisone Trial Group. J Pediatr 1995;126:515–23.

71. Greally P, Hussain MJ, Vergani D, et al. Interleukin-1α, soluble interleukin-2 receptor, and IgG concentrations in cystic fibrosis treated with prednisolone. Arch Dis Child 1994;71:35–9.

72. Dezateux C, Walters S, Balfour-Lynn I. Inhaled corticosteroids for cystic fibrosis. Cochrane Database Syst Rev 2000;(2):CD001915.

73. Konstan MW, Byard PJ, Hoppel CL, et al. Effect of high-dose ibuprofen in patients with cystic fibrosis. N Engl J Med 1995;332:848–54.

74. Sordelli DO, Macri CN, Maillie AJ, et al. A preliminary study on the effect of antiimflammatory treatment in cystic fibrosis patients with Pseudomonas aeruginosa lung infection. Int J Immunopathol Pharmacol 1994;7:109–17.

75. Konstan MW, Hoppel CL, Chai B, et al. Ibuprofen in children with cystic fibrosis: pharmacokinetics and adverse effects. J Pediatr 1991;118:956–64.

76. Kapur N, Chang AB. Oral non steroid anti-inflammatories for children and adults with bronchiectasis. Cochrane Database Syst Rev 2007;(4):CD006427.

77. Franco F, Sheikh A, Greenstone M. Short acting beta-2 agonists for bronchiectasis. Cochrane Database Syst Rev 2003;(3):CD003572.

78. Halfhide C, Evans HJ, Couriel J. Inhaled bronchodilators for cystic fibrosis. Cochrane Database Syst Rev 2005;(4):CD003428.

79. Chang CC, Morris PS, Chang AB. Influenza vaccine for children and adults with bronchiectasis. Cochrane Database Syst Rev 2007;(3):CD006218.

80. Chang CC, Singleton RJ, Morris PS, et al. Pneumococcal vaccines for children and adults with bronchiectasis. Cochrane Database Syst Rev 2007;(2):CD006316.

81. Corless JA, Warburton CJ. Leukotriene receptor antagonists for non-cystic fibrosis bronchiectasis. Cochrane Database Syst Rev 2000;(4):CD002174.

82. Corless JA, Warburton CJ. Surgery versus non-surgical treatment for bronchiectasis. Cochrane Database Syst Rev 2000;(4):CD002180.

Aspiration Lung Disease

Fernando M. de Benedictis, MD[a],*, Virgilio P. Carnielli, MD[b],
Diletta de Benedictis, MD[c]

KEYWORDS

- Aspiration • Gastroesophageal reflux • Lung disease
- Children

The term *aspiration lung disease* describes several clinical syndromes. At one end of the spectrum is massive aspiration, usually of gastric contents, that causes acute symptoms and, occasionally, respiratory failure, whereas at the other end of the spectrum is chronic lung aspiration (CLA), which is repeated passage of food, gastric reflux, or saliva into the subglottic airways that causes chronic or recurrent respiratory symptoms.[1–3]

CLA has myriad causes and related factors. Clinical findings mainly depend on the amount and nature of the aspirated material, the frequency of aspiration, and the host response. Over the past 2 decades, significant advances have been made in understanding the mechanisms underlying dysphagia, gastroesophageal function, and airway protective reflexes and new diagnostic techniques have been introduced. Despite this, characterizing the presence or absence of aspiration, and under what circumstances a child might be aspirating what, is extremely challenging, and many children are still not adequately diagnosed or treated for aspiration until permanent lung damage has occurred.

ACUTE LUNG ASPIRATION
Disease Mechanisms

Acute lung aspiration is essentially lung injury caused by inhalation of gastric contents. In 1946, Mendelson[4] described patients who aspirated when receiving general anesthesia and first proved that acid is toxic to the respiratory tract. Further studies in humans and animal models showed that aspiration of acidic contents (pH <2.5) into the

[a] Division of Pediatric Medicine, Department of Pediatrics, Salesi Children's University Hospital, 11 via Corridoni, 1-60123, Ancona, Italy
[b] Division of Neonatology, Department of Neonatal Medicine, Salesi Children's University Hospital, 11 via Corridoni, 1-60123, Ancona, Italy
[c] Department of Pediatrics, Postgraduate School of Pediatrics, S. Maria della Misericordia Hospital, University of Perugia, S. Andrea delle Fratte, 1-06156, Perugia, Italy
* Corresponding author.
E-mail address: debenedictis@ao-salesi.marche.it (F.M. de Benedictis).

Pediatr Clin N Am 56 (2009) 173–190
doi:10.1016/j.pcl.2008.10.013
0031-3955/08/$ – see front matter © 2009 Elsevier Inc. All rights reserved.

pediatric.theclinics.com

lungs causes mucosal desquamation, damage to alveolar lining cell and capillaries, and acute neutrophil inflammation. Impaired respiratory tract defenses predispose to secondary pulmonary infection, with the risk increasing with prolonged hospitalization, enteral tube feeding, endotracheal intubation, and use of antacid drugs.

Assessment and Diagnosis

The diagnosis of acute aspiration is mainly clinical and usually involves witnessed inhalation of vomit or tracheal suctioning of gastric contents. Even in the absence of such events, however, a high suspicion index should be maintained when clinical and radiographic findings are compatible with aspiration. Early bronchoscopy may help to define the type of aspiration (ie, liquid versus particulate material) and improve clinical assessment.[5]

Clinical signs of acute aspiration include coughing, wheezing, chest discomfort, and fever. More dramatically, cyanosis, pulmonary edema, and rapid progression to severe respiratory distress syndrome may occur in cases of massive aspiration. Although high mortality was once reported with massive aspiration, recent studies estimated a mortality rate of 5% in children and no deaths when three or fewer lobes were involved.[6]

Management

Apart from immediate unblocking of airways in case of massive aspiration and general supportive care measures, further aspiration must be prevented. The benefits of artificial airway and oral or nasogastric tube placement should be weighed with caution against the increased risk for aspiration because of their effect on swallowing. Administering antacids or sucralfate to raise the stomach pH increases bacterial colonization in the stomach but not in the respiratory tract, and thus does not increase the risk for ventilator-associated pneumonia.[7] The use of corticosteroids is controversial, with some studies proving efficacy, especially when given close to the time of massive aspiration, and others the opposite;[8] given such uncertainty, their use is not generally recommended. Finally, there is some evidence that bronchoalveolar lavage (BAL) with normal saline and surfactant may have clinical value in treating severe aspiration syndrome in children.[9]

Should deterioration occur with some or all of these measures, infection ought to be suspected. Although it does not usually play a primary role in aspiration of gastric contents, the rate of superimposed infection is high. Antibiotics should be withheld unless there are reasonably clear signs of infection. Antibiotic therapy should be selected on the basis of aspiration pneumonia bacteriology, which mainly depends on the presence or absence of preexisting disease, the patient's age, and prior use of antibiotics.[10]

CHRONIC LUNG ASPIRATION

Small-volume aspiration into the lungs is relatively common, even in healthy subjects when normal airway protective mechanisms are impaired, bypassed, or overwhelmed.[11] Whether intermittent or persistent, CLA may occur in some children only coincidentally with other stressors, such as upper respiratory tract infection.

CLA may present with chronic cough, wheeze, noisy breathing, choking during feeding, recurrent episodes of pneumonia or bronchitis, and failure to thrive.[12,13] Chronic aspiration often results in progressive lung disease, bronchiectasis, and respiratory failure and is a major cause of death in children with severe neurologic disorders.[14] There is no "gold standard" test for diagnosing CLA, and determining whether aspiration is a significant cause of respiratory disease remains a challenge in pediatric medicine.

Disease Mechanisms

In subjects with CLA, more than one mechanism may be involved and separating out mechanisms is often difficult. Pulmonary aspiration may occur as a result of swallowing dysfunction, gastroesophageal reflux (GOR), or inability to protect the airway adequately from oral secretions. Furthermore, a tracheoesophageal fistula should always be considered and excluded.[15]

Aspiration attributable to swallowing dysfunction

Normal swallowing, a complex process requiring coordinated voluntary and involuntary actions, involves the mouth, pharynx, larynx, and esophagus in different phases. The maturation of oral and pharyngeal anatomy and the evolution of the suckling process develop parallel to the development of the brain and the nervous system. Anatomic abnormalities and intrinsic dysfunction in the effectiveness, duration, or timing of any of these components can result in direct aspiration.

Although children with neurologic disease are at high risk for aspiration, the inability to coordinate swallowing can be a problem in normal infants, especially those born prematurely.[16] In such cases, cricopharyngeal incoordination is attributable to delayed maturation of swallowing reflexes; it has been suggested that it appears more frequently in young infants with bronchiolitis.[17] A recent retrospective study in children with documented swallowing dysfunction showed that multisystem involvement (ie, medical conditions affecting more than one organ system) was highly associated with aspiration pneumonia.[18]

Reflux aspiration

An association between GOR and respiratory symptoms is well documented,[19,20] but a causal relation is difficult to determine in an individual child.[21,22] Possible mechanisms involved in this relation are listed in **Box 1**. In a study evaluating the relation between aspiration and recurrent respiratory tract infections in children with neurologic disability, Morton and colleagues[23] found that oral and pharyngeal motor problems were the major cause of respiratory involvement and that GOR without a coexisting swallowing dysfunction was less likely to cause respiratory tract infection. Despite these findings emphasizing the role of swallowing dysfunction in children with neurologic disability, patients with GOR have significantly reduced laryngopharyngeal

---

Box 1
Mechanisms for the association of gastroesophageal reflux and respiratory disease

GOR causing respiratory disease

Aspiration

> Direct effect: tracheitis, bronchitis, pneumonia, atelectasis

> Indirect effect: inflammation predisposing to airway hyperreactivity

Reflex mechanism: esophagus-airway reflex

Respiratory disease causing GOR

> Diaphragm flattening and changes in transthoracic pressure gradient

> Decreased lower esophageal sphincter pressure attributable to medication (ie, theophylline)

> Additive effect of chest physiotherapy

sensitivity because of repeated exposure of mucosa to small amounts of acid; this could potentially result in an increased risk for aspiration.[24]

Salivary aspiration

Chronic saliva aspiration is the least commonly recognized form of aspiration and is usually not diagnosed before development of significant lung injury.[3] The oral cavity contains potentially pathogenic organisms that, when aspirated in sufficient quantity, can cause recurrent pneumonia or pulmonary abscess.[10] Most neurologically impaired children who aspirate saliva do so because of severe swallowing incoordination and reduced laryngopharyngeal sensitivity rather than excessive production of saliva.[25]

Assessment

As for any pediatric patient, clinical evaluation is the cornerstone of the general assessment in children with suspected aspiration. A careful evaluation of the patient's history and physical findings should enable the clinician to proceed with appropriate diagnostic studies in a rational staged fashion. Particular conditions that predispose the child to aspirate should be considered in the initial assessment (**Box 2**). In any case, because of the complex nature of chronic aspiration, a multidisciplinary approach is mandatory.

Clinical assessment

When aspiration is suspected, the case history should focus on the timing of symptoms in relation to feeding and position changes, choking, gagging, spitting or vomiting, excessive salivation, apnea, and bradycardia; coughing and wheezing should also be investigated in detail. Coughing and gagging may be minimal or absent in children with a depressed cough reflex, however, as in neurologically impaired subjects (ie, silent aspiration).

Dysmorphic features (ie, micrognathia, macroglossia), which may be associated with structural airway problems, and anatomic abnormalities (ie, cleft palate) should be carefully sought during the clinical examination. Observation of the child during feeding is essential to detect excess drooling, difficulty with sucking, or swallowing with or without associated coughing or choking and, occasionally, nasopharyngeal reflux.

Imaging studies

Plain chest radiographs and high-resolution computed thomography (HRCT) are commonly used in the evaluation of children suspected of aspiration. Although not diagnostic tests for aspiration, they are useful indicators of lung injury and may also document disease progression or resolution over time.[26,27]

Chest radiograph

On radiographs, CLA typically presents as hyperaeration, peribronchial thickening, subsegmental or segmental infiltrates, and atelectasis. Bronchiectasis may also be seen. Basilar and superior segments of lower lobes, in addition to posterior upper lobe segments, are most involved. Chest radiographs are not sufficiently sensitive to detect the subtle changes that occur in early lung injury, however.

High-resolution CT

Chest HRCT is more sensitive in the detection of early airway and parenchymal disease in pediatric patients. In a child with a suggestive history, the combination of airway and parenchymal findings in a distribution pattern that is consistent with aspiration can be interpreted as evidence of lung injury caused by CLA. Such findings as

Box 2
Conditions predisposing to aspiration lung disease

Anatomic

- Micrognathia
- Macroglossia
- Cleft palate
- Laryngeal cleft
- Tracheoesophageal fistula
- Vascular rings

Functional

- Achalasia (cricopharyngeal, esophageal)
- GOR
- Collagen vascular disease (scleroderma, dermatomyositis)
- Tumors, masses, foreign body

Mechanical

- Nasoenteric tube
- Endotracheal tube
- Tracheostomy

Neuromuscular

- Depressed consciousness (eg, general anesthesia, drug intoxication, head trauma, seizures, central nervous system infection)
- Prematurity (immaturity of swallowing)
- Cerebral palsy
- Increased intracranial pressure
- Vocal cord paralysis
- Dysautonomia
- Muscular dystrophy
- Myasthenia gravis
- Polyradiculoneuritis
- Werding-Hoffmann disease

bronchial thickening, air trapping, bronchiectasis, ground-glass opacities, and centrilobular opacities ("tree-in-bud"), although not specific for aspiration, are common in children who chronically aspirate and may indicate a diagnosis.

Diagnosis

By assessing oral motor skills, clinical evaluation of swallowing may provide important information to the clinician but is insufficient to assess aspiration risk accurately.[28] Over the years, new techniques have been introduced and their role for supporting the diagnosis of lung aspiration has been better defined. The accuracy of some diagnostic methods and comparison among them still need to be ascertained in children, however.

Aspiration attributable to swallowing dysfunction

Videofluoroscopic swallow study (VFSS) is considered the gold standard for assessing the oral, pharyngeal, and esophageal phases of swallowing. Although a normal VFSS cannot entirely rule out aspiration because it is episodic in nature, it visualizes an extensive range of swallowing abnormalities (ie, premature spillage of the food bolus before the swallow, delayed swallow reflex, postswallow residue, laryngeal penetration, aspiration into the trachea with or without cough clearance, impaired passage into the esophagus, regurgitation of swallowed food).[29] When the accuracy of clinical evaluation was compared with VFSS, a sensitivity of 92% and 33% in detecting aspiration on a clinical basis was found for fluids and solids, respectively.[30] The inter- and intraobserver reliability of VFSS for the different parameters of swallowing is generally poor, except for detection of penetration or aspiration events.[31] The strengths and limitations of VFSS, and of other techniques, are summarized in **Table 1**.

Fiberoptic endoscopic evaluation of swallowing (FEES) enables direct visualization of the oral and pharyngeal phases but does not reveal events after pharyngeal contraction.[32] FEES is as sensitive as VFSS and has similar,[33] or even superior,[34] inter- and intraobserver reliability rates in detecting laryngeal penetration or aspiration events. Because FEES and VFSS provide different information, they should be considered complementary in the clinical assessment of a patient with suspect aspiration. Indeed, both studies can optimally assess feeding procedures with different consistencies and the effectiveness of implemented swallowing techniques.

As a test for CLA of various types, a quantitative index of lipid-laden alveolar macrophages (LLAMs) in BAL samples was repeatedly calculated, but results were conflicting. The index often yielded positive values in subjects with non–aspiration-related acute or chronic lung diseases (ie, fat embolism, oil infusions, cystic fibrosis, bronchiolitis obliterans) or in healthy people.[35–44] Cutoffs ranged from 67 to 200, and each institution was advised to determine its own LLAM index cutoff value.[45] A major limitation for using LLAM as a marker of CLA caused by swallowing dysfunction is that GOR was not consistently evaluated as a possible confounder in the various studies.[46] **Table 2** illustrates the variability in assessments of the utility of a LLAM index in the diagnosis of CLA.

Reflux aspiration

Monitoring of esophageal pH for 24 hours has long been considered the standard diagnostic tool for GOR. This method is unable to recognize superimposed acid events that occur after a pH decrease but before pH normalization, however, which may constitute up to 38% of acid reflux events.[47] In addition, it does not document the nonacid reflux of all kinds of fluids from the stomach to the esophagus that can be aspirated and cause lung disease.[48] It is therefore unlikely that simple detection of acid reflux alone is adequate for the diagnostic evaluation of CLA.

Multichannel intraluminal impedance and pH monitoring (MII-pH) has been increasingly studied for its ability to detect anterograde and retrograde passage of acid, non-acid, and gaseous material. By measuring changes in electrical impedance at multiple levels of the esophagus, the movement of a fluid or air bolus is detected; pH is measured simultaneously, thus differentiating between acidic and nonacidic material.[49] MII-pH studies found that children with GOR have a high proportion of nonacid reflux, predominantly in postprandial periods.[47,48] Nonacid reflux detected by MII-pH highly correlated with persistent respiratory symptoms in young children on antacid medications, and may therefore be an important predictor of respiratory disease.[50] MII-pH also detects much more pharyngeal-level reflux than pH monitoring alone; indeed, most of these events are gaseous refluxes with and without minor pH decreases.[51]

Table 1
Summary of diagnostic tests of aspiration

Evaluation	Benefits	Limitations
Chest radiograph	Inexpensive and widely available	Insensitive to subtle changes of lung injury
HRCT	Sensitive in detecting lung injury Assesses progression of lung injury over time	Radiation exposure Expensive
VFSS	Evaluates all phases of swallowing Evaluates multiple consistencies	Limited evaluation of anatomy Radiation exposure Intra- and interobserver variability Expensive
FEES	Evaluates functional anatomy Evaluates multiple consistencies Assesses aspiration in children not feeding orally Can be performed at bedside No radiation exposure	Blind to events after pharyngeal contraction Intra- and interobserver variability Invasive Expensive
BAL	Evaluates anatomy of upper and lower airways Sampling for multiple cytologic and microbiologic tests	Poor reproducibility and difficult interpretation of LLAM index Invasive Expensive
Esophageal pH monitoring	Detects acid reflux events Normative data in children	Blind to most reflux events Poor relation between reflux and aspiration Somewhat invasive
Esophageal impedance monitoring	Detects acid and nonacid reflux events Detects proximal reflux events	Lack of normative data for children Somewhat invasive Expensive and cumbersome to interpret Not widely available
Gastroesophageal scintigraphy	Performed under physiologic conditions Low radiation exposure	Variable sensitivity Does not differentiate between direct and reflux aspiration
Barium esophagram	Useful in detecting anatomic problems May yield information on esophageal motility	Low sensitivity Evaluates one moment in time
Radionuclide salivagram	No need of food bolus challenge Low radiation exposure	Unknown sensitivity Evaluates one moment in time

Abbreviation: LLAM, lipid-laden alveolar macrophages.

Modified from Boesch RP, Daines C, Willging JP, et al. Advances in the diagnosis and management of chronic pulmonary aspiration in children. Eur Respir J 2006;28:850; with permission.

Table 2
Summary of evidence regarding lipid-laden alveolar macrophage index in children

Reference	Comparison Groups	Subjects (n)	Age Mean (Range)	LLAM Index Mean (Range)
Nussbaum et al[36]	Chronic pulmonary disorders without GOR	41	7 years (30 days–14 years)	8 (19%)[a]
	Chronic pulmonary disorders with GOR	74	6 years (23 days–12 years)	63 (85%)[a]
Colombo and Hallberg[37]	Not suspected of food aspiration	23	4.3 years (1 month–25 years)	21 (0–72)
	Suspected of food aspiration	22	2.2 years (1 month–12 years)	139 (86–241)
Moran et al[38]	Lactose assay negative	25	Newborns	121
	Lactose assay positive	18	Newborns	204
Bauer and Lyrene[39]	Not chronic pulmonary aspiration	87	2.8 years	44 (0–170)
	Chronic pulmonary aspiration	26	(2 weeks–15 years)	104 (20–233)
Knauer-Fischer and Ratjen[40]	Surgical controls	18	8.6 years (3–15 years)	60 (35–106)
	Pulmonary disease without aspiration	18	8.2 years (1–16 years)	119 (74–178)
Ahrens et al[41]	Surgical controls	20	5.3 years (18–175 months)	37 (5–188)
	Recurrent pneumonia without GOR	14	3.4 years (10–117 months)	29 (5–127)
	Chronic lung disease and GOR	32	3.4 years (6–21 months)	117 (10–956)
Sacco et al[42]	Respiratory symptoms, pH negative	9	4.6 years (16–136 months)	12 (3–50)
	Respiratory symptoms, pH positive	11	6.6 years (10–145 months)	52 (5–105)
Kazachkov et al[43]	Healthy adult controls	8	26 ± 4 years	1[b]
	Chronic respiratory symptoms	21	2.3 years (2–94 months)	7[b]
	CF, uninfected	24	3.5 years (1–143 months)	19[b]
Furuya et al[44]	No respiratory symptoms, no suspicion of aspiration	41	4.4 years (5–168 months)	108 (5–248)
	Pulmonary disease without suspicion of aspiration	30	5.1 years (1–192 months)	187 (50–291)
	Pulmonary disease and suspicion of aspiration	41	1.6 years (1–132 months)	233 (145–305)

Abbreviation: CF, cystic fibrosis.
[a] Number and percentage of patients who had LLAM in BAL fluid.
[b] Different semiquantitative method was used to calculate the LLAM index.

Because of these characteristics, MII-pH has the potential to become the new gold standard for identifying children at risk for reflux aspiration.[52] At present, the major limitation of this method is lack of normative pediatric data.

Studies attempting to compare LLAM index values in children with chronic respiratory symptoms with and without documented GOR showed even wider variability than studies for direct aspiration. As a confirmatory method for reflux aspiration, Moran and colleagues[38] used a lactose assay in the trachea of intubated neonates who were receiving lactose-containing orogastric feeds. They found that the LLAM index differentiates well between neonates with positive and negative assays. At an index threshold of 100, sensitivity and specificity were 100% and 22%, respectively, whereas at a threshold of 150, they were 73% and 84%, respectively. The relation between LLAM index and GOR as determined by MII-pH has not been investigated, but data would be useful, given the limitations of esophageal pH monitoring alone. Currently, there is insufficient evidence to support the diagnosis of reflux aspiration using the LLAM index, largely because of the difficulty in establishing a causal link between GOR and lung aspiration.[3]

Gastroesophageal scintigraphy ("milk scan") is regarded as a "physiologic" test for detecting reflux and aspiration. After ingestion of a meal mixed with technetium 99m sulfur colloid, serial images are taken to detect tracer activity in the lung parenchyma. Sensitivity is questionable, and it does not clearly differentiate between direct and reflux aspiration.[53–55] One recent study showed that pulmonary aspiration as demonstrated by overnight scintigraphy was common in children with refractory respiratory symptoms and suggested that GOR might be the underlying cause; interestingly, 76% of patients with abnormal scintigraphy had normal pH study results, whereas half of the patients with an abnormal pH study had aspiration.[56] This study confirms that a normal intraesophageal pH study does not rule out GOR, whereas an abnormal pH study does not necessarily confirm aspiration.

A barium esophagram was also used to evaluate GOR or aspiration. This test is not reliable because the brief observation time renders it relatively insensitive for both. The esophagram is most useful for detecting anatomic anomalies, including vascular rings and tracheoesophageal fistulae, and may yield qualitative information on esophageal motility.[57]

Salivary aspiration

In children who continue to have symptoms of aspiration despite cessation of oral feeding and GOR treatment, an evaluation of salivary aspiration is warranted. In contrast, children with significant sialorrhea; choking on secretions; severe neurologic impairment; laryngotracheoesophageal cleft; vocal cord paralysis; coloboma, heart defects, atresia choanae, retardation of growth and development, genitourinary problems, and ear abnormalities (CHARGE) association; Moebius, West or Pfeiffer syndrome; or congenital high airway obstruction syndrome (CHAOS) should undergo evaluation for salivary aspiration earlier in the diagnostic process because there is a much higher likelihood of salivary aspiration with these conditions.[3]

Radionuclide salivagrams are performed by placing a small quantity of radiotracer into the mouth and recording serial images until the oropharynx is cleared of the radiotracer. Activity in the major airways and lung parenchyma indicates aspiration. In retrospective studies, the prevalence of positive salivagrams in children suspected of aspiration is reported to range from 26% to 73%,[58–60] but, unfortunately, no confirmatory tests were performed. Although a radionuclide salivagram is considered the most sensitive test for salivary aspiration, further evaluation regarding its accuracy is needed.

FEES with sensory testing (ST) directly visualizes pooled laryngeal secretions, and impending aspiration is determined by diminished laryngeal sensitivity. Laryngeal sensitivity is quantified by applying graded bursts of air to the aryepiglottic fold and registering the threshold pressure that elicits the laryngeal reflex. As seen in adults, pediatric patients with an increased laryngopharyngeal sensory threshold have a significantly higher likelihood of laryngeal penetration and aspiration during a feeding assessment.[61,62]

Management

In general, current management decisions for children who aspirate have to optimize oral nutrition and hydration and reduce the risk for aspiration to preserve pulmonary integrity (**Box 3**; **Table 3**).

Aspiration attributable to swallowing dysfunction

Pediatric dysphagia is usually a complex disorder in which biologic (ie, structural abnormalities, neurologic or metabolic conditions) and behavioral aspects mutually interact.[63] A multidisciplinary approach with a team of pediatricians, otolaryngologists, neurologists, psychologists, gastroenterologists, pulmonologists, and surgeons is often necessary for management of this disorder.

For dysphagic subjects, an initial plan for feeding intervention can be started with the help of a specialized nurse during the VFSS or FEES. Compensatory strategies, such as positioning, chin tuck, and different consistency feeds, can be gradually implemented. Although restricting oral water ingestion is anecdotally accepted as a useful measure, no trials have adequately evaluated the pulmonary effects of this measure in children with primary aspiration of thin fluids.[64]

For children who are unable to ingest sufficient calories safely by mouth, percutaneous or surgical placement of a feeding gastrostomy or jejunostomy may be needed. Despite normal clinical history and preoperative radiologic and pH studies, GOR can become apparent in neurologically impaired children after gastrostomy tube placement. The benefit of a routine antireflux procedure at the time of gastrostomy tube placement in children with neurologic impairment is the subject of debate. Indeed, such a procedure may prevent postoperative GOR and help to avoid the need for a subsequent surgical procedure, but it is associated with high morbidity and mortality. Although there is little evidence that morbidity or mortality increased in patients without GOR who did not undergo preventive fundoplication, it is generally accepted that neurologically impaired children with symptomatic GOR and swallowing dysfunction should undergo an antireflux procedure at the time of feeding tube placement.[65] Previous exclusion of GOR is therefore needed to establish optimal intervention strategies.[66] Cricopharyngeal achalasia is a specific cause of CLA and may be resolved successfully by cricopharyngeal myotomy.[67]

Box 3
What do I do when a child with suspected aspiration presents?

1. Carefully evaluate for symptoms and signs of aspiration in addition to risk factors for aspiration (see text and **Boxes 1 and 2**). (grade: recommended with benefits, moderate; quality of evidence: cohort studies)

2. Perform diagnostic tests for aspiration (type of test; see **Tables 1 and 2**). (grade: recommended with benefits, moderate; quality of evidence: variable depending on type of tests)

3. Manage aspiration.

Table 3
Management of aspiration lung disease

Type of Intervention	Recommendation[a]	Grading of Recommendation	Quality of Supporting Evidence
Aspiration related to dysphagia			
Compensatory strategies (eg, positioning, chin tuck)	Probably recommended: trade-off	Moderate	Case series
Restriction of water	Not recommended: uncertain trade-off	Extremely low	Systematic review: no data in children
Gastrostomy/ jejunostomy	Recommended: benefits	Moderate	Case series
Reflux aspiration			
Dietary measures (eg, restricting fluids, thickened feeds)	Probably recommended: trade-off	Moderate	Case series and one RCT: limited to the effect on regurgitation
Prokinetic agents (domperidone, erythromycin)	Not recommended: uncertain trade-off	Low	RCTs: limited to the effect on GOR
Acid-reducing agents (H_2 antagonists, PPIs)	Probably recommended: trade-off	Moderate	Case series: limited to the effect on GOR
Fundoplication	Recommended: benefits	High	Case series
Salivary aspiration			
Anticholinergics	Not recommended: uncertain trade-off	Low	Case series and one DBPCT: limited to control of sialorrhea
Botulinum toxin	Probably recommended: uncertain trade-off	Moderate	case series and 1 RCT: limited to control of sialorrhea
Salivary gland duct ligation	Not recommended: uncertain trade-off	Low	Case series: limited to control of sialorrhea
Tracheostomy	Not recommended: uncertain trade-off	Low	Case series

For many interventions, there is little high-quality evidence in children, and even less with respect to magnitude of benefit on symptoms of aspiration.

Abbreviations: DBPCT, double-blind placebo-controlled trial; PPIs, proton pump inhibitors; RCT, randomized controlled trial.

[a] Recommendation involves a trade-off between benefits and harms and is based on diagnostic tests showing evidence of type of aspiration present.

Reflux aspiration

Dietary measures have been recommended for treatment of GOR and make good sense. They include restricting fluids and providing texture-modified diets or thickened feeds. In a randomized, placebo-controlled, crossover study, Wenzl and colleagues[68] showed that thickened feeding significantly decreased the frequency and amount of regurgitation. This effect was caused by reduction in the number and height of nonacid reflux, whereas the occurrence of acid reflux was not reduced. Unfortunately, the effect of dietary measures on CLA lacks rigorous scientific backing.

Alginate-containing antacids form a "raft" that floats on the surface of the stomach contents, which should reduce reflux. Recent assessment of the effect of such a measure on GOR questions its efficacy at preventing reflux.[69]

Over the years, different prokinetic agents have been used for treatment of GOR. With the withdrawal of cisapride and the unacceptable side effects of metoclopramide,[70] the common prokinetic agents include domperidone and erythromycin. Domperidone, a peripheral D_2-receptor antagonist that increases motility and gastric emptying, showed little efficacy in the reduction of reflux symptoms in children[71] and has not been evaluated for the treatment of reflux aspiration. Erythromycin increases gastrointestinal motility by acting directly on motilin (a hormone secreted into the gastrointestinal tract during times of fasting) receptors. Trials involving erythromycin at antimicrobial or low doses have mainly focused on it use in premature neonates and infants with feeding intolerance. Conflicting results in terms of efficacy were obtained.[72,73]

Gastric acid suppressants are widely used for treatment of GOR. Ranitidine, an antagonist of the H_2 receptors of gastric parietal cells, showed greater efficacy in patients with mild GOR than in patients with severe GOR.[74] Proton pump inhibitors (ie, omeprazole, lansoprazole) reduce gastric acid secretion and increase the intragastric pH; their superiority over H_2-receptor antagonists for treatment of GOR has been repeatedly demonstrated.[75] Although the efficacy of gastric acid suppressant has been established for esophagitis, neither safety nor efficacy has been clearly demonstrated for CLA.[76] For many children with GOR-related CLA, medical therapy does not reduce respiratory tract injury, which is not surprising, given the predominance of nonacid reflux in children.

Fundoplication is currently the antireflux procedure of choice in children with persistent or severe respiratory symptoms and reflux aspiration. GOR is eliminated in almost all patients, and respiratory symptoms improve in most.[77–79] Care must be taken to identify the presence of significant esophageal dysmotility before tightening the esophagogastric junction because this can result in significant accumulation of oral secretions in the esophagus and an increased risk for aspiration.[3] In children with neurologic impairment, some researchers recommend jejunostomy tube placement as a primary procedure or after fundoplication failure.[80,81] Although this procedure solves feeding problems and may improve the quality of life, reflux is not completely eliminated and aspiration may continue.

Salivary aspiration

In neurologically impaired children, oral anticholinergic agents are used to treat sialorrhea symptoms. Glycopyrrolate effectively reduced salivation,[82] but whether the reduction persists beyond a few weeks remains to be ascertained. No studies have investigated the effects of anticholinergic drugs on reducing CLA.

The effectiveness of salivary gland injection of botulinum toxin in controlling sialorrhea in children with cerebral palsy has been evaluated with good results, but further research is needed to understand the range of responses fully.[83–85] No study has addressed the effects on CLA-associated respiratory symptoms.

Other potential options for reducing oral secretions are bilateral submandibular and parotid duct ligation or submandibular gland excision with parotid duct ligation. Although both approaches were reported to be effective in children,[86,87] prospective trials are needed.

Children with salivary aspiration often receive tracheostomy because of their underlying medical conditions and for pulmonary toilette. Some studies suggested that the presence of a tracheostomy tube and impaired swallowing were associated,[88,89] but this aspect has not been sufficiently evaluated in children.

Laryngotracheal separation eliminates all continuity between the respiratory and digestive tracts by disconnecting the upper trachea from the larynx.[90] Although this procedure definitively eliminates aspiration, there are several adverse sequelae.

FUTURE DIRECTIONS

Because of the invasive nature of FEES, a promising new method of assessing vocal cord motion using glottic ultrasound was developed to evaluate dysphagia.[91] It may allow for the noninvasive study of pharyngeal and glottic reflexes that favor airway protection in infants. Further development of this technique is awaited.

Gastric pepsin assays on BAL fluid were evaluated as a specific test of GOR-related aspiration, with variable results.[92–94] Pepsin assay in saliva or sputum may provide a promising noninvasive method to test for the proximal reflux of gastric contents, but the experience with this technique is limited.[95]

At present, many questions still remain unanswered, such as how much aspiration is normal at different ages, whether different types of aspiration have different outcomes, and how aspiration during childhood might affect future lung function. More research is needed to shed further light on this heterogeneous and challenging condition of pediatric medicine.

ACKNOWLEDGMENT

The authors thank Consuelo Ramacogi for her help in preparing the manuscript.

REFERENCES

1. Colombo JL, Sammut PH. Aspiration syndromes. In: Taussig LM, Landau LI, editors. Pediatric respiratory medicine. St. Louis (MO): Mosby; 1999. p. 435–43.
2. Marick PE. Aspiration pneumonitis and aspiration pneumonia. N Engl J Med 2001;344(9):665–71.
3. Boesch RP, Daines C, Willging JP, et al. Advances in the diagnosis and management of chronic pulmonary aspiration in children. Eur Respir J 2006; 28(4):846–61.
4. Mendelson CL. The aspiration of the stomach contents into the lungs during obstetric anaesthesia. Am J Obstet Gynecol 1946;52:191–205.
5. Campinos L, Duvall G, Couturier M, et al. The value of early fibreoptic bronchoscopy after aspiration of gastric contents. Br J Anaesth 1983;55(11): 1103–5.
6. Hickling KG, Howard R. A retrospective survey of treatment and mortality in aspiration pneumonia. Intensive Care Med 1988;14(6):617–22.
7. Bonten MJ, Gaillard CA, van der Geest S, et al. The role of intragastric acidity and stress ulcus prophylaxis on colonization and infection in mechanically ventilated ICU patients. A stratified, randomized, double-blind study of sucralfate versus antacids. Am J Respir Crit Care Med 1995;152(6):1825–34.
8. de Benedictis FM, Canny GJ, Levison H. The role of corticosteroids in respiratory diseases of children. Pediatr Pulmonol 1996;22(1):44–57.
9. Marraro GA, Luchetti M, Spada C, et al. Selective medicated (normal saline and exogenous surfactant) bronchoalveolar lavage in severe aspiration syndrome in children. Pediatr Crit Care Med 2007;8(5):476–81.

10. Brook I, Finegold SM. Bacteriology of aspiration pneumonia in children. Pediatrics 1980;65(6):1115–20.
11. Gleeson K, Eggli DF, Maxwell SL. Quantitative aspiration during sleep in normal subjects. Chest 1997;111(5):1266–72.
12. Owayed AF, Campbell DM, Wang EEL. Underlying causes of recurrent pneumonia in children. Arch Pediatr Adolesc Med 2000;154(2):190–4.
13. Lodha R, Puranik M, Natchu UCM, et al. Recurrent pneumonia in children: clinical profile and underlying causes. Acta Paediatr 2002;91(11):1170–3.
14. Gillies JD, Seshia SS. Vegetative state following coma in childhood: evolution and outcome. Dev Med Child Neurol 1980;22(5):642–8.
15. Goyal A, Jones MO, Couriel JM, et al. Oesophageal atresia and tracheo-oesophageal fistula. Arch Dis Child Fetal Neonatal Ed 2006;91(5):381–4.
16. Sheikh S, Allen E, Shell R, et al. Chronic aspiration without gastroesophageal reflux as a cause of chronic respiratory symptoms in neurologically normal infants. Chest 2001;120(4):1190–5.
17. Khoshoo V, Edell D. Previously healthy infants may have increased risk of aspiration during syncytial viral bronchiolitis. Pediatrics 1999;104(6): 1389–90.
18. Weir K, McMahon S, Barry L, et al. Oropharyngeal aspiration and pneumonia in children. Pediatr Pulmonol 2007;42(11):1024–31.
19. Chen PH, Chang MH, Hsu SC. Gastroesophageal reflux in children with chronic recurrent bronchopulmonary infection. J Pediatr Gastroenterol Nutr 1991;13(1): 16–22.
20. Orenstein SR. An overview of reflux-associated disorders in infants: apnea, laryngospasm, and aspiration. Am J Med 2001;111(Suppl 3):60S–3S.
21. Harding SM. Recent clinical investigations examining the association of asthma and gastroesophageal reflux. Am J Med 2003;115(Suppl 3A): 39S–44S.
22. Weinberger M. Gastroesophageal reflux disease is not a significant cause of lung disease in children. Pediatr Pulmonol Suppl 2004;26:197–200.
23. Morton RE, Wheatley R, Minford J. Respiratory tract infections due to direct and reflux aspiration in children with severe neurodisability. Dev Med Child Neurol 1999;41(5):329–34.
24. Phua SY, McGarvey LP, Ngu MC, et al. Patients with gastro-oesophageal reflux disease and cough have impaired laryngopharyngeal mechanosensitivity. Thorax 2005;60(6):488–91.
25. Hussein I, Kershaw AE, Tahmassebi JF, et al. The management of drooling in children and patients with mental and physical disabilities: a literature review. Int J Paediatr Dent 1998;8(1):3–11.
26. Rossi UG, Owens CM. The radiology of chronic lung disease in children. Arch Dis Child 2005;90(6):601–7.
27. Kuhn JP, Brody AS. High-resolution CT of pediatric lung disease. Radiol Clin North Am 2002;40(1):89–110.
28. McCullough GH, Wertz RT, Rosenbek JC, et al. Inter- and intrajudge reliability of a clinical examination of swallowing on adults. Dysphagia 2000;15(2): 58–62.
29. Martin-Harris B, Logemann JA, McMahon S, et al. Clinical utility of the modified barium swallow. Dysphagia 2000;15(3):136–41.
30. DeMatteo C, Matovich D, Hjartarson A. Comparison of clinical and videofluoroscopic evaluation of children with feeding and swallowing difficulties. Dev Med Child Neurol 2005;47(3):149–57.

31. Stoeckli SJ, Huisman TA, Seifert B, et al. Interrater reliability of videofluoroscopic swallow evaluation. Dysphagia 2003;18(1):53–7.
32. Leder SB, Karas DE. Fiberoptic endoscopic evaluation of swallowing in the pediatric population. Laryngoscope 2000;110(7):1132–6.
33. Colodny N. Interjudge and intrajudge reliabilities in fiberoptic endoscopic evaluation of swallowing (FEES) using the penetration-aspiration scale: a replication study. Dysphagia 2002;17(4):308–15.
34. Kelly AM, Drinnan MJ, Leslie P. Assessing penetration and aspiration: how do videofluoroscopy and fiberoptic endoscopic evaluation of swallow compare? Laryngoscope 2007;117(10):1723–7.
35. Corwin RW, Irwin RS. The lipid-laden alveolar macrophage as a marker of aspiration in parenchymal lung disease. Am Rev Respir Dis 1985;132(3):576–81.
36. Nussbaum E, Maggi JC, Mathis R, et al. Association of lipid-laden macrophages and gastroesophageal reflux in children. J Pediatr 1987;110(2):190–4.
37. Colombo JL, Hallberg TK. Recurrent aspiration in children: lipid-laden alveolar macrophage quantitation. Pediatr Pulmonol 1987;3(2):86–9.
38. Moran JR, Block SM, Lyerly AD, et al. Lipid-laden alveolar macrophage and lactose assay as markers of aspiration in neonates with lung disease. J Pediatr 1988;112(4):643–5.
39. Bauer ML, Lyrene RK. Chronic aspiration in children: evaluation of the lipid-laden macrophage index. Pediatr Pulmonol 1999;28(2):94–100.
40. Knauer-Fischer S, Ratjen F. Lipid-laden macrophages in bronchoalveolar lavage fluid as a marker for pulmonary aspiration. Pediatr Pulmonol 1999;27(6):419–22.
41. Ahrens P, Noll C, Kitz R, et al. Lipid-laden alveolar macrophages (LLAM): a useful marker of silent aspiration in children. Pediatr Pulmonol 1999;28(2):83–8.
42. Sacco O, Fregonese B, Silvestri M, et al. Bronchoalveolar lavage and esophageal pH monitoring data in children with "difficult to treat" respiratory symptoms. Pediatr Pulmonol 2000;30(4):313–9.
43. Kazachkov MY, Muhlebach MS, Livasy CA, et al. Lipid-laden macrophage index and inflammation in bronchoalveolar lavage fluids in children. Eur Respir J 2001;18(5):790–5.
44. Furuya ME, Moreno-Cordova V, Ramirez-Figueroa JL, et al. Cutoff value of lipid laden alveolar macrophages for diagnosing aspiration in infants and children. Pediatr Pulmonol 2007;42(5):452–7.
45. Colombo JL, Hallberg TK. Pulmonary aspiration and lipid-laden macrophages: in search of gold (standards). Pediatr Pulmonol 1999;28(2):78–82.
46. Ding Y, Simpson PM, Schellhase DE, et al. Limited reliability of lipid-laden macrophage index restricts its use as a test for pulmonary aspiration: comparison with a simple semiquantitative assay. Pediatr Dev Pathol 2002;5(6):551–8.
47. Shay SS, Johnson LF, Richter JE. Acid reflux: a review, emphasizing detection by impedance, manometry, and scintigraphy, and the impact on acid clearing pathophysiology as well as interpreting the pH record. Dig Dis Sci 2003;48(1):1–9.
48. Wenzl TG, Moroder C, Trachterna M, et al. Esophageal pH monitoring and impedance measurement: a comparison of two diagnostic tests for gastroesophageal reflux. J Pediatr Gastroenterol Nutr 2002;34(5):519–23.
49. Condino AA, Sondheimer J, Pan Z, et al. Evaluation of infantile acid and nonacid gastroesophageal reflux using combined pH monitoring and impedance measurement. J Pediatr Gastroenterol Nutr 2006;42(1):16–21.
50. Rosen R, Nurko S. The importance of multichannel intraluminal impedance in the evaluation of children with persistent respiratory symptoms. Am J Gastroenterol 2004;99(12):2452–8.

51. Kawamura O, Aslam M, Rittmann T, et al. Physical and pH properties of gastro-esophagopharyngeal refluxate: a 24-hour simultaneous ambulatory impedance and pH monitoring study. Am J Gastroenterol 2004;99(6):1000–10.

52. Tutuian R, Castell DO. Use of multichannel intraluminal impedance to document proximal esophageal and pharyngeal nonacidic reflux episodes. Am J Med 2003; 115(Suppl 3A):119S–23S.

53. McVeagh P, Howman-Giles R, Kemp A. Pulmonary aspiration studied by radionuclide milk scanning and barium swallow roentgenography. Am J Dis Child 1987; 141(8):917–21.

54. Fawcett HD, Hayden CK, Adams JC, et al. How useful is gastroesophageal reflux scintigraphy in suspected childhood aspiration? Pediatr Radiol 1988;18(4): 311–3.

55. Baikie G, South MJ, Reddihough DS, et al. Agreement of aspiration tests using barium videofluoroscopy, salivagram, and milk scan in children with cerebral palsy. Dev Med Child Neurol 2005;47(2):86–93.

56. Ravelli AM, Panarotto MB, Verdoni L, et al. Pulmonary aspiration shown by scintigraphy in gastroesophageal reflux-related respiratory disease. Chest 2006; 130(5):1520–6.

57. Meyers WF, Roberts CC, Jhonson DG, et al. Value of tests for evaluation of gastroesophageal reflux in children. J Pediatr Surg 1985;20(5):515–20.

58. Bar-Sever Z, Connolly LP, Treves ST. The radionuclide salivagram in children with pulmonary disease and a high risk of aspiration. Pediatr Radiol 1995;25(Suppl 1): S180–3.

59. Levin K, Colon A, DiPalma J, et al. Using the radionuclide salivagram to detect pulmonary aspiration and esophageal dysmotility. Clin Nucl Med 1993;18(2):110–4.

60. Cook SP, Lawless S, Mandell GA, et al. The use of the salivagram in the evaluation of severe and chronic aspiration. Int J Pediatr Otorhinolaryngol 1997;41(3):353–61.

61. Thompson DM. Laryngopharyngeal sensory testing and assessment of airway protection in pediatric patients. Am J Med 2003;115(Suppl 3A):166S–8S.

62. Perlman PW, Cohen MA, Setzen M, et al. The risk of aspiration of pureed food as determined by flexible endoscopic evaluation of swallowing with sensory testing. Otolaryngol Head Neck Surg 2004;130(1):80–3.

63. Burklow KA, Phelps AN, Schultz JR, et al. Classifying complex pediatric feeding disorders. J Pediatr Gastroenterol Nutr 1998;27(2):143–7.

64. Weir K, McMahon S, Chang AB. Restriction of oral intake of water for aspiration lung disease in children. Cochrane Database Syst Rev 2005;4: CD005303.

65. Burd RS, Price MR, Whalen TV. The role of protective antireflux procedures in neurologically impaired children: a decision analysis. J Pediatr Surg 2002; 37(3):500–6.

66. Del Buono R, Wenzl TG, Rawat D, et al. Acid and nonacid gastro-oesophagel reflux in neurologically impaired children: investigation with the multiple intraluminal impedance procedure. J Pediatr Gastroenterol Nutr 2006;43(3):331–5.

67. Muraji T, Takamizawa S, Satoh S, et al. Congenital cricopharyngeal achalasia: diagnosis and surgical management. J Pediatr Surg 2002;37(5):E12.

68. Wenzl TG, Schneider S, Scheele F, et al. Effects of thickened feeding on gastroesophageal reflux in infants: a placebo-controlled crossover study using intraluminal impedance. Pediatrics 2003;111(4):e355–9.

69. Del Buono R, Wenzel TG, Ball G, et al. Effect of Gaviscon Infant on gastro-oesophageal reflux in infants assessed by combined intraluminal impedance/pH. Arch Dis Child 2005;90(5):460–3.

70. Chicella MF, Batres LA, Heesters MS, et al. Prokinetic drug therapy in children: a review of current options. Ann Pharmacother 2005;39(4):706–11.

71. Pritchard DS, Baber N, Stephenson T. Should domperidone be used for the treatment of gastro-oesophageal reflux in children? Systematic review of randomized controlled trials in children aged 1 month to 11 years old. Br J Clin Pharmacol 2005;59(6):725–9.

72. Costalos C, Gounaris A, Varhalama E, et al. Erythromycin as a prokinetic agent in preterm infants. J Pediatr Gastroenterol Nutr 2002;34(1):13–5.

73. Ng SC, Gomez JM, Rajaduri VS, et al. Establishing enteral feeding in preterm infants with feeding intolerance: a randomized controlled study of low-dose erythromycin. J Pediatr Gastroenterol Nutr 2003;37(5):554–8.

74. Kelly DA. Do H2 receptor antagonists have a therapeutic role in childhood? J Pediatr Gastroenterol Nutr 1994;19(3):270–6.

75. Keady S. Update on drugs for gastro-oesophageal reflux disease. Arch Dis Child Educ Pract Ed 2007;92(4):ep114–8.

76. Hassal E. Decisions in diagnosing and managing chronic gastroesophageal reflux disease in children. J Pediatr 2005;146(Suppl 3):S3–12.

77. Mattioli G, Sacco O, Repetto P, et al. Necessity for surgery in children with gastro-oesophageal reflux and supraoesophageal symptoms. Eur J Pediatr Surg 2004; 14(1):7–13.

78. Kawahara H, Okuyama H, Kubota A, et al. Can laparoscopic antireflux surgery improve the quality of life in children with neurologic and neuromuscular handicaps? J Pediatr Surg 2004;39(12):1761–4.

79. Esposito C, Langer JC, Schaarschmidt K, et al. Laparoscopic antireflux procedures in the management of gastroesophageal reflux following esophageal atresia repair. J Pediatr Gastroenterol Nutr 2005;40(3):349–51.

80. Wales PW, Diamond IR, Dutta S, et al. Fundoplication and gastrostomy versus image-guided gastrojejunal tube for enteral feeding in neurologically impaired children with gastroesophageal reflux. J Pediatr Surg 2002;37(3):407–12.

81. Esposito C, Settimi A, Centonze A, et al. Laparoscopic-assisted jejunostomy: an effective procedure for the treatment of neurologically impaired children with feeding problems and gastroesophageal reflux. Surg Endosc 2005;19(4):501–4.

82. Mier RJ, Bachrach SJ, Lakin RC, et al. Treatment of sialorrhea with glycopyrrolate: a double-blind, dose-ranging study. Arch Pediatr Adolesc Med 2000;154(12): 1214–8.

83. Jongerius PH, van den Hoogen FJ, van Limbeek J, et al. Effect of botulinum toxin in the treatment of drooling: a controlled clinical trial. Pediatrics 2004;114(3): 620–7.

84. Hassin-Baer S, Scheuer E, Buchman AS, et al. Botulinum toxin injections for children with excessive drooling. J Child Neurol 2005;20(2):120–3.

85. Reid SM, Johnstone BR, Wetsbury C, et al. Randomized trial of botulinum toxin injections into the salivary glands to reduce drooling in children with neurological disorders. Dev Med Child Neurol 2008;50:123–8.

86. Gerber ME, Gaugler MD, Myer CM 3rd, et al. Chronic aspiration in children. When are bilateral submandibular gland excision and parotid duct ligation indicated? Arch Otolaryngol Head Neck Surg 1996;122(12):1368–71.

87. Stern Y, Feinmesser R, Collins M, et al. Bilateral submandibular gland excision with parotid duct ligation for treatment of sialorrhea in children: long-term results. Arch Otolaryngol Head Neck Surg 2002;128(7):801–3.

88. Elpern EH, Scott MG, Petro L, et al. Pulmonary aspiration in mechanically ventilated patients with tracheostomies. Chest 1994;105(2):563–6.

89. Abraham SS, Wolf EL. Swallowing physiology of toddlers with long-term tracheostomies: a preliminary study. Dysphagia 2000;15(3):206–12.
90. Takamizawa S, Tsugawa C, Nishijima E, et al. Laryngotracheal separation for intractable aspiration pneumonia in neurologically impaired children: experience with 11 cases. J Pediatr Surg 2003;38(6):975–7.
91. Jadcherla SR, Gupta A, Stoner E, et al. Pharyngeal swallowing: defining pharyngeal and upper esophageal sphincter relationships in human neonates. J Pediatr 2007;151(6):597–603.
92. Krishnan U, Mitchell JD, Messina I, et al. Assay of tracheal pepsin as a marker of reflux aspiration. J Pediatr Gastroenterol Nutr 2002;35(3):303–8.
93. Farrell S, McMaster C, Gibson D, et al. Pepsin in bronchoalveolar lavage fluid: a specific and sensitive method of diagnosing gastro-oesophageal reflux-related pulmonary aspiration. J Pediatr Surg 2006;41(2):289–93.
94. Starosta V, Kitz R, Hartl D, et al. Bronchoalveolar pepsin, bile acids, oxidation, and inflammation in children with gastroesophageal reflux disease. Chest 2007; 132(5):1557–64.
95. Potluri S, Friedenberg F, Parkman HP, et al. Comparison of a salivary/sputum pepsin assay with 24-hour esophageal pH monitoring for detection of gastric reflux into the proximal esophagus, oropharynx, and lung. Dig Dis Sci 2003;48(9): 1813–7.

Asthma in Childhood

Paul D. Robinson, MBChB, MRCPCH, FRACP[a,b,]*,
Peter Van Asperen, MBBS, MD, FRACP[a,b]

KEYWORDS

• Asthma • Pediatrics • Management

Asthma is the most common chronic disease in childhood, with a prevalence of 10% to 30%.[1] Many of the current recommendations for management of asthma in children are based on studies in the adult asthmatic population, and there is a paucity of published pediatric data. The available literature can be divided into two main age groups, children younger than 12 years, and those aged 12 years and older (adults and adolescents). Although adult and adolescent asthma are comparable, adult asthma is different from pediatric asthma (age < 12 years) in many important ways, and consequently it may not be appropriate to extrapolate adult evidence to pediatric management. This article reviews the available pediatric evidence and provides evidence-based recommendations for management, based on recent American Thoracic Society grading recommendations (**Table 1**).[2] A number of guidelines exist for asthma management, but for consistency this article refers primarily to the National Asthma Council guidelines, recently updated and published in Australia.[3] Management of asthma is divided into the management of acute exacerbations (**Tables 1–5**) and interval management (**Tables 6–10**).

DIAGNOSIS AND MISDIAGNOSIS

Wheeze and dyspnea, with or without cough, are the core symptoms of asthma, but because these individual respiratory symptoms are common in children, asthma frequently is misdiagnosed. Parents may misinterpret other respiratory sounds, such as stridor and rattle, as wheeze. The relationship between cough and asthma also is complex.[4] Isolated persistent cough is rarely asthma. A number of important differential diagnoses exist and should be considered (see **Table 2**)[3,5] if other features of asthma are not present or if an inappropriate response to treatment is seen. A more detailed discussion of each of these conditions is beyond the scope of this article.

[a] Department of Respiratory Medicine, The Children's Hospital at Westmead, Westmead, Sydney, Australia
[b] The Children's Hospital at Westmead Clinical School, Discipline of Paediatrics and Child Health, Faculty of Medicine, University of Sydney, Westmead, Sydney, Australia
* Corresponding author. Department of Respiratory Medicine, The Children's Hospital at Westmead, Locked Bag 4001, Westmead, NSW, 2145, Sydney, Australia.
E-mail address: paulr3@chw.edu.au (P.D. Robinson).

Pediatr Clin N Am 56 (2009) 191–226
doi:10.1016/j.pcl.2008.10.008
pediatric.theclinics.com
0031-3955/08/$ – see front matter. Crown Copyright © 2009 Published by Elsevier Inc. All rights reserved.

Table 1
The American Thoracic Society grading recommendations

Grade of Recommendation	Clarity of Risk/Benefit	Quality of Supporting Evidence	Implications
Strong recommendation: High-quality evidence	Benefits clearly outweigh harms and burdens or vice versa	Consistent evidence from well-performed randomized, controlled trials or exceptionally strong evidence from unbiased observational studies	Recommendation can apply to most patients in most circumstances. Further research is very unlikely to change our confidence in the estimate of effect.
Strong recommendation: Moderate-quality evidence	Benefits clearly outweigh harms and burdens or vice versa	Evidence from randomized, controlled trials with important limitations (inconsistent results, methodologic flows, indirect or imprecise), or unusually strong evidence from unbiased observational studies	Recommendation can apply to most patients in most circumstances. Further research (if performed) is likely to have an important impact on our confidence in the estimate of effect and may change the estimate.
Strong recommendation: Low-quality evidence	Benefits clearly outweigh harms and burdens or vice versa	Evidence for at least one critical outcome from observational studies, from randomized, controlled trials with serious flaws, or indirect evidence	Recommendation may change when higher-quality evidence becomes available. Further research (if performed) is likely to have an important impact on our confidence in the estimate of effect and is likely to charge the estimate.
Strong recommendation: Very low-quality evidence (very rarely applicable)	Benefits clearly outweigh harms and burdens or vice versa	Evidence for a least one of the critical outcomes from unsystematic clinical observations or very indirect evidence	Recommendation may change when higher-quality evidence becomes available; any estimate of effect, for at least one critical outcome, is very uncertain.
Weak recommendation: High-quality evidence	Benefits closely balanced with harms and burdens	Consistent evidence from well-performed randomized, controlled trials or exceptionally strong evidence from unbiased observational studies	The best action may differ depending on circumstances, patient characteristics, or societal values. Further research is very unlikely to change our confidence in the estimate of effect.

Weak recommendation: Moderate-quality evidence	Benefits closely balanced with harms and burdens	Evidence from randomized, controlled trials with important limitations (inconsistent results, methodologic flaws, indirect or imprecise), or unusually strong evidence from unbiased observational studies	Alternative approaches are likely to be better for some patients under some circumstances. Further research (if performed) is likely to have an important impact on our confidence in the estimate of effect and may change the estimate.
Weak recommendation: Low-quality evidence	Uncertainty in the estimates of benefits, harms, and burdens; benefits may be closely balanced with harms and burdens	Evidence for at least one critical outcome from observations studies, from randomized, controlled trials with serious flaws, or indirect evidence	Other alternatives may be equally reasonable. Further research is very likely to have an important impact on our confidence in the estimate of effect and is likely to change the estimate.
Weak recommendation: Very low quality evidence	Major uncertainty in the estimates of benefits, harms, and burdens; benefits may or may not be balanced with harms and burdens	Evidence for at least one critical outcome from unsystematic clinical observations or very indirect evidence	Other alternatives may be equally reasonable. Any estimate of effect, for at least one critical outcome, is very uncertain.

From Schunemann HJ, Jaeschke R, Cook DJ, et al. An official ATS statement: grading the quality of evidence and strength of recommendations in ATS guidelines and recommendations. Am J Respir Crit Care Med 2006;174:612; with permission. Copyright © 2006, American Thoracic Society.

Table 2
Important differential diagnoses in pediatric asthma

Condition	Characteristics
Transient infant wheezing (eg, recurrent bronchiolitis)	Onset in infancy No associated atopy Associated with maternal smoking
Cystic fibrosis	Recurrent wheeze and failure to thrive
Primary ciliary dyskinesia	Associated recurrent otitis media and sinusitis Initial oxygen requirement postnatally Situs inversus in 50%
Chronic bronchitis (viral or bacterial)	Persistent moist cough in combination with wheeze Purulent sputum suggests bacterial cause
Structural abnormality (eg, tracheomalacia, bronchomalacia)	Onset usually from or shortly after birth but occasionally later
Vocal cord dysfunction	High-pitched inspiratory stridor and dyspnea May be spontaneous or exercise induced Blunting of inspiratory volume loop on spirometry
Inhaled foreign body	Sudden onset Differential air entry or wheeze on examination
Cardiac failure	Associated with congenital or acquired heart disease (eg, dilated cardiomyopathy after viral infection)
Eosinophilic lung disorders including allergic bronchopulmonary aspergillosis	Skin prick test positivity to *Aspergillus fumigatus* Raised serum IgE Infiltrates on chest radiograph
Anxiety causing hyperventilation	No wheeze audible Spirometry at the time of symptoms may help distinguish
Exertional dyspnea	No respiratory symptoms other than with exercise Exercise testing may distinguish
Milk aspiration/cough during feeds	Symptomatic particularly with liquids Associated with developmental delay

Data from National Asthma Council Australia. Asthma management handbook. 2006. Available at: www.nationalasthma.org.au; and Weinberger M, Abu-Hasan M. Pseudo-asthma: when cough, wheezing, and dyspnea are not asthma. Pediatrics 2007;120:855–64.

MANAGEMENT OF ACUTE ASTHMA
Assessing Severity

Assessment of severity (see **Table 3**) determines subsequent treatment. The evidence and grading of the approach and options of managing acute asthma are summarized in **Table 4**. Treatment of acute asthma is based on the underlying pathophysiology, attempting to reverse bronchoconstriction, airway inflammation, and mucus production.

Oxygen

If a patient is in acute distress, oxygen (to maintain oxygen saturations $\geq$ 95%) and a short-acting beta-2 agonist (SABA) should be given immediately. Subsequent salbutamol administration may precipitate further desaturation via pulmonary vasodilatation in areas of poorly ventilated lung. The value of initial oxygen saturation as a predictor of

Table 3
Initial assessment of acute asthma

Symptom	Mild	Moderate	Severe or Life-Threatening[a]
Confused/drowsy	No	No	Agitated or altered consciousness
Oximetry on presentation (SaO$_2$)	94%	94%–90%	Less than 90%
Talks in	Sentences	Phrases	Words or unable to speak
Pulse rate	Less than 100 beats/min	100–200 beats /min	More than 200 beats/min
Central cyanosis	Absent	Absent	Likely to be present
Wheeze intensity	Variable	Moderate to loud	Often quiet
PEF[b]	More than 60% predicted or personal best	40%–60% predicted or personal best	Less than 40% predicted or personal best or unable to perform
FEV$_1$	More than 60% predicted	40%–60% predicted	Less than 40% predicted or unable to perform

[a] Any of these features indicates that the episode is severe. The absence of any feature does not exclude a severe attack.
[b] Children under 7 years old are unlikely to perform PEF or spirometry reliably during an acute episode. These tests usually are not used in the assessment of acute asthma in children.
From National Asthma Council Australia. Asthma management handbook. 2006. Available at: www.nationalasthma.org.au; with permission.

subsequent hospitalization remains controversial.[6,7] Intensity of wheeze is a poor predictor.

Beta-2 Agonists

Selective beta-2 agonists (salbutamol) have been the mainstay of acute asthma management since the late 1970s. Frequency of administration is determined by the severity of the exacerbation (see **Table 5**). Continuous use of SABA has been shown to be more effective than intermittent regimens in severe exacerbations[8] and to reduce hospitalization (RR, 0.64; 95% confidence interval [CI], 0.5–0.9), resulting in a modest improvement in lung function at 2 to 3 hours. This benefit was not seen in mild or moderate asthma. Only one of the eight relatively small randomized, control trials (RCTs) included was pediatric[9] (n = 70, age 2–18 years) and studied children who had moderate to severe asthma. It found no difference in hospitalization rates or time spent in the emergency department. Excluded from the analysis was an RCT in a more severe pediatric asthma cohort (n = 17) admitted to intensive care, which demonstrated a benefit in clinical status and hospital stay.[10] A meta-analysis of 25 RCTs, including 21 pediatric studies and more than 2000 children,[11] demonstrated that in acute asthma spacers were as effective as nebulizers in limiting hospitalization rates and reducing the time spent in emergency department (−0.47 hours; 95% CI, −0.58 to −0.37). The role of spacers in life-threatening asthma has yet to be investigated.

Table 4
Grading of evidence and recommendations for acute asthma management in children

Medication	Recommendation	Grading of Recommendation (Based on Evidence of Benefit)	Quality of Supporting Evidence
SABA	Recommended as first-line bronchodilator	Strong	High
Anticholinergics	Multiple doses beneficial in severe asthma	Strong	Moderate
Corticosteroids			
Inhaled	May be an alternative in mild asthma. High dose required if given.	Strong	Moderate
Oral	Beneficial in acute asthma not responding to SABA	Strong	High
Intravenous salbutamol	Beneficial in severe or life-threatening asthma	Strong	Moderate
Intravenous aminophylline	Alternative to IV salbutamol in severe or life-threatening asthma	Strong	Moderate
Magnesium sulfate			
Inhaled	Unclear role in severe asthma	Weak	Moderate
Intravenous	Beneficial in severe or life-threatening asthma	Strong	High
Heliox	May have a role in medication delivery but insufficient evidence to recommend currently	Weak	Moderate
Noninvasive ventilation	May have a role in life-threatening asthma to prevent intubation	Weak	Low
Leukotriene receptor antagonists	May have a role in mild to moderate acute asthma but further studies are required	Weak	Low
Antibiotics	No indication for routine use	Weak	Low
Education	Recommended but little evidence for improved outcome	Weak	High
Physiotherapy	May be of benefit in resolving stage of hypersecretory asthma	Weak	Low
Spacers	Spacer delivery of inhaled medications is recommended for all but life-threatening acute asthma	Strong	High

Anticholinergic Agents

Anticholinergic agents (ipratropium bromide, atropine sulfate) produce a weaker bronchodilation response with a slower onset of action (30–90 minutes versus 5–15 minutes)[12] but, by relieving cholinergic bronchomotor tone and secretions, have a beneficial effect when added to beta-agonist therapy in acute asthma. Meta-analysis of eight high-quality pediatric RCTs demonstrated that a single dose of an anticholinergic agent was insufficient to reduce hospital admission rate for any grade of severity (although in severe attacks persisting to 120 minutes, a benefit in lung function was seen).[13] In severe exacerbations in school-age children, multiple doses reduced hospital admission rates by 25% (number needed to treat [NNT], 7; 95% CI, 5–20) and additional bronchodilator use by 19%. No benefit was seen for mild attacks. The suggested benefit in moderate acute asthma may be skewed by the response in the severe subset and is insufficient to allow recommendation. There is a paucity of studies in children of preschool age.

The role of anticholinergics in wheezy children under the age of 2 years, excluding those who have bronchiolitis and chronic lung disease of prematurity, remains questionable. Parental preference and improvement in some (eg, clinical scores at 24 hours, additional treatment) but not all outcomes (eg, respiratory rate, need for oxygen supplementation, hospital stay), when given with or without beta-agonist, are not sufficient to recommend the use of an anticholinergic agent in this population.[14]

Corticosteroids

Although bronchoconstriction is best targeted with beta-2 agonists, the airway edema and secretions that accompany an acute exacerbation respond to systemic corticosteroid therapy. Considerable research effort has concentrated on the best route of administration, timing, and dose of corticosteroid. Corticosteroids are recommended for asthma exacerbations that are incompletely responsive to inhaled beta-agonists.

Doubling the dose of inhaled corticosteroids (ICS) at the onset of an exacerbation is ineffective in improving lung function and controlling symptoms (n = 28, age 6–14 years).[15] A review of published pediatric studies concluded that ICS given at high doses (eg, 1600 µg/d of budesonide) seem to have a modest benefit compared with placebo but are inferior to oral corticosteroids (OCS) in preventing hospitalization in more severe attacks.[16] The most commonly used OCS is prednisolone, often chosen because of its palatability[17] rather than because of comparative OCS data. Only one pediatric RCT has examined differing doses of prednisolone, in a mild to moderate severity cohort, and found no difference between 0.5, 1.0, and 2.0 mg/kg/d.[18] Meta-analysis of adult RCT data in severe asthma has shown no benefit from higher doses of corticosteroids, although these trials primarily examined intravenous (IV) administration.[19] At present, the recommended dose of oral prednisolone is 1 mg/kg every 12 to 24 hours (maximum dose, 50 mg) depending on progress.[20] The optimal duration of treatment also is unclear. A single dose of OCS on admission has failed to show consistent benefit.[21,22] A recent pediatric RCT comparing 3- and 5-day courses demonstrated equivalent efficacy.[23] Currently a 3-day course is recommended, lengthened to 5 days in more severe exacerbations.[20]

Early administration of OCS, within the first hour of arrival, has been shown to reduce admission rates in children (three RCTs; OR, 0.24; 95% CI, 0.11–0.53).[24] To date, however, parent-initiated OCS has not been demonstrated to improve outcomes, as evaluated by unscheduled medical visits,[25] but further trials are required to establish firm recommendations. OCS in children are as effective as parenteral dosing,[26] are more cost effective, and are more convenient but rely on the child's

Table 5
Initial management of children who have acute asthma

Treatment	Mild Episode	Moderate Episode	Severe or Life-Threatening Episode
Hospital admission necessary	Probably not required	Probably required	Yes
			Consider intensive care
Supplementary oxygen	Probably not required	May be required. Monitor Sao$_2$	Required. Monitor Sao$_2$. Arterial blood gases may be required.
Salbutamol (100 μg per puff)[a]	4–6 puffs (children < 6 years) or 8–12 puffs (children ≥ 6 years). Review in 20 minutes	6 puffs (children < 6 years) or 12 puffs (children ≥ 6 years) If initial response is inadequate, repeat at 20-minute intervals for two further doses; then give every 1–4 hours.	6 puffs (children < 6 years) or 12 puffs (children ≥ 6 years) every 20 minutes for three doses in first hour. If episode is life threatening, use continuous nebulized salbutamol. If no response, bolus IV salbutamol (15 μg/kg) over 10 minutes, then 1 μg/kg/min thereafter.
Ipratropium (20 μg per puff)	Not necessary	Optional	2 puffs (children < 6 years) or 4 puffs (children ≥ 6 years) every 20 minutes for three doses in first hour or use nebulized ipratropium
Systemic corticosteroids	Yes (consider)	Oral prednisolone (1 mg/kg daily for up to 3 days)	Oral prednisolone (1 mg/kg/dose) daily for up to 5 days Methylprednisolone IV (1 mg/kg) every 6 hours on day 1, every 12 hours on day 2, then daily

Magnesium	No	No	Magnesium sulfate 50% 0.1 mL/kg (50 mg/kg) IV over 20 minutes, then 0.06 mL/kg/h (30 mg/kg/h): target serum 1.5–2.5 mmol/L
Aminophylline	No	No	Only in intensive care: loading dose: 10 mg/kg; maintenance: 1.1 mg/kg/h if < 9 years or 0.7 mg/kg/h if ≥ 9 years
Chest radiograph	Not necessary unless focal signs present	Not necessary unless focal signs present	Necessary if no response to initial therapy or pneumothorax is suspected
Observations	Observe for 20 minutes after dose	Observe for 1 hour after last dose	Arrange for admission to hospital

[a] In children who have severe acute asthma that does not respond to initial treatment with inhaled SABA, bolus IV salbutamol (15 µg/kg) is effective and can avoid the need for continuous IV salbutamol and ICU admission.

From National Asthma Council Australia. Asthma management handbook. 2006. Available at: www.nationalasthma.org.au; with permission.

Table 6
Assessment of severity of interval asthma

Severity Level	Daytime Symptoms Between Exacerbations	Night-Time Symptoms Between Exacerbations	Exacerbations	PEF or FEV$_1$[a]	PEF Variability[b]
Infrequent intermittent	None	None	Brief, mild Occur < every 4–6 weeks	> 80% predicted	< 20%
Frequent intermittent	None	None	> Two per month	At least 80% predicted	< 20%
Mild persistent	More than once per week but not every day	More than twice per month but not every week	May affect activity and sleep	At least 80% predicted	20%–30%
Moderate persistent	Daily	More than once per week	At least twice per week; restrict activity or affect sleep	60%–80% predicted	> 30%
Severe persistent	Continual	Frequent	Frequent; restrict activity	≤ 60% predicted	> 30%

An individual's asthma pattern (infrequent intermittent, frequent intermittent, mild persistent, or severe persistent) is determined by the level in the table that corresponds to the most severe feature present. Other features associated with that pattern need not be present.

[a] Predicted values are based on age, sex, and height.
[b] Difference between morning and evening values.

From National Asthma Council Australia. Asthma management handbook. 2006. Available at: www.nationalasthma.org.au; with permission.

Table 7
Assessment of asthma control

Parameters	Level of Control		
	Good	Fair	Poor
Daytime symptoms	None	< 3 days/wk	≥ 3 days/wk
Night-time symptoms	Not wakened	≤ 1 night/wk	> 1 night/wk
Physical activity	Normal	Normal	Restricted
Exacerbations	None	Mild, infrequent	Moderate, severe frequent
Missed school/work because of asthma	None	None	Any
Reliever use[a]	None	< 3 doses/wk	≥ 3 doses/wk
[b]FEV$_1$ [b]FEV$_1$/FVC	Normal	≥ 90% personal best	< 90% personal best
[b]PEF	Normal	≥ 90% personal best	< 90% personal best

[a] Does not include one dose per day for prevention of exercise-induced symptoms.
[b] Applicable to adults and older children. Lung function parameters are not appropriate measures of asthma control in younger children.

From National Asthma Council Australia. Asthma management handbook. 2006. Available at: www.nationalasthma.org.au; with permission.

tolerating and retaining the dose. IV corticosteroids should be used in patients who are unlikely to tolerate OCS (ie, children experiencing severe exacerbation). Benefit is seen by 4 to 6 hours.[24] A single dose of oral or intramuscular (IM) dexamethasone (0.6 mg/kg to a maximum of 15–18 mg) was comparable to a 5-day course of oral prednisolone (2 mg/kg/d) in three pediatric RCTs (total n = 324),[27,28,29] although systemic side effects may be more common with IM long-acting corticosteroids.[17] OCS also have been shown to reduce relapse rates,[24] although this meta-analysis included only one pediatric RCT.[30] High-dose ICS regimens on discharge from hospital have shown efficacy similar to OCS but are not as cost effective.[31]

Intravenous Bronchodilators

First-line IV bronchodilator therapy in severe acute asthma not improving with inhaled beta-agonist and OCS therapy remains controversial. Guidelines recommend IV salbutamol as the first-line agent; it is preferred because of its better safety profile, but the lack of clear evidence has led to the continuing widespread use of aminophylline.[32]

Intravenous salbutamol

IV salbutamol has been shown to improve clinical outcome in comparison with placebo in individual pediatric RCTs both as an infusion[33] and as a bolus of 15 µg/kg.[34,35] Although an attempted meta-analysis of the adult and pediatric data failed to demonstrate improvement,[36] the conclusions of this meta-analysis have been criticized.[37]

Intravenous aminophylline

Meta-analysis of seven pediatric RCTs (n = 380 patients, mean age 5–9 years) in severe acute asthma demonstrated improvements in lung function and clinical symptoms with IV aminophylline infusion,[38] but the analysis is affected significantly by the results of the largest RCT (n = 179), the only RCT to show benefit.[39] A recent pediatric RCT (n = 44) directly comparing aminophylline and salbutamol (an IV salbutamol bolus of 15 µg/kg versus IV aminophylline infusion) demonstrated no difference in efficacy in the first 2 hours of treatment[37] but found a 30% reduction in hospital stay in the aminophylline group. Repeat IV aminophylline boluses have demonstrated no additional benefit over standard treatment (n = 60, age 2–5 years).[40]

Magnesium sulfate

Magnesium is a potential therapeutic agent in asthma because of its bronchodilating effect on smooth muscle cells[41] and reduction of the neutrophilic burst associated with inflammation.[42] In a meta-analysis of five pediatric RCTs (n = 182, age 1–18 years), IV magnesium sulfate decreased hospitalizations (OR, 0.29; 95% CI, 0.14–0.59; NNT, 4; 95% CI, 3–8) and improved pulmonary function and symptom scores, despite variation in dosage (25–75 mg/kg).[43] Another predominantly adult meta-analysis that included two pediatric RCTs (n = 78 subject age 1–18 years in a total of 665 subjects) confirmed its safe and beneficial role in severe acute asthma.[44] Meta-analysis of trials of inhaled magnesium sulfate, including two pediatric RCTs (n = 102), demonstrated significant improvements in lung function only in severe acute asthma and no difference in hospitalization.[45] The comparative benefit of bolus IV salbutamol and bolus IV magnesium sulfate is yet to be established.

Other Therapies

Heliox (helium/oxygen mixture) has lower gas density and higher viscosity, decreasing flow resistance and enhancing airway penetration. A meta-analysis including three pediatric RCTs demonstrated a potential benefit for heliox as a stand-alone therapy in severe acute asthma, but sample sizes were small.[46] In a recent pediatric RCT

Table 8
Table of grading of evidence and recommendations for interval asthma management in children

Medication	Recommendation	Grading of Recommendation (Based on Evidence of Benefit)	Quality of Supporting Evidence
Cromones (sodium cromoglycate and nedocromil sodium)	Alternative to inhaled corticosteroid in frequent intermittent and mild persistent asthma. May be beneficial in exercise-induced asthma.	Weak	Moderate
Leukotriene receptor antagonists	Beneficial as sole therapy in frequent intermittent or mild persistent asthma. May be beneficial in exercise-induced asthma or allergic rhinitis.	Strong	High
Corticosteroids			
Inhaled corticosteroids	Recommended for persistent asthma	Strong	High
Oral corticosteroids	Severe asthma not responsive to maximal inhaled therapy	Weak	Very weak
Long-acting beta-agonists	Should be considered as an add-on therapy	Weak	Moderate
Steroid-weaning agents			
Immunosuppressive agents	No evidence of efficacy in pediatric patients	Weak	Very low
Intravenous immunoglobulin	Limited role in pediatric asthma. May be beneficial if co-existent immunodeficiency	Weak	Low
Omalizumab	Role in asthma management is not well defined in pediatrics. Expensive	Weak	Moderate

Allergen immunotherapy (subcutaneous)	Potential benefit in children suspected of having allergen-triggered disease, when allergen avoidance has been ineffective or is not possible	Weak	Strong
Macrolides	Some adult data but no evidence of efficacy in pediatric asthma	Weak	Very low
Xanthines	Alternative in mild persistent asthma when inhaled corticosteroids are not available	Weak	Strong
Ketotifen	Alternative in mild persistent asthma when inhaled corticosteroids are not available	Weak	Moderate
Dietary manipulation	Current evidence does not support use in asthma	Weak	Low
Complementary alternative medicine	Current evidence does not support use in asthma	Weak	Low
Allergen avoidance	Some patients may benefit, but there is insufficient evidence to recommend routinely	Weak	High
Prevention strategies			
Primary	Current evidence does not support the use of preventative strategies in asthma	Weak	High
Secondary		Weak	Moderate
Tertiary		Weak	High
Vaccination (influenza and pneumococcus)		Weak	Moderate
Education	Recommended for all asthma patients	Strong	High
Psychotherapy	May be beneficial in a subset of patients	Weak	Moderate

Table 9
Management algorithm for chronic asthma

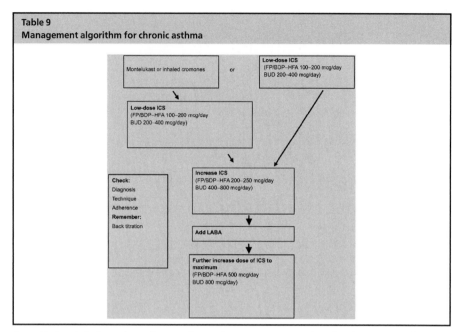

From National Asthma Council Australia. Asthma management handbook. 2006. Available at: www.nationalasthma.org.au; with permission.

(n = 30, age 2–18 years), however, heliox used as a facilitator of aerosol delivery in moderate to severe exacerbations provided significant improvement in clinical scores at 2 to 4 hours and improved discharge rates at 12 hours.[47]

Continuous positive airways pressure often is used in an attempt to avoid intubation and ventilation in exhausted patients who have life-threatening asthma. Its role in asthma remains controversial despite interesting and promising results. Significant improvements in hospitalization rate, discharge from emergency department, pulmonary function, and respiratory rate have been reported by the sole RCT included in a recent adult meta-analysis.[48] There have been no RCTs to date in pediatric populations, although published case reports of benefit exist.[49]

Table 10
Equivalent corticosteroid dosing

Dose Level	Daily ICS Dose			
	CIC[a]	BDP–HFA[b]	FP[b]	BUD[b]
Low	80–160 µg	100–200 µg	100–200 µg	200–400 µg
Medium	160–320 µg	200–400 µg	200–400 µg	400–800 µg
High	≥ 320 µg	> 400 µg	> 400 µg	> 800 µg

Abbreviations: BDP-HFA, beclomethasone dipropionate; BUD, budesonide; CIC, ciclesonide; FP, fluticasone propionate.
[a] Ex actuator dose.
[b] Ex valve dose.
From National Asthma Council Australia. Asthma management handbook. 2006. Available at: www.nationalasthma.org.au; with permission.

Leukotrienes are proinflammatory mediators involved in both early and late asthmatic airway responses to allergen challenge. Leukotriene receptor antagonists (LTRAs) inhibit a part of the asthmatic inflammatory response that is relatively unaffected by OCS[50] and also provide some degree of bronchodilation. Onset of benefit has been shown to occur at 10 minutes with IV administration and within 2 hours with oral administration.[51] An RCT in preschool children demonstrated benefit in respiratory rate and symptoms scores for up to 4 hours and reduced OCS use at 1 hour (20.8% versus 38.5%) in comparison with placebo when LTRAs were given with the first dose of SABA.[52] A short course of LTRAs (given for 7 days or until symptoms had resolved for 48 hours) introduced at the first sign of an asthma exacerbation has been shown to have a beneficial effect in intermittent asthma, with a modest reduction in health care utilization, symptoms, and time off school/work.[53] Although these results are promising, the current evidence is insufficient to recommend the routine use of LTRAs in acute asthma.

There is a paucity of evidence to support the use of antibiotics in the routine management of acute asthma,[54] because most exacerbations are triggered by viral infections. Antibiotics should be reserved for cases in which infection with an antibiotic-responsive organism (bacterial, Mycoplasma) is suspected.

Other Aspects of Treatment

Chest radiographs are indicated only for first presentations of asthma, when there are atypical clinical features (to investigate for important differential diagnoses) or focal signs on examination (collapse, consolidation, or pneumothorax), or when there are severe exacerbations with a lack of response to initial treatment.

The difficulty of performing reproducible spirometry and peak expiratory flow (PEF) in young children means that, despite being listed in severity-assessment guidelines, lung function tests rarely are used during the initial assessment of acute asthma in children.

Arterial blood gases also rarely are used in pediatrics, apart from life-threatening exacerbations.[3] Free-flowing venous blood gases, taken at the time of intravenous cannulation, provide an accurate assessment of PCO_2, which may indicate impending exhaustion if in the normal range (35–45 mm Hg).

Education of parents and children attending the emergency department with acute exacerbations is part of routine management in many centers, although on systematic review an improvement in subsequent emergency department visits, hospitalization, or unscheduled medical reviews was not demonstrated, despite eight pediatric RCTs and large numbers (n = 1407).[55]

Physiotherapy should be avoided in the acute phase of an asthma exacerbation because of the danger of precipitating clinical deterioration[56] but may be of benefit in hypersecretory asthma in the recovery phase once bronchoconstriction has improved.[57]

INTERVAL ASTHMA MANAGEMENT
Assessing Severity

The grading of interval asthma severity and subsequent treatment are based on the clinical features present before commencing treatment (see **Table 6**). This approach, however, does not allow for re-evaluation of severity once treatment has been started, and control then is defined as the extent to which clinical features have been removed by treatment (see **Table 7**). It is important to exclude modifiable factors, such as poor adherence, incorrect inhaler technique, and smoking in adolescents, before this assessment. Another important consideration is that asthma symptoms are not specific for asthma. The goals of management are a combination of good current control (control of symptoms, no exercise limitation, and normal lung function, if the patient is old enough to perform the test) and minimizing future risk (preventing decline in lung function, preventing future exacerbations, and avoiding medication side effects). The evidence for interval management of asthma is summarized in **Table 8**.

Specific practice points relevant to pediatric asthma management are highlighted in the National Asthma Council guidelines:[3]

- It often is not possible to eradicate transient infant wheeze or intermittent viral-induced wheezing in young children, and dose increases in an attempt to treat this aspect are inappropriate.
- One should avoid inappropriate dose increases made in an attempt to eradicate cough completely.
- Cough should not be used as a marker of control, in the absence of other symptoms.
- Symptoms are as reliable as PEF measurement in the monitoring of asthma control.

PHARMACOLOGIC MANAGEMENT
Preventive Medications

The necessity and choice of preventive medications is determined by the initial severity assessment or the degree of control on the current medication (see **Tables 4** and **5**).

Nonsteroidal Agents

Nonsteroidal preventive medications include sodium cromoglycate, nedocromil sodium, and LTRAs. All three are currently recommended as alternatives to ICS for frequent intermittent or mild persistent asthma.[3]

The use of sodium cromoglycate stretches back 35 years but has decreased substantially with the emergence of ICS, and recent systematic reviews (25 RCTs, 17 of which were in a pediatric population) have demonstrated its inferiority to ICS.[58] Its role in asthma remains contentious, however, after initial meta-analyses (24 pediatric RCTs, n = 1024), which concluded that insufficient evidence existed for benefit over placebo, were strongly criticized.[59] Subsequent re-analysis of the data has demonstrated a beneficial effect, particularly in older children who have asthma.[60] Having been withdrawn from the British Thoracic Society guidelines in 2003, it has since been reinstated as "effective in children aged 5–12," but is not named in the corresponding guideline.

Nedocromil sodium is also a cromone, a disodium salt of a pyranoquinolone dicarboxylic acid developed as an anti-inflammatory agent for the treatment of asthma.[61] A recent systematic review of 15 pediatric RCTs (n = 1422) concluded that the benefits in lung function and symptom outcomes suggested by short-term studies was not replicated consistently in longer-term trials. Despite its better side-effect profile, the lack of direct comparison with ICS in RCTs has meant the evidence needed to clarify its position in the treatment of chronic asthma is lacking.[62] This lack of data is in contrast to the adult literature, which shows it to be an effective treatment for asthma.[63]

The role of LTRAs such as montelukast and zafirlukast in interval asthma management is of particular interest in pediatrics because montelukast can be administered as a once-daily oral agent, potentially aiding compliance.[64] In a preschool cohort (age 2–5 years) of 549 children who had predominantly virally induced intermittent asthma, regular LTRA use reduced the rate of exacerbation over a 12-month treatment period by 31.9% (1.60/year versus 2.34/year) and also reduced the need for ICS.[65] A short course of a LTRA introduced at the first sign of infection also has been shown to have benefit.[53] Regular low-dose ICS is not effective in reducing the exacerbation rate or severity in this asthma subgroup,[66] and parent-initiated OCS does not reduce hospitalization rates in preschoolers.[67] No direct comparison of LTRA and a short-course of high-dose ICS, which may have a beneficial role, has been published to date. Although the published data for zafirlukast in adolescents and adults largely mirror those of montelukast, there is a paucity of data available in pediatric populations.

In persistent asthma, the greatest benefit seems to be in cases of mild severity.[68] Large RCTs in preschool (n = 689)[69] and school-age (n = 336)[70] children have demonstrated benefit in symptoms, SABA and OCS use, and lung function (in those old enough to perform the test). These improvements were not documented for the subgroups that had moderate persistent asthma within these studies. For mild persistent asthma, LTRA offers a clinical alternative to ICS, although ICS has a better effect on lung function parameters.[71] ICS remains the more cost-effective option.[72,73] In moderate persistent asthma, low-dose ICS is superior to LTRA, when the two are compared directly, over a range of outcomes.[72,74,75,76] The clinical characteristics of children more likely to respond to LTRAs are not clearly defined, but children who have more frequent symptoms, increased inflammatory markers, and poorer lung function are more likely to respond to ICS.[75,77] Although a predominantly adult systematic review (only 2 of 27 RCTs were pediatric) found modest improvements (equivalent to increasing the ICS dose) when a LTRA was used as an add-on therapy to ICS,[78] this finding was not replicated in a recent pediatric RCT, which showed a increased exacerbation rate in the add-on group.[76] LTRAs may have a modest steroid-sparing effect.[78] The equivalent data are lacking in pediatrics. A meta-analysis of data concluding that the effect of an add-on LTRA was inferior to that of long-acting beta-agonists (LABA)[79] contained only one pediatric RCT in abstract form, which has been published since then[80] (n = 80 of 6476). No formal comparison pediatric RCTs have been published to date. There is emerging evidence of genetic polymorphisms that may influence the response to LTRAs.[81]

Allergic rhinitis may coexist with asthma. LRTAs are superior to placebo,[82] equivalent to antihistamines,[83] but inferior to nasal ICS in the treatment of allergic rhinitis.[84] A unified approach to treating the airway inflammation of both conditions is recommended. Treatment of allergic rhinitis with nasal corticosteroids also has shown a trend to improved asthma symptoms and forced expiratory volume in 1 second (FEV_1) which did not reach statistical significance (14 RCTs, 3 of which were pediatric).[85] A recent adult RCT of asthmatics who had allergic rhinitis has demonstrated a pronounced benefit of LRTA added to ICS, greater than the benefit achieved by doubling the dose of ICS.[86]

Inhaled Corticosteroids

ICS have formed the cornerstone of modern asthma management. Although not shown to be effective in patients who have episodic virally induced exacerbations,[66] the beneficial effect of ICS in persistent asthma has been established for some time.[87] A number of different ICS have been used, from the first ICS, beclomethasone, to budesonide and, more recently, fluticasone, ciclesonide, and mometasone. (Initial chlorofluorocarbon [CFC]-propelled metered-dose inhalers [MDI] have been reformulated using hydroxyfluoroalkane [HFA] propellant, because of concerns about the environmental impact of CFCs.)

Efficacy

Beclomethasone dipropionate was introduced in 1972. A meta-analysis of eight solely pediatric RCTs (n = 744, age $\geq$ 5 years) and four further RTCs that included children found beclomethasone to be superior to placebo with respect to FEV_1, symptoms, and likelihood of exacerbations when used for at least 4 weeks.[88] Beclomethasone seems to have a flat dose–response curve at higher doses,[89] based on two main RCTs, one of which was pediatric[90] (n = 177, age 6–16 years) comparing 400 μg/d versus 800 μg/d. The overall documented benefits in FEV_1 are small, however, and are of uncertain clinical significance, because there was no benefit in symptoms or exacerbation rate. No differences between the doses were shown in the pediatric trial. Previously reported ability to wean OCS dose with beclomethasone must be interpreted in the context of the time when the RCT was conducted (1970s) and the availability of other treatment options. Subsequent development of a HFA-propelled beclomethasone MDI, with its improved solubility and smaller particle size delivery, has led to improved drug delivery with consequent lower dose requirements.

Budesonide was introduced in 1980. Systematic review (11 pediatric RCTs, n = 926) demonstrated clear benefit over placebo in mild to moderate persistent asthma.[91] No dose-dependent effect above 100 to 200 μg/d was found for mild persistent asthma (seven pediatric RCTs, n = 726),[92] but an apparent further benefit (4% benefit in predicted FEV_1) in moderate-severe persistent asthma at doses of 800 μg/d has been reported in the only pediatric RCT examining this subgroup.[93] No pediatric RCTs have examined doses above 800 μg/d. A number of guidelines recommend use at the same dosage as CFC beclomethasone, but there is a lack of quality RCT data to support this recommendation (six pediatric RCTs of generally small numbers, with the number of subjects ranging from 10 to 41).[94]

Fluticasone was developed in 1990 and is available as an HFA-MDI and dry powder inhaler (DPI), both alone and in combination with salmeterol. Systematic review (75 RCTs including 8 pediatric RTCs, 5 of which had large sample sizes) has confirmed the benefit of fluticasone in mild to moderate asthma with minimal additional benefit from higher doses.[95] The finding of additional benefit of higher doses and an OCS-sparing effect in severe asthma is based on adolescent and adult data and is not definitive,[96] because no pediatric RCTs examined doses higher than 500 μg/d or included children taking daily OCS. An equivalent or slightly superior effect to budesonide or CFC-beclomethasone at half the dose was demonstrated on systematic review (75 RCTs, 16 pediatric).[97] A newer HFA-beclomethasone aerosol has been recommended at the same dose as fluticasone and was found to be equivalent in an essentially adult meta-analysis.[98] The only pediatric RCT comparison to date (n = 280, age 5–12 years) also has demonstrated equivalent effect.[99]

The two newest ICS are mometasone and ciclesonide. Mometasone is not currently available as an MDI in Australia but has US Food and Drug Administration (FDA) approval for children age 12 years and older. Ciclesonide is licensed in Australia for children 12 years and older and in June 2008 became available for children age 4 years and older, in line with the current FDA approval. Both drugs are approved for once-daily use. Mometasone was introduced in 1999, and evidence from a number of adult studies, some of which included adolescents, suggests a dose-dependent effect up to 400 μg/d in moderate persistent asthma, with no apparent benefit at higher doses.[100,101] An OCS-sparing effect has been documented at doses of 800/1600 μg/d.[102] Once-daily administration seems to be as effective as twice-daily administration at the same total daily dose. The one pediatric RCT to date in 296 children (age 4–11 years) who had mild to moderate persistent asthma showed benefit over placebo, with equal efficacy of 100 μg once-daily (evening) dosing and 100 μg twice-daily regimens.[103] Ciclesonide is the newest ICS. It has a small particle size with higher lung deposition (52%) and lower oropharyngeal deposition (38%).[104] It is delivered as a prodrug, des-ciclesonide, and is converted to the active drug primarily in the lungs. Initial pediatric RCTs have shown efficacy equal to that of budesonide, at half the budesonide dose, to 320 μg of ciclesonide administered once daily,[105,106] and to equivalent doses of fluticasone.[107] Once-daily dosing seems to be effective.[105,106,108]

Safety

Although ICS remain the treatment of choice for chronic asthma, there are concerns about systemic side effects, such as hypothalamic-pituitary-adrenal axis suppression and effects on linear growth, particularly at higher doses. On meta-analysis, beclomethasone administered at a dose of 200 μg twice daily for 7 to 12 months in mild to moderate persistent asthma has been shown to cause a decrease in linear growth of 1.54 cm/y in children.[109] In the Childhood Asthma Management Plan (CAMP) study, budesonide at doses of 200 to 400 μg/d caused a significant reduction in growth velocity, of 1.0 to 1.5 cm, over 3 to 5 years of treatment.[110] Catch-up growth seems to occur in subsequent years if a lower maintenance dose is used,[111] and final adult height was unaffected in a follow-up of the CAMP cohort.[112] Fluticasone, at half the budesonide and beclomethasone dose, seems to have a comparable safety profile, although firm conclusions are difficult.[97] Adrenal suppression, as detected by urinary cortisol levels, has been demonstrated at 800 to 3200 μg of budesonide,[92] and high doses of fluticasone have been implicated in most (30 of 33) cases of adrenal crisis caused by ICS.[113] Local side effects, such as oral candidiasis, pharyngitis, and hoarse voice can occur with these ICS but generally are not a major issue in children, particularly if the drug is delivered via a spacer, which limits oropharyngeal deposition. Oral candidiasis occurred in approximately 5% of patients taking fluticasone[95] and increased at higher doses.[96] Mometasone seems to have a similar safety profile. The ideal ICS should have high pulmonary deposition and residency time, low systemic bioavailability, and rapid systemic clearance.[114] Ciclesonide with its low oral conversion rate (< 20%), very low systemic bioavailability (< 1%), rapid degradation, high clearance rate, and high plasma protein binding (> 99%) results in negligible systemic levels.[115] No adrenal suppression with ciclesonide has been reported to date, even at high doses, and the rate of local side effects is much better than with fluticasone.[116]

Low-dose ICS have been shown often to provide optimal control for mild persistent asthma and to reduce the risk of severe asthma exacerbations. When commencing ICS therapy, initial low-dose ICS (see **Table 10**) is as effective as an initial high dose and subsequent down titration (23 RCTs, including 5 pediatric and 4 infant RCTs).[117]

Long-Acting Beta-Agonists

LABAs have a mechanism of action similar to that of SABA, but prolonged activation of beta-2 receptors in bronchial smooth muscle results in a prolonged duration of action of up to 12 hours. LABA monotherapy is inferior to ICS in mild to moderate asthma.[118] In addition, no benefit in asthma control was documented when a LABA was added to maintenance ICS in a moderate asthma cohort.[90] (The negative finding in this study may reflect the actual population studied, rather than the intended target population, because the children in the study were controlled as well on low-dose ICS as on a doubled dose of ICS or added LABA.) This lack of response to LABA in children is very different from the response observed in adults;[119,120] in adults, LABA has demonstrated benefits in a number of asthma control measures both in patients being treated with ICS[121] and in

ICS-naïve patients.[122] The apparent increase in exacerbations and lack of protective effect with LABA use in pediatric populations has been well documented.[119,123]

Concern about the safety of LABA has arisen also. Meta-analysis of RCTs with LABA use longer than 3 months has documented an increased risk of severe and life-threatening exacerbations, as well as increased asthma-related deaths, in both adult and pediatric populations.[124] Particular populations identified as being at risk were African Americans and steroid-naïve patients. This concern led the US FDA Pulmonary and Allergy Drugs Advisory Committee to strengthen its warning on all LABAs.[125] Precipitating tachyphylaxis with regular LABA therapy and subsequent lack of response to SABAs during exacerbations is a further concern. Currently, LABA therapy is recommended only as add-on therapy for patients who have moderate persistent asthma and who remain symptomatic despite moderate-dose ICS. The exact recommended dose of ICS above which LABA treatment can be considered in children remains unclear, because of the small number of available pediatric RCTs.[90,121] Until more evidence exists to delineate better the indications for LABA therapy, including the underlying mechanism for the different observed response in children, these recommendations should be followed strictly.

There currently are two choices of combination inhaler: salmeterol/fluticasone available in an MDI and a DPI and eformoterol/ budesonide in an inspiratory flow-driven suspension inhaler. Patient preference for the type of device may influence the physician's decision when evaluating the choice of combination therapy. The fast onset of eformoterol, comparable to that of SABAs, has led to the development of a therapeutic strategy with a single combination medication (eformoterol/budesonide), used as both preventer and reliever medication. This has been demonstrated to reduce exacerbation rates in both adults and children (n = 2760),[126] with pediatric benefit confirmed by subanalysis of the pediatric data (n = 341).[127] Although not yet incorporated into guidelines, this approach remains a promising management strategy that may offer improved compliance and a therapeutic option for adolescents who have difficult-to-control, severe persistent asthma. The drug currently is not approved in Australia for children under age 12 years.

Oral Corticosteroids and Other Immunosuppressive Agents

Five percent to 10% of persons who have severe persistent asthma are not responsive to maximal inhaled therapy[128] and depend on OCS for adequate control. Although some data comparing ICS and OCS dosages in adults are available,[129] equivalent data for the pediatric population are lacking, and the side effects associated with regular OCS are a concern. Potential side effects of regular OCS include osteoporosis, hypertension, and secondary diabetes mellitus. A number of second-line immunosuppressive agents ("steroid-sparing agents") have been evaluated. Attempted systematic reviews of the efficacy of azathioprine,[130] chloroquine,[131] colchicine,[132] cyclosporine,[133] dapsone,[134] methotrexate[135] and gold[136] have been limited by a small number, if any, of acceptable RCTs. No pediatric RCTs have been included. Small but statistically significant decreases in OCS have been demonstrated with gold, methotrexate, and cyclosporine, but the clinical significance of this observed dose response is unclear, especially given the additional side-effect profile of the immunosuppressive drugs themselves. The longest study to date investigating methotrexate, 10 mg weekly for 1 year in adults, reported a 55% reduction in OCS dose (compared with 4% in placebo) but no benefit in bone metabolism.[137]

Immunoglobulins and Omalizumab Therapy

A number of small studies have examined the role of intravenous immunoglobulin (IVIG) as a steroid-sparing agent. The positive results of initial open-label studies have not been replicated in subsequent RCTs including children,[138,139] and its role in asthma has been restricted. There also are safety concerns: one RCT was terminated prematurely after 3 of 16 patients in the high-dose IVIG arm (2 mg/kg monthly for 7 months) developed aseptic meningitis.[139] IVIG may play a role in a subset patients who have severe asthma with associated specific antibody deficiency,[140] but further research is needed.

Omalizumab is a humanized monoclonal antibody that forms complexes with circulating free IgE and represents a potential therapy for allergic disease. It currently is the only monoclonal antibody approved for asthma treatment and is included at step 5 in the current Global Initiative for Asthma guidelines (2006). Its true role in asthma management remains unclear, however. As an add-on therapy to ICS, omalizumab demonstrated benefits in symptom control and exacerbation rates in persistent asthma of varying severity,[141] but no benefit in exacerbation rate or steroid dose was seen in persons receiving regular OCS therapy. Only one RCT[142] has been conducted to date in children under age 12 years (range, 5–12 years) who had mild to moderate persistent asthma, and the results were similar. Omalizumab is an expensive drug, and its cost effectiveness remains debated.[143,144] Further studies are needed in the pediatric population for better clarification of patients likely to respond. The modest ICS-sparing effect also needs to be compared formally with cheaper alternatives such as the addition of LABA and LTRA.

Allergen Immunotherapy

Allergen immunotherapy is an evolving field, with both subcutaneous immunotherapy (SCIT) and sublingual immunotherapy (SLIT) desensitization now available for common aeroallergens such as pollen, house dust mite (HDM), and cat. Although immunotherapy has been shown to be an effective treatment for insect allergy and allergic rhinitis, its effectiveness and utility in the treatment of asthma are controversial.

On meta-analysis, in comparison with placebo, SCIT led to a reduction in asthma symptoms and use of asthma medication, as well as allergen-specific bronchial hyper-responsiveness, but had no consistent effect on lung function (75 RCTs, including 38 RCTs limited to or including pediatric patients).[145] It remains unclear how SCIT performs against other available therapies; the only comparison RCT, performed in adults, suggests a response inferior to the response to ICS.[146] In a pediatric-specific meta-analysis (nine RCTs including 441 children), SLIT was shown to be effective in reducing asthma scores and reducing the need for rescue medication, but positive findings were confined to SLIT with HDM extract, not in children treated with pollen or grass extract.[147] No directly comparative studies in pediatric asthma have been performed, although SLIT has been reported to be about 50% as efficacious as SCIT for the treatment of allergic rhinitis in adults.[148] Of note, all SCIT and SLIT studies to date included only patients who had mild/moderate asthma and examined monotherapy, not polytherapy with an allergen mixture. Although allergen immunotherapy may provide therapeutic benefit in patients who have an identified extrinsic, clinically unavoidable allergen, the risk of potentially fatal anaphylaxis (although rare) should be considered carefully and discussed with the parents if SCIT is being considered. SLIT has very few reported serious side effects and can be delivered at home. There currently is insufficient evidence to recommend SLIT or SCIT as a standard treatment for pediatric asthma.

Other Anti-Inflammatory Medications

A number of agents with potential anti-inflammatory actions have been identified, including macrolides, xanthines, and ketotifen. Small RCTs of macrolide therapy, including one pediatric RCT (n = 19),[149] have suggested a beneficial effect, but further studies are necessary to delineate which patients are most likely to benefit.[150] Xanthines (eg, theophylline) have been shown on meta-analysis to improve symptom control and SABA use compared with placebo and seem to be similar in efficacy to sodium cromoglycate but inferior to ICS (n = 2734, 34 pediatric RCTs).[151] Concern regarding a potential negative impact on behavior and concentration has limited its use, although these data are inconclusive; this concern is likely to be less of an issue now that lower doses are being used.[151] Ketotifen, an antihistamine, has been shown to improve asthma control in predominantly atopic, mild to moderate childhood asthma when used alone or in combination with other therapies (meta-analysis of 26 pediatric RCTs).[152] Benefit needs to be weighed against side effects such as sedation and weight gain.

Other Medications

Gastroesophageal reflux is common in asthma[153,154] and often is asymptomatic.[154] Pediatric RCTs of gastroesophageal reflux treatment have documented statistically significant improvements in clinical scores with treatment, but the clinical significance is unclear.[154,155]

Exercise-Induced Asthma

SABA administration before exercise confers significant protection for up to 3 hours.[156] A number of potential preventive therapies also have been shown to be effective for symptoms not adequately controlled with this approach. ICS given for at least 4 weeks were shown on meta-analysis (six RCTs of which four were pediatric, total n = 123, 102 pediatric subjects) to attenuate the fall in FEV_1 associated with exercise.[157] There currently is insufficient evidence to draw conclusions about shorter durations of ICS treatment. Also of note, in a population with mild persistent asthma,[158] there was a pronounced decrease in the exercise-induced fall in FEV_1 with 400 μg/d budesonide compared with 100 μg g/d, suggesting that a higher ICS dose may be needed to negate exercise symptoms despite good control of other symptoms. Nonsteroidal alternatives include sodium cromoglycate, nedocromil sodium, and LTRA. On meta-analysis (n = 280, 60% pediatric), nedocromil sodium has shown a consistent benefit in exercise-induced symptoms in both adults and children age 6 years and older.[159] LRTAs have a beneficial effect in exercise-induced asthma in children, with a significant reduction in FEV_1 fall[160,161,162,163] and onset of action within two doses.[162] Recently a head-to-head comparison between different therapies has been performed in a pediatric RCT (age 6–18 years, n = 80), which confirmed the beneficial effect of regular therapy and suggested that the best protection is offered by montelukast, either alone or in combination with budesonide.[164]

NONPHARMACOLOGIC MANAGEMENT
Dietary

Epidemiologic studies have attempted to explain the increasing prevalence of allergic diseases, especially in developed countries, and have examined a number of possible dietary factors. Attempted meta-analysis of calorie-controlled diets[165] and selenium supplementation[166] was limited by a lack of well-designed RCTs (only one was identified for either condition). Other RTCs, for fish oil supplements,[167] low or excluded salt,[168] tartrazine exclusion,[169] and vitamin C supplementation,[170] included between six and nine RCTs (two or fewer were pediatric) and failed to demonstrate any benefit.

Complementary Alternative Medicine

Complementary alternative medicine (CAM) is used commonly in pediatric asthma, with an estimated 50% to 60% of children using CAM at any one time.[171] (Only half of the cohort volunteered this information to their physician.) A lack of high-quality RCTs and heterogeneity of practice has hampered meta-analysis. There currently is no evidence to support the role of acupuncture,[172] homeopathy,[173] manual therapy,[174] or various breathing techniques[175,176] in chronic asthma. A recent RCT of breathing techniques in adults and adolescents who had mild persistent asthma documented impressive reductions in SABA use and ICS dose, although the lack of a true control arm makes it hard to rule out a trial effect.[177] Inspiratory muscle training in adults has demonstrated significant improvement in maximum inspiratory pressure, but the most of the research has been conducted by a single research group, and the clinical significance remains unclear.[178] A number of pediatric studies of physical fitness training in chronic asthmatics have successfully demonstrated improved cardiorespiratory fitness without deterioration in respiratory symptoms,[179] but whether improved fitness translates into better quality of life or lung function remains unclear. This finding, however, reinforces the overall aim of management in pediatric asthma, namely to allow the child to live as normal a life as possible, including full participation in activity.

Allergen Avoidance

Meta-analysis of studies using allergen-avoidance measures, including HDM reduction measures,[180] humidity control,[181] use of ionizers,[182] pet allergen control,[183] non-feather bedding,[184] and speleotherapy,[185] have failed to document any benefit in asthma control.

Asthma Prevention

Asthma prevention can be divided into primary (preventing onset of established risk factors), secondary (preventing development of asthma once established risk factors have developed) and tertiary prevention (care of established asthma and preventing exacerbations).

Potential environmental factors in asthma are supported by marked geographic and temporal variation in asthma prevalence.[1] Initial studies of environmental manipulation were promising, with HDM and food allergen avoidance measures in the first 12 months of life resulting in decreased sensitization and asthma diagnosis persisting until the age of 8 years in a high-risk birth cohort in the Isle of Wight.[186] Subsequent larger, multifaceted studies in Canada and Australia have failed to reproduce these results. The Canadian Childhood Asthma Primary Prevention Study showed a benefit in asthma symptoms but not bronchial hyper-responsiveness at 7 years,[187] whereas the Australian Childhood Asthma Prevention Study failed to show any clinical benefit at 5 years despite a 61% reduction in HDM and successful dietary manipulation.[188] Other current studies at earlier stages have yet to report positive results. The balance of evidence at present does not support the benefit of avoidance of allergens in early life on the subsequent development of asthma.

Breastfeeding currently is recommended for the first 6 months of life. There are a number of advantages to breastfeeding, but its protective role against allergic disease remains controversial. Although studies of formula-fed infants have reported higher rates of allergic disease, evidence does not support a protective effect on allergy and asthma. A recent large RCT in a birth cohort (n = 17,046) documented no protective effect at age 6.5 years of prolonged or exclusive breast feeding.[189] The link between antenatal and postnatal exposure to environmental tobacco smoke and subsequent increased risk of asthma is well established.[190] No RCTs have been performed to date, but avoidance of environmental tobacco smoke is strongly recommended.

The Early Treatment of the Atopic Child study reported no overall benefit of prolonged cetirizine (H1 receptor antagonist) treatment in infants who had atopic dermatitis at 18-month posttreatment follow-up. Benefit was seen only in sensitized subgroups, persisting to 36 months in grass pollen–sensitized infants but only transiently in those sensitized to HDM.[191] A subsequent study, the Early Prevention of Asthma in Atopic Children study, specifically targeted these subgroups but failed to show any benefit (UCB Pharma SA Belgium, unpublished data).

The rationale for tertiary prevention studies is the observation that a large number of persistent asthma cases start early in life,[192] but the three trials conducted to date, at differing ages or stages of "asthma development," have had disappointing results. Intermittent courses of ICS[193] and maintenance ICS,[194] for varying durations, in infants who had recurrent wheeze demonstrated no difference in asthma prevalence. The Childhood Asthma Management Program examined the effects of prolonged ICS or nedocromil sodium treatment for 4 to 6 years in a large group of school-age (5–12 years) children who had mild to moderate persistent asthma. Although ICS resulted in better symptom control, there was only a mild benefit in bronchial hyper-responsiveness and no effect on lung function outcome at the end of treatment.[110]

Vaccination in asthma may prevent exacerbations and serious complications such as pneumonia. Current guidelines recommend influenza vaccination for all children who have asthma, but there is a lack of pediatric evidence to support this recommendation.[195,196] In practice, vaccine coverage remains low despite the recommendation.[197] Pneumococcal vaccine has yet to demonstrate proven benefit in RCTs[198] but is now part of the routine vaccination schedule in many countries.

Other Aspects of Care

Education is a fundamental part of pediatric asthma management, including specific components of care (eg, training in the optimal use of medications), review of inhaler technique, and understanding of individualized written asthma-management plans. Education in self-management strategies does improve asthma outcomes,[199] including morbidity, but does not seem to improve quality of life.[200] Child-centered education seems to offer greater benefit than caregiver-focused education.[200] Written asthma-management plans, targeting symptom-based management rather than PEF, are effective in reducing exacerbation rates.[201,202] Having health care workers of patients' ethnic groups may be beneficial in improving asthma outcomes.[203] The evidence to support the role of family therapy or other psychologic interventions is limited,[204,205] but it may be a useful adjunct to care in certain children.

Spacers are required to deliver MDI medication effectively to younger children and are recommended to optimize delivery for older children, particularly in preventive therapy and in acute asthma. Small-volume spacers can be used from infancy with facemasks and from age 3 years with mouthpieces. Large-volume spacers can be used from 5 years of age. DPIs can be considered from the age of 6 years; breath-actuated devices are more appropriate from the age of 8 years, depending on the abilities and development of the individual child.[3]

Noninvasive methods to monitor airway inflammation, including exhaled nitric oxide, exhaled breath condensate, and induced sputum eosinophils, have shown benefits in adults.[206] The first pediatric longitudinal studies now have been published. These studies show a benefit in asthma control, and although there is not yet definitive evidence for incorporating these measures into asthma-management guidelines, these methods are promising tools for future management.[206,207]

SUMMARY

Pediatric asthma is a common condition with a large health care burden. Despite the large number of RCTs and meta-analyses conducted, there is a paucity of pediatric evidence on which to base appropriate management guidelines, and data from adult RCTs should not be extrapolated inappropriately to this younger age group. Consensus guidelines based on a combination of available evidence and expert opinion do exist, however, and these guidelines will continue to evolve as more conclusive pediatric evidence becomes available. Although these guidelines should form the basis of pediatric asthma management, important differential diagnoses and potentially modifiable factors also should be considered before commencing or escalating treatment. Recommendations based on the available pediatric evidence are summarized in **Tables 4** and **8**.

REFERENCES

1. Asher MI, Montefort S, Bjorksten B, et al. Worldwide time trends in the prevalence of symptoms of asthma, allergic rhinoconjunctivitis, and eczema in childhood: ISAAC phases one and three repeat multicountry cross-sectional surveys. Lancet 2006;368:733–43.
2. Schunemann HJ, Jaeschke R, Cook DJ, et al. An official ATS statement: grading the quality of evidence and strength of recommendations in ATS guidelines and recommendations. Am J Respir Crit Care Med 2006;174:605–14.
3. National Asthma Council Australia. Asthma management handbook. Melbourne: National Asthma Council Australia Ltd.; 2006.
4. van Asperen PP. Cough and asthma. Paediatr Respir Rev 2006;7:26–30.
5. Weinberger M, Abu-Hasan M. Pseudo-asthma: when cough, wheezing, and dyspnea are not asthma. Pediatrics 2007;120:855–64.
6. Geelhoed GC, Landau LI, Le Souef PN. Evaluation of SaO_2 as a predictor of outcome in 280 children presenting with acute asthma. Ann Emerg Med 1994;23:1236–41.
7. Keahey L, Bulloch B, Becker AB, et al. Initial oxygen saturation as a predictor of admission in children presenting to the emergency department with acute asthma. Ann Emerg Med 2002;40:300–7.
8. Camargo CA Jr, Spooner CH, Rowe BH. Continuous versus intermittent beta-agonists for acute asthma. Cochrane Database Syst Rev 2003;(4):Art. No.: CD001115. DOI:10.1002/14651858.CD001115.
9. Khine H, Fuchs SM, Saville AL. Continuous vs intermittent nebulized albuterol for emergency management of asthma. Acad Emerg Med. 1996;3:1019–24.
10. Papo MC, Frank J, Thompson AE. A prospective, randomized study of continuous versus intermittent nebulized albuterol for severe status asthmaticus in children. Crit Care Med 1993;21:1479–86.
11. Cates CJ, Crilly JA, Rowe BH. Holding chambers (spacers) versus nebulisers for beta-agonist treatment of acute asthma. Cochrane Database Syst Rev 2006;(2):Art. No.: CD000052. DOI:10.1002/14651858.CD000052.pub2.
12. Sears MR. Inhaled beta agonists. Ann Allergy 1992;68:446.
13. Plotnick LH, Ducharme FM. Combined inhaled anticholinergics and beta2-agonists for initial treatment of acute asthma in children. Cochrane Database Syst Rev 2000;(3):Art. No.: CD000060. DOI:10.1002/14651858.CD000060.

14. Everard ML, Bara A, Kurian M, et al. Anticholinergic drugs for wheeze in children under the age of two years. Cochrane Database Syst Rev 2005;(3):Art. No.: CD001279. DOI:10.1002/14651858.CD001279.pub2.

15. Garrett J, Williams S, Wong C, et al. Treatment of acute asthmatic exacerbations with an increased dose of inhaled steroid. Arch Dis Child 1998;79:12–7.

16. Hendeles L, Sherman J. Are inhaled corticosteroids effective for acute exacerbations of asthma in children? J Pediatr 2003;142:S26–32.

17. Hendeles L. Selecting a systemic corticosteroid for acute asthma in young children. J Pediatr 2003;142:S40–4.

18. Langton HS, Hobbs J, Reid F, et al. Prednisolone in acute childhood asthma: clinical responses to three dosages. Respir Med 1998;92:541–6.

19. Manser R, Reid D, Abramson M. Corticosteroids for acute severe asthma in hospitalised patients. Cochrane Database Syst Rev 2001;(1):Art. No.: CD001740. DOI:10.1002/14651858.CD001740.

20. van Asperen PP, Mellis CM, Sly PD. The role of corticosteroids in the management of childhood asthma. Med J Aust 2002;176:168–73.

21. Storr J, Barrell E, Barry W, et al. Effect of a single oral dose of prednisolone in acute childhood asthma. Lancet 1987;1:879–82.

22. Ho L, Landau LI, Le Souef PN. Lack of efficacy of single-dose prednisolone in moderately severe asthma. Med J Aust 1994;160:701–4.

23. Chang AB, Clark R, Thearle D, et al. Longer better than shorter? A multicentre randomised contriol trial (RCT) of 5 vs 3 days of oral prednisolone for acute asthma in children. Respirology 2007;12:A67 (12th Congress of the APSR/2nd Joint Congress of the APSR/ACCP, 30 November–4 December, Queensland, Australia).

24. Rowe BH, Spooner C, Ducharme FM, et al. Early emergency department treatment of acute asthma with systemic corticosteroids. Cochrane Database Syst Rev 2001;(1):Art. No.: CD002178. DOI:10.1002/14651858.CD002178.

25. Vuillermin P, South M, Robertson C. Parent-initiated oral corticosteroid therapy for intermittent wheezing illnesses in children. Cochrane Database Syst Rev 2006;(3):CD005311. DOI:10.1002/14651858.CD005311.pub2.

26. Becker JM, Arora A, Scarfone RJ, et al. Oral versus intravenous corticosteroids in children hospitalized with asthma. J Allergy Clin Immunol 1999;103:586–90.

27. Altamimi S, Robertson G, Jastaniah W, et al. Single-dose oral dexamethasone in the emergency management of children with exacerbations of mild to moderate asthma. Pediatr Emerg Care 2006;22:786–93.

28. Gries DM, Moffitt DR, Pulos E, et al. A single dose of intramuscularly administered dexamethasone acetate is as effective as oral prednisone to treat asthma exacerbations in young children. J Pediatr 2000;136:298–303.

29. Gordon S, Tompkins T, Dayan PS. Randomized trial of single-dose intramuscular dexamethasone compared with prednisolone for children with acute asthma. Pediatr Emerg Care 2007;23:521–7.

30. Deshpande A, McKenzie SA. Short course of steroids in home treatment of children with acute asthma. Br Med J (Clin Res Ed) 1986;293:169–71.

31. Edmonds ML, Camargo CA Jr, Brenner BE, et al. Replacement of oral corticosteroids with inhaled corticosteroids in the treatment of acute asthma following emergency department discharge: a meta-analysis. Chest 2002;121:1798–805.

32. Parr JR, Salama A, Sebire P. A survey of consultant practice: intravenous salbutamol or aminophylline for acute severe childhood asthma and awareness of potential hypokalaemia. Eur J Pediatr 2006;165:323–5.

33. Kirby C. Comparison of intravenous and inhaled salbutamol in severe acute asthma. Pediatr Rev Commun 1988;3:67–77.
34. Browne GJ, Penna AS, Phung X, et al. Randomised trial of intravenous salbutamol in early management of acute severe asthma in children. Lancet 1997;349: 301–5.
35. Browne GJ, Lam LT. Single-dose intravenous salbutamol bolus for managing children with acute severe asthma in the emergency department: reanalysis of data. Pediatr Crit Care Med 2002;3:117–23.
36. Travers A, Jones AP, Kelly K, et al. Intravenous beta2-agonists for acute asthma in the emergency department. Cochrane Database Syst Rev 2001;(1):Art. No.: CD002988. DOI:10.1002/14651858.CD002988.
37. Roberts G, Newsom D, Gomez K, et al. Intravenous salbutamol bolus compared with an aminophylline infusion in children with severe asthma: a randomised controlled trial. Thorax 2003;58:306–10.
38. Mitra A, Bassler D, Watts K, et al. Intravenous aminophylline for acute severe asthma in children over two years receiving inhaled bronchodilators. Cochrane Database Syst Rev 2005;(2):Art. No.: CD001276. DOI:10.1002/14651858. CD001276.pub2.
39. Yung M, South M. Randomised controlled trial of aminophylline for severe acute asthma. Arch Dis Child 1998;79:405–10.
40. Silveira DR, Piva JP, Jose Cauduro MP, et al. Early administration of two intravenous bolus of aminophylline added to the standard treatment of children with acute asthma. Respir Med 2008;102:156–61.
41. Gourgoulianis KI, Chatziparasidis G, Chatziefthimiou A, et al. Magnesium as a relaxing factor of airway smooth muscles. J Aerosol Med 2001;14:301–7.
42. Cairns CB, Kraft M. Magnesium attenuates the neutrophil respiratory burst in adult asthmatic patients. Acad Emerg Med 1996;3:1093–7.
43. Cheuk DK, Chau TC, Lee SL. A meta-analysis on intravenous magnesium sulphate for treating acute asthma. Arch Dis Child 2005;90:74–7.
44. Rowe BH, Bretzlaff JA, Bourdon C, et al. Intravenous magnesium sulfate treatment for acute asthma in the emergency department: a systematic review of the literature. Ann Emerg Med 2000;36:181–90.
45. Blitz M, Blitz S, Beasely R, et al. Inhaled magnesium sulfate in the treatment of acute asthma. Cochrane Database Syst Rev 2005;(4):Art. No.: CD003898. DOI:10.1002/14651858.CD003898.pub4.
46. Rodrigo G, Pollack C, Rodrigo C, et al. Heliox for nonintubated acute asthma patients. Cochrane Database Syst Rev 2006;(4):Art. No.: CD002884. DOI:10.1002/ 14651858.CD002884.pub2.
47. Kim IK, Phrampus E, Venkataraman S, et al. Helium/oxygen-driven albuterol nebulization in the treatment of children with moderate to severe asthma exacerbations: a randomized, controlled trial. Pediatrics 2005;116: 1127–33.
48. Ram FSF, Wellington SR, Rowe B, et al. Non-invasive positive pressure ventilation for treatment of respiratory failure due to severe acute exacerbations of asthma. Cochrane Database Syst Rev 2005;(3):Art. No.: CD004360. DOI:10.1002/ 14651858.CD004360.pub3.
49. Haggenmacher C, Biarent D, Otte F, et al [Non-invasive bi-level ventilation in paediatric status asthmaticus]. Arch Pediatr 2005;12:1785–7 [in French].
50. Dworski R, Fitzgerald GA, Oates JA, et al. Effect of oral prednisone on airway inflammatory mediators in atopic asthma. Am J Respir Crit Care Med 1994; 149:953–9.

51. Camargo CA Jr, Smithline HA, Malice MP, et al. A randomized controlled trial of intravenous montelukast in acute asthma. Am J Respir Crit Care Med 2003;167: 528–33.

52. Harmanci K, Bakirtas A, Turktas I, et al. Oral montelukast treatment of preschool-aged children with acute asthma. Ann Allergy Asthma Immunol 2006;96:731–5.

53. Robertson CF, Price D, Henry R, et al. Short-course montelukast for intermittent asthma in children: a randomized controlled trial. Am J Respir Crit Care Med 2007;175:323–9.

54. Graham V, Lasserson TJ, Rowe BH. Antibiotics for acute asthma. Cochrane Database Syst Rev 2001;(2):Art. No.: CD002741. DOI:10.1002/14651858.CD002741.

55. Haby MM, Waters E, Robertson CF, et al. Interventions for educating children who have attended the emergency room for asthma. Cochrane Database Syst Rev 2001;(1):Art. No.: CD001290. DOI:10.1002/14651858.CD001290.

56. Echeverria ZL, Tomico DR, Bracamonte BT, et al. Status asthmaticus: is respiratory physiotherapy necessary? Allergol Immunopathol (Madr) 2000;28:290–1.

57. Asher MI, Douglas C, Airy M, et al. Effects of chest physical therapy on lung function in children recovering from acute severe asthma. Pediatr Pulmonol 1990;9:146–51.

58. Guevara JP, Ducharme FM, Keren R, et al. Inhaled corticosteroids versus sodium cromoglycate in children and adults with asthma. Cochrane Database Syst Rev 2006;(2):Art.No.: CD003558. DOI:10.1002/14651858.CD003558.pub2.

59. van der Wouden JC, Tasche MJA, Bernsen RMD, et al. Sodium cromoglycate for asthma in children. Cochrane Database Syst Rev 2003;(3):Art. No.: CD002173. DOI:10.1002/14651858.CD002173.

60. Stevens MT, Edwards AM, Howell JB. Sodium cromoglicate: an ineffective drug or meta-analysis misused? Pharm Stat. 2007;6:123–37.

61. Rainey DK. Evidence for the anti-inflammatory activity of nedocromil sodium. Clin Exp Allergy 1992;22:976–9.

62. Sridhar AV, McKean M. Nedocromil sodium for chronic asthma in children. Cochrane Database Syst Rev 2006;(3):Art. No.: CD004108. DOI:10.1002/14651858.CD004108.pub2.

63. Edwards AM, Stevens MT. The clinical efficacy of inhaled nedocromil sodium (Tilade) in the treatment of asthma. Eur Respir J 1993;6:35–41.

64. Maspero JF, Duenas-Meza E, Volovitz B, et al. Oral montelukast versus inhaled beclomethasone in 6- to 11-year-old children with asthma: results of an open-label extension study evaluating long-term safety, satisfaction, and adherence with therapy. Curr Med Res Opin 2001;17:96–104.

65. Bisgaard H, Zielen S, Garcia-Garcia ML, et al. Montelukast reduces asthma exacerbations in 2- to 5-year-old children with intermittent asthma. Am J Respir Crit Care Med 2005;171:315–22.

66. McKean M, Ducharme F. Inhaled steroids for episodic viral wheeze of childhood. Cochrane Database Syst Rev 2000;(1):Art. No.: CD001107. DOI:10.1002/14651858.CD001107.

67. Oommen A, Lambert PC, Grigg J. Efficacy of a short course of parent-initiated oral prednisolone for viral wheeze in children aged 1-5 years: randomised controlled trial. Lancet 2003;362:1433–8.

68. Becker A, Swern A, Tozzi CA, et al. Montelukast in asthmatic patients 6 years–14 years old with an FEV1 > 75%. Curr Med Res Opin 2004;20:1651–9.

69. Knorr B, Franchi LM, Bisgaard H, et al. Montelukast, a leukotriene receptor antagonist, for the treatment of persistent asthma in children aged 2 to 5 years. Pediatrics 2001;108:E48.

70. Knorr B, Matz J, Bernstein JA, et al. Montelukast for chronic asthma in 6- to 14-year-old children: a randomized, double-blind trial. Pediatric Montelukast Study Group. JAMA 1998;279:1181–6.

71. Garcia Garcia ML, Wahn U, Gilles L, et al. Montelukast, compared with fluticasone, for control of asthma among 6- to 14-year-old patients with mild asthma: the MOSAIC study. Pediatrics 2005;116:360–9.

72. Ostrom NK, Decotiis BA, Lincourt WR, et al. Comparative efficacy and safety of low-dose fluticasone propionate and montelukast in children with persistent asthma. J Pediatr 2005;147:213–20.

73. Stempel DA, Kruzikas DT, Manjunath R. Comparative efficacy and cost of asthma care in children with asthma treated with fluticasone propionate and montelukast. J Pediatr 2007;150:162–7.

74. Sorkness CA, Lemanske RF, Jr., Mauger DT, et al. Long-term comparison of 3 controller regimens for mild-moderate persistent childhood asthma: the Pediatric Asthma Controller Trial. J Allergy Clin Immunol 119:64–72, 200.

75. Zeiger RS, Szefler SJ, Phillips BR, et al. Response profiles to fluticasone and montelukast in mild-to-moderate persistent childhood asthma. J Allergy Clin Immunol 2006;117:45–52.

76. Jat GC, Mathew JL, Singh M. Treatment with 400 microg of inhaled budesonide vs 200 microg of inhaled budesonide and oral montelukast in children with moderate persistent asthma: randomized controlled trial. Ann Allergy Asthma Immunol 2006;97:397–401.

77. Szefler SJ, Phillips BR, Martinez FD, et al. Characterization of within-subject responses to fluticasone and montelukast in childhood asthma. J Allergy Clin Immunol 2005;115:233–42.

78. Ducharme F, Schwartz Z, Kakuma R. Addition of anti-leukotriene agents to inhaled corticosteroids for chronic asthma. Cochrane Database Syst Rev 2004;(1):Art. No.: CD003133. DOI:10.1002/14651858.CD003133.pub2.

79. Ducharme FM, Lasserson TJ, Cates CJ. Long-acting beta2-agonists versus anti-leukotrienes as add-on therapy to inhaled corticosteroids for chronic asthma. Cochrane Database Syst Rev 2006;(4):Art. No.: CD003137. DOI:10.1002/14651858.CD003137.pub3.

80. Stelmach I, Grzelewski T, Bobrowska-Korzeniowska M, et al. A randomized, double-blind trial of the effect of anti-asthma treatment on lung function in children with asthma. Pulm Pharmacol Ther 2007;20:691–700.

81. Morrow T. Implications of pharmacogenomics in the current and future treatment of asthma. J Manag Care Pharm. 2007;13:497–505.

82. Razi C, Bakirtas A, Harmanci K, et al. Effect of montelukast on symptoms and exhaled nitric oxide levels in 7- to 14-year-old children with seasonal allergic rhinitis. Ann Allergy Asthma Immunol 2006;97:767–74.

83. Chen ST, Lu KH, Sun HL, et al. Randomized placebo-controlled trial comparing montelukast and cetirizine for treating perennial allergic rhinitis in children aged 2-6 yr. Pediatr Allergy Immunol 2006;17:49–54.

84. Nayak A, Langdon RB. Montelukast in the treatment of allergic rhinitis: an evidence-based review. Drugs 2007;67:887–901.

85. Taramarcaz P, Gibson PG. Intranasal corticosteroids for asthma control in people with coexisting asthma and rhinitis. Cochrane Database Syst Rev 2003;(3):Art. No.: CD003570. DOI:10.1002/14651858.CD003570.

86. Price DB, Swern A, Tozzi CA, et al. Effect of montelukast on lung function in asthma patients with allergic rhinitis: analysis from the COMPACT trial. Allergy 2006;61:737–42.

87. Calpin C, Macarthur C, Stephens D, et al. Effectiveness of prophylactic inhaled steroids in childhood asthma: a systemic review of the literature. J Allergy Clin Immunol 1997;100:452–7.
88. Adams NP, Bestall JB, Malouf R, et al. Beclomethasone versus placebo for chronic asthma. Cochrane Database Syst Rev 2005;(1):Art. No.: CD002738. DOI:10.1002/14651858.CD002738.pub2.
89. Adams N, Bestall J, Jones P. Beclomethasone at different doses for chronic asthma. Cochrane Database Syst Rev 1999;(4):Art. No.: CD002879. DOI:10.1002/14651858.CD002879.
90. Verberne AA, Frost C, Duiverman EJ, et al. Addition of salmeterol versus doubling the dose of beclomethasone in children with asthma. The Dutch Asthma Study Group. Am J Respir Crit Care Med 1998;158:213–9.
91. Adams N, Bestall J, Jones PW. Budesonide versus placebo for chronic asthma in children and adults. Cochrane Database Syst Rev 1999;(4):Art. No.: CD003274. DOI:10.1002/14651858.CD003274.
92. Adams N, Bestall J, Jones P. Budesonide at different doses for chronic asthma. Cochrane Database Syst Rev 2000;(2):Art. No.: CD003271. DOI:10.1002/14651858.CD003271.
93. Shapiro G, Bronsky EA, LaForce CF, et al. Dose-related efficacy of budesonide administered via a dry powder inhaler in the treatment of children with moderate to severe persistent asthma. J Pediatr 1998;132:976–82.
94. Adams N, Bestall JM, Jones PW. Beclomethasone versus budesonide for chronic asthma. Cochrane Database Syst Rev 2000;(1):Art. No.: CD003530. DOI:10.1002/14651858.CD003530.
95. Adams NP, Bestall JC, Lasserson TJ, et al. Fluticasone versus placebo for chronic asthma in adults and children. Cochrane Database Syst Rev 2005;(4):Art. No.: CD003135. DOI:10.1002/14651858.CD003135.pub3.
96. Adams NP, Bestall JC, Jones PW, et al. Fluticasone at different doses for chronic asthma in adults and children. Cochrane Database Syst Rev 2005;(3):Art. No.: CD003534. DOI:10.1002/14651858.CD003534.pub2.
97. Adams N, Lasserson TJ, Cates CJ, et al. Fluticasone versus beclomethasone or budesonide for chronic asthma in adults and children. Cochrane Database Syst Rev 2007;(4):Art. No.: CD002310. DOI:10.1002/14651858.CD002310.pub4.
98. Lasserson TJ, Cates CJ, Jones A-B, et al. Fluticasone versus HFA-beclomethasone dipropionate for chronic asthma in adults and children. Cochrane Database Syst Rev 2006;(2):Art. No.: CD005309. DOI:10.1002/14651858.CD005309.pub3.
99. van Aalderen WM, Price D, De Baets FM, et al. Beclomethasone dipropionate extrafine aerosol versus fluticasone propionate in children with asthma. Respir Med 2007;101:1585–93.
100. O'Connor B, Bonnaud G, Haahtela T, et al. Dose-ranging study of mometasone furoate dry powder inhaler in the treatment of moderate persistent asthma using fluticasone propionate as an active comparator. Ann Allergy Asthma Immunol 2001;86:397–404.
101. Bernstein DI, Berkowitz RB, Chervinsky P, et al. Dose-ranging study of a new steroid for asthma: mometasone furoate dry powder inhaler. Respir Med 1999;93:603–12.
102. Fish JE, Karpel JP, Craig TJ, et al. Inhaled mometasone furoate reduces oral prednisone requirements while improving respiratory function and health-related quality of life in patients with severe persistent asthma. J Allergy Clin Immunol 2000;106:852–60.

103. Berger WE, Milgrom H, Chervinsky P, et al. Effects of treatment with mometasone furoate dry powder inhaler in children with persistent asthma. Ann Allergy Asthma Immunol 2006;97:672–80.
104. Richter K, Kanniess F, Biberger C, et al. Comparison of the oropharyngeal deposition of inhaled ciclesonide and fluticasone propionate in patients with asthma. J Clin Pharmacol 2005;45:146–52.
105. von Berg A, Engelstatter R, Minic P, et al. Comparison of the efficacy and safety of ciclesonide 160 microg once daily vs. budesonide 400 microg once daily in children with asthma. Pediatr Allergy Immunol 2007;18:391–400.
106. Vermeulen JH, Gyurkovits K, Rauer H, et al. Randomized comparison of the efficacy and safety of ciclesonide and budesonide in adolescents with severe asthma. Respir Med 2007;101:2182–91.
107. Pedersen S, Garcia Garcia ML, Manjra A, et al. A comparative study of inhaled ciclesonide 160 microg/day and fluticasone propionate 176 microg/day in children with asthma. Pediatr Pulmonol 2006;41:954–61.
108. Gelfand EW, Georgitis JW, Noonan M, et al. Once-daily ciclesonide in children: efficacy and safety in asthma. J Pediatr 2006;148:377–83.
109. Sharek PJ, Bergman DA, Ducharme F. Beclomethasone for asthma in children: effects on linear growth. Cochrane Database Syst Rev 1999;(3):Art. No.: CD001282. DOI:10.1002/14651858.CD001282.
110. Long-term effects of budesonide or nedocromil in children with asthma. The Childhood Asthma Management Program Research Group. N Engl J Med 2000;343:1054–63.
111. Anthracopoulos MB, Papadimitriou A, Panagiotakos DB, et al. Growth deceleration of children on inhaled corticosteroids is compensated for after the first 12 months of treatment. Pediatr Pulmonol 2007;42:465–70.
112. Agertoft L, Pedersen S. Effect of long-term treatment with inhaled budesonide on adult height in children with asthma. N Engl J Med 2000;343:1064–9.
113. Todd GR, Acerini CL, Ross-Russell R, et al. Survey of adrenal crisis associated with inhaled corticosteroids in the United Kingdom. Arch Dis Child 2002;87:457–61.
114. Gulliver T, Morton R, Eid N. Inhaled corticosteroids in children with asthma: pharmacologic determinants of safety and efficacy and other clinical considerations. Paediatr Drugs 2007;9:185–94.
115. Rohatagi S, Luo Y, Shen L, et al. Protein binding and its potential for eliciting minimal systemic side effects with a novel inhaled corticosteroid, ciclesonide. Am J Ther. 2005;12:201–9.
116. Abdullah AK, Khan S. Evidence-based selection of inhaled corticosteroid for treatment of chronic asthma. J Asthma 2007;44:1–12.
117. Powell H, Gibson PG. High dose versus low dose inhaled corticosteroid as initial starting dose for asthma in adults and children. Cochrane Database Syst Rev 2003;(4):Art. No.: CD004109. DOI:10.1002/14651858.CD004109.pub2.
118. Verberne AA, Frost C, Roorda RJ, et al. One year treatment with salmeterol compared with beclomethasone in children with asthma. The Dutch Paediatric Asthma Study Group. Am J Respir Crit Care Med 1997;156:688–95.
119. Bisgaard H. Effect of long-acting beta2 agonists on exacerbation rates of asthma in children. Pediatr Pulmonol 2003;36:391–8.
120. Bisgaard H, Szefler S. Long-acting beta2 agonists and paediatric asthma. Lancet 2006;367:286–8.

121. Ni Chroinin M, Greenstone IR, Danish A, et al. Long-acting beta2-agonists versus placebo in addition to inhaled corticosteroids in children and adults with chronic asthma. Cochrane Database Syst Rev 2005;(4):Art. No.: CD005535. DOI:10.1002/14651858.CD005535.

122. Ni Chroinin M, Greenstone IR, Ducharme FM. Addition of inhaled long-acting beta2-agonists to inhaled steroids as first line therapy for persistent asthma in steroid-naive adults. Cochrane Database Syst Rev 2004;(4):Art. No.: CD005307. DOI:10.1002/14651858.CD005307.

123. Walters EH, Gibson PG, Lasserson TJ, et al. Long-acting beta2-agonists for chronic asthma in adults and children where background therapy contains varied or no inhaled corticosteroid. Cochrane Database Syst Rev 2007;(1):Art. No.: CD001385. DOI:10.1002/14651858.CD001385.pub2.

124. Salpeter SR, Buckley NS, Ormiston TM, et al. Meta-analysis: effect of long-acting beta-agonists on severe asthma exacerbations and asthma-related deaths. Ann Intern Med 2006;144:904–12.

125. Chowdhury BA. Division Director Memorandum: overview of the FDA background materials prepared for the meeting to discuss the implications of the available data related to the safety of long acting beta-agonist bronchodilators. 2005. Available at: http://www.fda.gov/ohrms/dockets/ac/05/briefing/2005-414881_03_01-FDA-Div-Dir-Memo.pdf. Accessed April 2008.

126. O'Byrne PM, Bisgaard H, Godard PP, et al. Budesonide/formoterol combination therapy as both maintenance and reliever medication in asthma. Am J Respir Crit Care Med 2005;171:129–36.

127. Bisgaard H, Le Roux P, Bjamer D, et al. Budesonide/formoterol maintenance plus reliever therapy: a new strategy in pediatric asthma. Chest 2006;130:1733–43.

128. Robinson DS, Campbell DA, Durham SR, et al. Systematic assessment of difficult-to-treat asthma. Eur Respir J 2003;22:478–83.

129. Mash B, Bheekie A, Jones PW. Inhaled versus oral steroids for adults with chronic asthma. Cochrane Database Syst Rev 2001;(1):Art. No.: CD002160. DOI:10.1002/14651858.CD002160.

130. Dean T, Dewey A, Bara A, et al. Azathioprine as an oral corticosteroid sparing agent for asthma. Cochrane Database Syst Rev 2003;(4):Art. No.: CD003270. DOI:10.1002/14651858.CD003270.pub2.

131. Dewey A, Dean T, Bara A, et al. Chloroquine as a steroid sparing agent for asthma. Cochrane Database Syst Rev 2003;(4):Art. No.: CD003275. DOI:10.1002/14651858.CD003275.

132. Dewey A, Dean T, Bara A, et al. Colchicine as an oral corticosteroid sparing agent for asthma. Cochrane Database Syst Rev 2003;(3):. DOI:10.1002/14651858.CD003273.

133. Evans DJ, Cullinan P, Geddes DM, et al. Cyclosporin as an oral corticosteroid sparing agent in stable asthma. Cochrane Database Syst Rev 2000;(4):Art. No.: CD002993. DOI:10.1002/14651858.CD002993.

134. Dewey A, Bara A, Dean T, et al. Dapsone as an oral corticosteroid sparing agent for asthma. Cochrane Database Syst Rev 2002;(4):Art. No.: CD003268. DOI:10.1002/14651858.CD003268.

135. Davies H, Olson L, Gibson P. Methotrexate as a steroid sparing agent for asthma in adults. Cochrane Database Syst Rev 1998;(3):Art. No.: CD000391. DOI:10.1002/14651858.CD000391.

136. Evans DJ, Cullinan P, Geddes DM, et al. Gold as an oral corticosteroid sparing agent in stable asthma. Cochrane Database Syst Rev 2000;(4):Art. No.: CD002985. DOI:10.1002/14651858.CD002985.

137. Comet R, Domingo C, Larrosa M, et al. Benefits of low weekly doses of methotrexate in steroid-dependent asthmatic patients. A double-blind, randomized, placebo-controlled study. Respir Med 2006;100:411–9.

138. Niggemann B, Leupold W, Schuster A, et al. Prospective, double-blind, placebo-controlled, multicentre study on the effect of high-dose, intravenous immunoglobulin in children and adolescents with severe bronchial asthma. Clin Exp Allergy 1998;28:205–10.

139. Kishiyama JL, Valacer D, Cunningham-Rundles C, et al. A multicenter, randomized, double-blind, placebo-controlled trial of high-dose intravenous immunoglobulin for oral corticosteroid-dependent asthma. Clin Immunol 1999;91:126–33.

140. Schwartz HJ, Hostoffer RW, McFadden ER Jr, et al. The response to intravenous immunoglobulin replacement therapy in patients with asthma with specific antibody deficiency. Allergy Asthma Proc 2006;27:53–8.

141. Walker S, Monteil M, Phelan K, et al. Anti-IgE for chronic asthma in adults and children. Cochrane Database Syst Rev 2006;(2):Art. No.: CD003559. DOI:10.1002/14651858.CD003559.pub3.

142. Milgrom H, Berger W, Nayak A, et al. Treatment of childhood asthma with anti-immunoglobulin E antibody (omalizumab). Pediatrics 2001;108:E36.

143. Wu AC, Paltiel AD, Kuntz KM, et al. Cost-effectiveness of omalizumab in adults with severe asthma: results from the Asthma Policy Model. J Allergy Clin Immunol 2007;120:1146–52.

144. Brown R, Turk F, Dale P, et al. Cost-effectiveness of omalizumab in patients with severe persistent allergic asthma. Allergy 2007;62:149–53.

145. Abramson MJ, Puy RM, Weiner JM. Allergen immunotherapy for asthma. Cochrane Database Syst Rev 2003;(4):Art. No.: CD001186. DOI:10.1002/14651858.CD001186.

146. Shaikh WA. Immunotherapy vs inhaled budesonide in bronchial asthma: an open, parallel, comparative trial. Clin Exp Allergy 1997;27:1279–84.

147. Penagos M, Passalacqua G, Compalati E, et al. Metaanalysis of the efficacy of sublingual immunotherapy in the treatment of allergic asthma in pediatric patients, 3 to 18 years of age. Chest 2008;133:599–609.

148. Nelson HS. Allergen immunotherapy: where is it now? J Allergy Clin Immunol 2007;119:769–79.

149. Kamada AK, Hill MR, Ikle DN, et al. Efficacy and safety of low-dose troleandomycin therapy in children with severe, steroid-requiring asthma. J Allergy Clin Immunol 1993;91:873–82.

150. Sharma S, Jaffe A, Dixon G. Immunomodulatory effects of macrolide antibiotics in respiratory disease: therapeutic implications for asthma and cystic fibrosis. Paediatr Drugs 2007;9:107–18.

151. Seddon P, Bara A, Ducharme FM, et al. Oral xanthines as maintenance treatment for asthma in children. Cochrane Database Syst Rev 2006;(1):Art. No.: CD002885. DOI:10.1002/14651858.CD002885.pub2.

152. Bassler D, Mitra A, Ducharme FM, et al. Ketotifen alone or as additional medication for long-term control of asthma and wheeze in children. Cochrane Database Syst Rev 2004;(1):Art. No.: CD001384. DOI:10.1002/14651858.CD001384.pub2.

153. Andze GO, Luks FI, Bensoussan AL, et al [Role of surgical treatment of gastroesophageal reflux in children with severe asthma]. Pediatrie 1991;46:451–4 [in French].

154. Tucci F, Resti M, Fontana R, et al. Gastroesophageal reflux and bronchial asthma: prevalence and effect of cisapride therapy. J Pediatr Gastroenterol Nutr 1993;17:265–70.

155. Gustafsson PM, Kjellman NI, Tibbling L. A trial of ranitidine in asthmatic children and adolescents with or without pathological gastro-oesophageal reflux. Eur Respir J 1992;5:201–6.
156. Shapiro GG, Kemp JP, DeJong R, et al. Effects of albuterol and procaterol on exercise-induced asthma. Ann Allergy 1990;65:273–6.
157. Koh MS, Tee A, Lasserson TJ, et al. Inhaled corticosteroids compared to placebo for prevention of exercise induced bronchoconstriction. Cochrane Database Syst Rev 2007;(3):Art. No.: CD002739. DOI:10.1002/14651858.CD002739.pub3.
158. Pedersen S, Hansen OR. Budesonide treatment of moderate and severe asthma in children: a dose-response study. J Allergy Clin Immunol 1995;95:29–33.
159. Spooner CH, Saunders LD, Rowe BH. Nedocromil sodium for preventing exercise-induced bronchoconstriction. Cochrane Database Syst Rev 2002;(1):Art. No.: CD001183. DOI:10.1002/14651858.CD001183.
160. Pearlman DS, Ostrom NK, Bronsky EA, et al. The leukotriene D4-receptor antagonist zafirlukast attenuates exercise-induced bronchoconstriction in children. J Pediatr 1999;134:273–9.
161. Melo RE, Sole D, Naspitz CK. Exercise-induced bronchoconstriction in children: montelukast attenuates the immediate-phase and late-phase responses. J Allergy Clin Immunol 2003;111:301–7.
162. Kemp JP, Dockhorn RJ, Shapiro GG, et al. Montelukast once daily inhibits exercise-induced bronchoconstriction in 6- to 14-year-old children with asthma. J Pediatr 1998;133:424–8.
163. Kim JH, Lee SY, Kim HB, et al. Prolonged effect of montelukast in asthmatic children with exercise-induced bronchoconstriction. Pediatr Pulmonol 2005;39:162–6.
164. Stelmach I, Grzelewski T, Majak P, et al. Effect of different antiasthmatic treatments on exercise-induced bronchoconstriction in children with asthma. J Allergy Clin Immunol 2008;121:383–9.
165. Cheng J, Tao Pan, Ye GH, et al. Calorie controlled diet for chronic asthma. Cochrane Database Syst Rev 2003;(2):Art. No.: CD004674. DOI:10.1002/14651858.CD004674.pub2.
166. Allam MF, Lucena RA. Selenium supplementation for asthma. Cochrane Database Syst Rev 2004;(2):Art. No.: CD003538. DOI:10.1002/14651858.CD003538.pub2.
167. Thien FCK, De Luca S, Woods R, et al. Dietary marine fatty acids (fish oil) for asthma in adults and children. Cochrane Database Syst Rev 2002;(2):Art. No.: CD001283. DOI:10.1002/14651858.CD001283.
168. Ram FSF, Ardern KD. Dietary salt reduction or exclusion for allergic asthma. Cochrane Database Syst Rev 2004;(2):Art. No.: CD000436. DOI:10.1002/14651858.CD000436.pub2.
169. Ram FS, Ardern KD. Tartrazine exclusion for allergic asthma. Cochrane Database Syst Rev 2001;(4):Art. No.: CD000460. DOI:10.1002/14651858.CD000460.
170. Ram FSF, Rowe BH, Kaur B. Vitamin C supplementation for asthma. Cochrane Database Syst Rev 2004;(3):Art. No.: CD000993. DOI:10.1002/14651858.CD000993.pub2.
171. Shenfield G, Lim E, Allen H. Survey of the use of complementary medicines and therapies in children with asthma. J Paediatr Child Health 2002;38:252–7.
172. McCarney RW, Brinkhaus B, Lasserson TJ, et al. Acupuncture for chronic asthma. Cochrane Database Syst Rev 2003;(3):Art. No.: CD000008. DOI:10.1002/14651858.CD000008.pub2.
173. McCarney RW, Linde K, Lasserson TJ. Homeopathy for chronic asthma. Cochrane Database Syst Rev 2004;(1):Art. No.: CD000353. DOI:10.1002/14651858.CD000353.pub2.

174. Hondras MA, Linde K, Jones AP. Manual therapy for asthma. Cochrane Database Syst Rev 2005;(2):Art. No.: CD001002. DOI:10.1002/14651858.CD001002.pub2.

175. Holloway E, Ram FSF. Breathing exercises for asthma. Cochrane Database Syst Rev 2004;(1):Art. No.: CD001277. DOI:10.1002/14651858.CD001277.pub2.

176. Dennis J, Cates CJ. Alexander technique for chronic asthma. Cochrane Database Syst Rev 2000;(2):Art.No.:CD000995. DOI:10.1002/14651858.CD000995.

177. Slader CA, Reddel HK, Spencer LM, et al. Double blind randomised controlled trial of two different breathing techniques in the management of asthma. Thorax 2006;61:651–6.

178. Ram FSF, Wellington SR, Barnes NC. Inspiratory muscle training for asthma. Cochrane Database Syst Rev 2003;(3):Art. No.: CD003792. DOI:10.1002/14651858.CD003792.

179. Ram FSF, Robinson SM, Black PN, et al. Physical training for asthma. Cochrane Database Syst Rev 2005;(4):Art. No.: CD001116. DOI:10.1002/14651858.CD001116.pub2.

180. Gøtzsche PC, Johansen HK, Schmidt LM, et al. House dust mite control measures for asthma. Cochrane Database Syst Rev 2004;(4):Art. No.: CD001187. DOI:10.1002/14651858.CD001187.pub2.

181. Singh M, Bara A, Gibson P. Humidity control for chronic asthma. Cochrane Database Syst Rev 2002;(1):Art. No.: CD003563. DOI:10.1002/14651858.CD003563.

182. Blackhall K, Appleton S, Cates CJ. Ionisers for chronic asthma. Cochrane Database Syst Rev 2003;(2):Art. No.: CD002986. DOI:10.1002/14651858.CD002986.

183. Kilburn S, Lasserson TJ, McKean M. Pet allergen control measures for allergic asthma in children and adults. Cochrane Database Syst Rev 2001;(1):Art. No.: CD002989. DOI:10.1002/14651858.CD002989.

184. Campbell F, Gibson P. Feather versus non-feather bedding for asthma. Cochrane Database Syst Rev 2000;(4):Art. No.: CD002154. DOI:10.1002/14651858. CD002154.

185. Beamon S, Falkenbach A, Fainburg G, et al. Speleotherapy for asthma. Cochrane Database Syst Rev 2001;(2):Art. No.: CD001741. DOI:10.1002/14651858. CD001741.

186. Arshad SH, Bateman B, Sadeghnejad A, et al. Prevention of allergic disease during childhood by allergen avoidance: the Isle of Wight prevention study. J Allergy Clin Immunol 2007;119:307–13.

187. Chan-Yeung M, Ferguson A, Watson W, et al. The Canadian childhood asthma primary prevention study: outcomes at 7 years of age. J Allergy Clin Immunol 2005;116:49–55.

188. Marks GB, Mihrshahi S, Kemp AS, et al. Prevention of asthma during the first 5 years of life: a randomized controlled trial. J Allergy Clin Immunol 2006;118: 53–61.

189. Kramer MS, Matush L, Vanilovich I, et al. Effect of prolonged and exclusive breast feeding on risk of allergy and asthma: cluster randomised trial. BMJ 2007;335:815.

190. DiFranza JR, Aligne CA, Weitzman M. Prenatal and postnatal environmental tobacco smoke exposure and children's health. Pediatrics 2004;113:1007–15.

191. Warner JO. A double-blinded, randomized, placebo-controlled trial of cetirizine in preventing the onset of asthma in children with atopic dermatitis: 18 months' treatment and 18 months' posttreatment follow-up. J Allergy Clin Immunol 2001;108:929–37.

192. Yunginger JW, Reed CE, O'Connell EJ, et al. A community-based study of the epidemiology of asthma. Incidence rates, 1964–1983. Am Rev Respir Dis 1992;146:888–94.

193. Bisgaard H, Hermansen MN, Loland L, et al. Intermittent inhaled corticosteroids in infants with episodic wheezing. N Engl J Med 2006;354:1998–2005.

194. Murray CS, Woodcock A, Langley SJ, et al. Secondary prevention of asthma by the use of Inhaled Fluticasone propionate in Wheezy infants (IFWIN): double-blind, randomised, controlled study. Lancet 2006;368:754–62.

195. Cates CJ, Jefferson TO, Bara AI, et al. Vaccines for preventing influenza in people with asthma. Cochrane Database Syst Rev 2003;(4):Art. No.: CD000364. DOI:10.1002/14651858.CD000364.pub2.

196. Carroll W, Burkimsher R. Is there any evidence for influenza vaccination in children with asthma? Arch Dis Child 2007;92:644–5.

197. Influenza vaccination coverage among children with asthma—United States—2004–05 influenza season. MMWR Morb Mortal Wkly Rep 2007;56:193–6.

198. Sheikh A, Alves B, Dhami S. Pneumococcal vaccine for asthma. Cochrane Database Syst Rev 2002;(1):Art. No.: CD002165. DOI:10.1002/14651858.CD002165.

199. Wolf FM, Guevara JP, Grum CM, et al. Educational interventions for asthma in children. Cochrane Database Syst Rev 2002;(4):Art. No.: CD000326. DOI:10.1002/14651858.CD000326.

200. Cano-Garcinuno A, Diaz-Vazquez C, Carvajal-Uruena I, et al. Group education on asthma for children and caregivers: a randomized, controlled trial addressing effects on morbidity and quality of life. J Investig Allergol Clin Immunol 2007;17:216–26.

201. Bhogal S, Zemek R, Ducharme FM. Written action plans for asthma in children. Cochrane Database Syst Rev 2006;(3):Art. No.: CD005306. DOI:10.1002/14651858.CD005306.pub2.

202. Wensley D, Silverman M. Peak flow monitoring for guided self-management in childhood asthma: a randomized controlled trial. Am J Respir Crit Care Med 2004;170:606–12.

203. Chang AB, Taylor B, Masters IB, et al. Indigenous healthcare worker involvement for indigenous adults and children with asthma. Cochrane Database Syst Rev 2007;(4):Art.No.: CD006344. DOI:10.1002/14651858.CD006344.pub2.

204. Yorke J, Fleming S, Shuldham C. Psychological interventions for children with asthma. Cochrane Database Syst Rev 2005;(4):Art. No.: CD003272. DOI:10.1002/14651858.CD003272.pub2.

205. Yorke J, Shuldham C. Family therapy for asthma in children. Cochrane Database Syst Rev 2005;(2):Art.No.:CD000089. DOI:10.1002/14651858.CD000089.pub2.

206. Petsky HL, Kynaston JA, Turner C, et al. Tailored interventions based on sputum eosinophils versus clinical symptoms for asthma in children and adults. Cochrane Database Syst Rev 2007;(2):. DOI:10.1002/14651858.CD005603.pub2.

207. Zacharasiewicz A, Erin EM, Bush A. Noninvasive monitoring of airway inflammation and steroid reduction in children with asthma. Curr Opin Allergy Clin Immunol 2006;6:155–60.

Congenital Airway Lesions and Lung Disease

Ian Brent Masters, MBBS, FRACP, PhD

KEYWORDS

- Laryngomalacia • Tracheobronchomalacia
- Cystic adenomatoid malformation

THE RELEVANCE OF CONGENITAL AIRWAY AND LUNG LESIONS FOR PEDIATRICIANS

Congenital airway and cystic lung lesions are not common in pediatrics.[1–3] Despite the low incidence of these lesions, pediatricians are likely to encounter this type of disorder through common respiratory symptoms and signs (respiratory noises, tachypnea, and cough). For pediatricians, pediatric pulmonologists, radiologists, otolaryngologists, thoracic surgeons, and intensive care staff, the management and care of children who have these lesions can require considerable expenditures of time and other resources within a tertiary care center.[4,5] Specifically, most children who have suspected airway lesions require a laryngoscopy and bronchoscopy and detailed radiologic assessments, and some need intensive care and/or operative management.[6,7] Even though there are no published health economics data for this level of care, the health care costs for the diagnostic and long-term management of these disorders are likely to be large.

Congenital lesions related to the lung can be classified as (1) parenchymal, (2) airway, (3) vascular (arterial/venous), and (4) lymphatic lesions. Upper airway structural disorders are the most common disorders encountered, with laryngomalacia being the most common; subglottic stenosis, subglottic hemangiomas, subglottic cystic lesions, vocal cord paralysis, and webs are less common. The lower airway disorders are the malacia disorders, airway stenoses, hypoplastic disorders or small airways, ectopic and accessory bronchi, bronchial atresia, and diverticulum and airway distortion disorders.[1–3] Finally, parenchymal lung lesions such as cystic adenomatoid malformation, sequestrations, foregut malformations, and congenital lobar emphysema also can be seen as structural lesions of the distal airways and parenchyma.[8]

Queensland Children's Respiratory Centre, Royal Children Hospital, Herston, 4029, Brisbane, Queensland, Australia
E-mail address: brent_masters@health.qld.gov.au

Pediatr Clin N Am 56 (2009) 227–242
doi:10.1016/j.pcl.2008.10.006
0031-3955/08/$ – see front matter © 2009 Elsevier Inc. All rights reserved.

Pulmonary vascular and lymphatic anomalies include pulmonary arteriovenous malformations[9] and primary and secondary lymphangiectasia disorders.[10–12]

This article describes some of the many diagnostic and management issues that surround the most common of these disorders: laryngomalacia, tracheobronchomalacia disorders, and the cystic lesions, particularly cystic adenomatoid malformation. Management of these conditions generally is not evidenced based, but most of the current approaches to care have stood the test of time and have very good outcomes.

LARYNGOMALACIA
Incidence

The incidence of laryngomalacia is not known, but it has long been recognized as the most common cause of chronic or persistent stridor in infants. Laryngomalacia also may occur in late-onset forms in the child and adult populations with various levels of associated feeding difficulties, disordered breathing during sleep, and exercise-induced laryngeal obstruction.[13–15]

Pathogenesis

The pathogenesis of laryngomalacia is not known, but familial cases and cases associated with a variety of syndromes have been described,[16–20] thus suggesting a potential genetic basis.

The morphologic descriptions of laryngomalacia consist of an omega-shaped epiglottis, short aryepiglottic folds, and varying degrees of arytenoid and arytenoid mucosal prolapse and of posterior displacement of the epiglottis. Laryngomalacia has been classified as type 1, 2, and 3, depending the involvement of the three components.[21,22] The functional elements of these changes have resulted in many theories about the cause of laryngomalacia, but it is possible that both the anatomic appearances and functional elements result from genetic factors producing abnormalities and maturational delays in the sensorineural function of the larynx, because symptoms resolve in most children by 2 years of age.[23]

Classification of Laryngomalacia

Laryngomalacia generally is classified by its laryngoscopic appearance. In the most commonly used classification, prolapse of the mucosa overlying the arytenoid cartilages is designated type 1; foreshortened aryepiglottic folds are designated type 2; and posterior displacement of the epiglottis is designated type 3. Various combinations of these types may be seen,[21] and concomitant pharyngeal collapse also may occur.[24] In addition to this classification, clinical classifications have been used to help direct therapy. In neonates and infants these classifications have centered on stridor, the severity of airway obstruction, and the impact on respiratory function and general well being, development, and growth.[25] In late-onset groups, from childhood to adulthood, laryngomalacia has been described by its association with feeding disorders (feeding-disordered laryngomalacia), sleep-disordered breathing (sleep-disordered laryngomalacia), and exercise (exercise-induced laryngomalacia).[15]

Evidence-based management of laryngomalacia

Evidence-based management recommendations using integrated and validated algorithms for diagnosis and management are lacking for almost all aspects of care of laryngomalacia. Despite these apparent deficits, current management of laryngomalacia depends on an accurate diagnosis and an assessment of the clinical impact on respiratory function and general features of growth and neurodevelopmental status. In addition, concomitant management of reflux-related diseases is helpful in some patients.[26] The following general approach to the assessment and management of stridor and laryngomalacia is suggested:

1. Define the timing of the stridor (eg, inspiratory, expiratory, biphasic)
2. Classify the severity of obstruction
3. Assess for concomitant factors
   - Syndromes
   - Chronic cough
   - Swallowing difficulties, general growth such as weight gain
   - Cutaneous disorders
   - Neurodevelopmental status of the infants

When stridor is inspiratory, the degree of obstruction is minimal, and there are no concomitant factors, management should be expectant observation over time.

If other factors are found, referral to a pediatric pulmonologist or otolaryngologist is recommended. The ongoing management for the different severities of laryngomalacia is described in the following sections.

Mild laryngomalacia Mild laryngomalacia is characterized by isolated, intermittent, cogwheel inspiratory stridor with minimal work of breathing (recession/retractions) and normal growth and development. Symptoms and signs such as concomitant coughing, wheezing, vocal changes, swallowing or feeding difficulties, skin lesions, and cardiovascular or constitutional symptoms invariably denote other disorders. In most infants signs resolve progressively over the first 2 years of life. Parental reassurance and regular follow-up assessments should be performed to support the parent and to ensure appropriate resolution of the child's problems.

Moderate laryngomalacia Moderate laryngomalacia is characterized by continual stridor and significant work of breathing (recession/retractions) without other constitutional symptoms and signs. Children should have a chest radiograph and an airway assessment with laryngoscopy and bronchoscopy. Radiographic investigations in the form of airway fluoroscopy screening are of limited specific diagnostic value (evidence grade = very low). A barium-swallow esophagogram may provide important specific diagnostic information concerning the swallow mechanisms, particularly when vascular rings and slings are suspected (evidence grade = very low). Laryngoscopy and bronchoscopy provide the specifics of diagnosis that surround the differential diagnoses of lingual cysts, vocal cord disorders, hemangiomas and cysts, and tracheobronchial abnormalities. In most children, symptoms resolve by 2 years of age. Once the diagnosis has been affirmed by the diagnostic procedures, parental reassurance and regular follow-up assessments should be performed to support the parents and ensure appropriate progress and resolution of the child's problems.

Severe laryngomalacia Severe laryngomalacia is characterized by continuous inspiratory stridor, increased work or breathing, varying degrees of respiratory failure (severe obstruction) requiring oxygen therapy and/or airway support, and constitutional symptoms such as failure to thrive or developmental delay. Surgical interventions are likely to be required. The surgical interventions are predominantly aryepiglottoplasties (supraglottoplasty) performed by a variety of techniques including laser (evidence grade = low).[15,21,23,27] Tracheostomy is rarely required. Once the diagnosis has been affirmed by the diagnostic procedures and interventions have taken place, regular follow-up assessments should be performed to support the parents and ensure appropriate progress and resolution of the child's problems. Supraglottoplasty does not necessarily result in a total and sustained loss of stridor, but it usually reduces the work of breathing appreciably. Successful feeding may be slower to recover (**Table 1**).[21,27]

TRACHEOBRONCHOMALACIA DISORDERS
Incidence

The incidence of tracheobronchomalacia disorders is thought to range between 1:1500 and 1:2500 children.[29,30] Despite this relatively low incidence, these lesions are encountered commonly in pediatric bronchoscopic practices, particularly when investigating stridulous, recurrent, or persistent wheezy and "rattly" conditions and chronic cough, especially in association with congenital heart disease and syndromic conditions.[20,31,32] Marchant and colleagues[33] have shown that a significant number of children who have isolated chronic cough also have malacia disorders. In addition Chang and colleagues[34] have shown that an unusual quality of cough, such as a vibratory or brassy cough, has high levels of association with bronchoscopically proven malacia. Despite these advances in knowledge, incorrect diagnoses brought about by attributing these disorders to asthma are common in both pediatric[35,36] and adult practice.[37] Therefore it is likely that the estimated incidence of malacia of 1:1500 to 1:2500 significantly underestimates the true incidence. Consequently, pediatricians need to remain vigilant and cognizant of this diagnosis.

Pathogenesis

The pathogenesis of tracheobronchomalacia disorders is not known, but indirect associative evidence indicates that it is likely that these disorders develop during fetal life around 5 to 8 weeks after conception.[38–41]

Molecular genetic studies of fetal lung and airway development indicate signaling pathway abnormalities involving a variety of genes[42] including the *Hox*, *Shh*, and *Gli* genes.[43–49] The *Sox9* gene is essential to the formation of cartilage both spatially and temporally,[5] and *Shh* (sonic hedgehog) expression is important to the formation of cartilage rings.[40]

In addition, alterations in the timing of expression or in the compounds that form the structural support of the airway cartilage—the collagens and aggrecans—could alter the mechanical properties of tracheal cartilage.[50–54] Type II collagen has the dominant role in tensile properties of cartilage, whereas type I collagen seems to be more important in shaping the airway.[51,53–55] The aggrecans, which offer the airway cartilage compressive resilience, are vulnerable to proteases, including the metalloproteases that abound during fetal lung growth and development.[50,52,56] Lysyl oxidases,

Table 1			
Outline of the evidence for management of laryngomalacia			
Medication/Intervention	Recommendation	Grading of Recommendation (Based on Evidence of Benefit)	Quality of Supporting Evidence
Airway fluoroscopy screen[28]	Not recommended	Low	Low
Supraglottoplasty[27]	Recommended in severe cases only	Moderate	Low
Investigation for GOR[26]	Recommended in symptomatic patients	Moderate	Low

a copper-dependent extracellular enzyme group, are important to the tensile properties of collagen because they catalyze the formation of lysine and hydroxy-lysine cross-links in collagen.[57] Bone morphogenetic protein expression also is important for lysyl oxidase gene expression and activation, and it currently is thought to be important in tracheoesophageal fistula and malacia.[42,58–63]

The anatomic distribution of different collagen types within the large airways complicates the issues further, because collagen type I, II, and III patterns of distribution do change temporarily and regionally from the neonatal period to childhood.[64] Just how gene expression controls these transitions is not known, but, again, alterations to these processes could render the airway vulnerable, both temporally and spatially, to the formation of malacia lesions.

Classification of Malacia Lesions

The term "malacia" is derived from Greek word "malakia," meaning "soft." In the respiratory context it infers a sustained softening of the airway cartilage that results in a dynamic change in the appearance of the airway during the respiratory cycle or during forced breathing maneuvers.[4] Malacia has been classified in a variety of ways, but none has been accepted universally. These classifications include major airway collapse,[4] excessive dynamic airway collapse,[37,65] and tracheal dyskinesia;[66–68] where a 50% reduction in cross-sectional area is considered significant.[69] Qualified descriptions (eg, "consistent with innominate artery compression" or "Eiffel Tower appearance consistent with double aortic arch")[70–72] and the designations "primary malacia" and "secondary malacia" also are used.[73,74]

The degree of malacia is measured best with bronchoscopy assessment at the end-expiratory point when the lumen is at its narrowest.[4,75–79] Tracheomalacia can be defined and measured using CT,[80–86] but this approach has a number of limitations in pediatrics, and publications are limited to anecdotal case reports.[87–91] Bronchomalacia (lobar and segmental) is not well defined by CT.

Evidence-based management of tracheobronchomalacia

Diagnosis Essentially, the management of tracheobronchomalacia disorders is based on expert opinion derived from anecdotal experiences using the levels of severity of the symptoms and signs, the bronchoscopic appearance of the lesions across the respiratory cycle, and other investigations to define the spectrum of illness from mild to severe. Currently, diagnostic and management algorithms are being developed, but none has been tested rigorously (evidence grade = very low).[65,92] These approaches

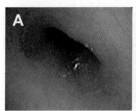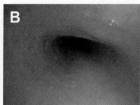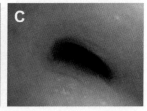

Fig. 1. Bronchoscopic images of malacia (tracheomalacia) taken with the bronchoscope held 10 mm from the anterior aspect of the lesion in low-light conditions to enhance the visual definition of the lesion. (*A*) Anterior flattening of the trachea at the junction of the middle and lower third of the trachea. (*B*) Anterior flattening with anterior slope from left to right. (*C*) Tracheomalacia: saber or triangular shape.

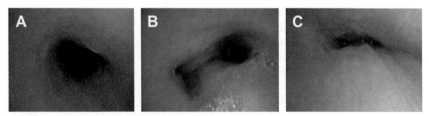

Fig. 2. Tracheomalacia. (*A*) Note localized anterior flattening at the junction of the mid and lower thirds of the trachea with maintenance of the posterior shape. (*B*) Note the anterior flattening at the carina and lateral to medial apposition of the origin of left main stem bronchus. (*C*) Note anterior flattening and some bulging of the pars with anterior-to-posterior apposition of surfaces on the right side.

are necessary, because the loss of cross-sectional area in the lesions does not seem to correlate well with symptoms and signs (evidence grade = moderate).[79,93]

The diagnosis should be considered in children who have persistent or protracted recurrent airway symptoms (persistent or recurrent "wet" cough, unusual cough, expiratory stridor, wheeze, rattliness or rattly respirations, dyspnea/respiratory distress), recurrent protracted bacterial bronchitis, pneumonia (particularly with atypical radiographic features such as persistent or recurrent collapse), localized gas trapping, and unusual radiographic densities. Suspicion of this diagnosis also should be increased in children who have syndromes involving cardiac disorders, non-cystic fibrosis bronchiectatic states, and "asthmalike states" in which there has not been an adequate response to medications (evidence grade = moderate).[33,94–97] All children in whom the diagnosis is suspected should have simple radiographic assessments, and some will require bronchoscopic assessments and more invasive and detailed radiographic assessments such as a contrast swallow, CT with contrast, or MRI (evidence grade = very low).

Mild tracheobronchomalacia The mild end of the tracheobronchomalacia spectrum usually ranges from trivial rattly respirations and intermittent illnesses to more troublesome recurrent bronchitic illnesses, recurrent croup, recurrent cough, and wheezy illnesses.[33,66–68,94,95] Even in this group of children, unpredictable and severe obstructive episodes may require intensive care management. The management of patients who have recurrent bronchitis or protracted bronchitis has not been studied in any formal sense,[98] but there is little doubt that these illnesses have a significant

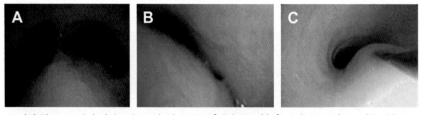

Fig. 3. (*A*) The pars is bulging into the lumen of right and left main stem bronchi with excessive dynamic collapse or tracheal dyskinesia. (*B*) Crescent-shaped tracheomalacia with extension to and complete occlusion of the right main stem bronchi. (*C*) H-shaped tracheoesophageal fistula with a catheter and posterior malacia. The catheter was passed through the working channel of the bronchoscope and placed into and through the fistula. In this case the pars was "heaped up" in the extrathoracic trachea before the passage of the catheter.

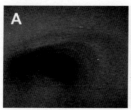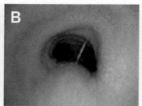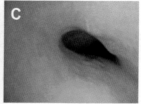

Fig. 4. Tracheomalacia. (*A*) Note the anterior flattening forming a triangular appearance from left to right. (*B*) Eiffel tower or equilateral triangular appearance consistent with double aortic arch. (*C*) Note the anterior flattening forming a triangular appearance from right to left.

effect on the psychologic functioning of both the child and families involved[99] (evidence grade = high). Antibiotics and chest physiotherapy along with conventional asthma medications, particularly bronchodilators and oral steroids, are the commonly used modes of treatment[36] (evidence grade = very low). Evidence-based information is lacking for these modes of treatment except salbutamol[100] (evidence grade = low), for which the benefits of outcome are inconclusive. Because children treated with oral steroids may experience significant side effects, this practice, in particular, should be evaluated thoroughly by evidence-based methodologies.

Moderate tracheobronchomalacia For children who have intermittent severe obstruction or moderate sustained obstruction, management usually involves supportive therapies such as subnasal oxygen and continuous positive airway pressure (CPAP) or bi-level positive airway pressure (BiPAP) during sleep and with intercurrent illness (evidence grade = very low).[101–104]

Severe tracheobronchomalacia At the severe end of the spectrum, with sustained and life-threatening airway obstruction that necessitates intensive care management with intubation, surgery has been the most common approach because of its potential to be curative without the need for ongoing supportive care.[105] The surgical approaches include aortopexy,[105–107] tracheopexy, stent placement,[7] correction of vascular deformities, and correction of existing cardiac defects, when possible.[108–112] The outcome of these approaches has been defined by case series; these approaches generally result in functional improvement even though the anatomic repair sometimes is incomplete or nonsustained. Many difficulties have been reported with stent

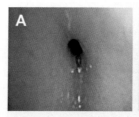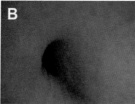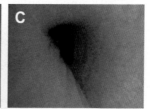

Fig. 5. Bronchomalacia: left main stem malacia. (*A*) Proximal. Note a rotated view and complete closure of the medial aspect of the left main stem (anterior/posterior surface apposition). (*B*) Midpoint. Note incomplete closure of the left main stem (superior/inferior surface apposition) forming a crescent appearance. (*C*) Distal. Note incomplete closure of the left main stem (superior/inferior surface apposition) forming a triangular appearance with the left upper lobe visible at 12 o'clock.

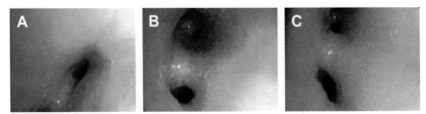

Fig. 6. Bronchomalacia. (*A*) Left upper lobe is flattened to produce a slit like appearance. (*B*) The left lower lobe has a circumferential appearance, while the left upper lobe appears normal but small. (*C*) Crescent-like appearance of left lower lobe orifice.

placement, and benefits do not necessarily justify the potential problems in maintenance and removal.[7] Not all reports of surgery have included ventilated patients, and none of the surgical series has reported any detailed clinical assessments of severity or quantified measurements of the malacia. It is difficult to attribute the entire outcome of the operations to the reduction in airway resistance, particularly because the cross-sectional area of lesions does not correlate well with measured illness profiles,[79,93] and in infants who have malacia a complex interrelationship exists between lung volumes and flow and resistance measurements (evidence grade = moderate).[103] Despite these operative approaches, some children require long-term tracheostomy and pressure support in the form of CPAP or BiPAP. Deaths also have been recorded within this group of severely ill patients.[113]

Advice to parents and caregivers The advice provided to parents and other health workers is important for the ongoing management of children who have malacia disorders. Parents often seem to have little or no understanding of the condition, especially when a child has a long-standing diagnosis of asthma. Therefore this author bases the general advice to parents and children around improving understanding of the disorder through visual imagery by using bronchoscopic images such as those in **Figs. 1** through **8**. In addition, the association between the dynamics of the lesions and symptoms and signs of the illness is explained. Furthermore, the natural history is explained. In particular, the caregivers are informed that the lesions tend to improve with increasing age and that only a small percentage of lesions remain the same or deteriorate over time, but the characteristics of the lesions that improve are not known (evidence grade = very low).[79] Generally children who have malacia have higher relative risks of respiratory illness, greater symptom levels, and a tendency to more protracted recovery than normal controls during infancy and early childhood (evidence

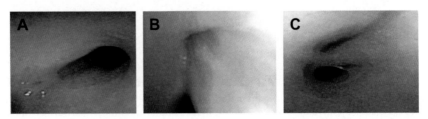

Fig. 7. Bronchomalacia. (*A*) Right main stem is flattened in the anterior/posterior aspects to produce a key-hole appearance. (*B*) Right upper lobe is crescent shaped with complete closure. (*C*) Right middle lobe has a slitlike appearance with the airway almost completely closed.

Table 2
Outline of the evidence for management of tracheobronchomalacia disorders

Medication/Intervention	Recommendation	Grading of Recommendation (Based on Evidence of Benefit)	Quality of Supporting Evidence
Inhaled beta-2 agonists[100]	Not routinely recommended	Moderate	Low
Inhaled or oral corticosteroids[36]	Not routinely recommended	Low	Low
Antibiotics[114]	Recommended for protracted bronchitis	Low	Low
Physiotherapy	Recommended	Low	Low
Surgery[105,106,115]	Recommended in severe cases	Low	Low

grade = moderate).[93] Treatment options and their limitations also are explained and reiterated during reviews (evidence grade = very low). Regular patient reviews also may have an important role in reducing anxieties, in reducing ad hoc medical visits and hospitalizations, and in regulating or removing unnecessary therapies (evidence grade = very low) (**Table 2**).[99]

CYSTIC LUNG DISORDERS

Cystic lung disorders include cystic adenomatoid malformation, extra lobar sequestration, bronchopulmonary foregut malformations, bronchial atresia, and lobar emphysema. There is considerable overlap among these conditions.[116,117]

Cricoid shelf

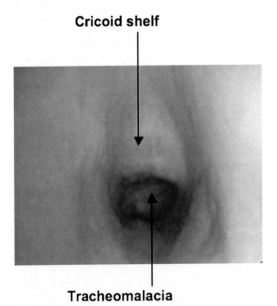

Tracheomalacia

Fig. 8. Secondary tracheomalacia. Anterior cartilages are depressed to the posterior trachea by the angle of the tracheostomy tube.

Incidence

The incidence of cystic lesions of the lung is not known, and the lesions may be subclinical across life, but they generally are regarded as rare.[8,118–120]

Pathogenesis

Molecular genetic evidence indicates congenital cyst adenomatoid malformation (c-CAM) and other cystic disorders are associated with aberrations in signaling pathway genes, in particular *Hoxb-5*, which is important for the proliferation and patterning of the last seven subdivisions of the smaller airways,[121] fibroblast growth factor,[122] and fatty acid binding protein.[123]

Classification

c-CAM is classified pathologically by the diameter of the cystic lesions. Type 1 cysts are 2 to 10 mm in diameter, type 2 cysts are 0.5 to 2 mm, and type 3 cysts are microscopic glandlike and bronchiole-like structures.[118] These cystic structures may be liquid or gas filled. There is no specific clinical classification, but they may be identified as a result of antenatal ultrasound assessments, in utero problems such a hydrops and pleural effusions, respiratory distress in the neonatal period with either radiodensities or gas-trapping radiologic appearances, atypical or recurrent pneumonia/abscess, gas-leak disorders, or as incidental or unsuspected radiologic findings in children and adults.[8,120]

Evidence-based management of congenital cystic lung disorders

Management depends on the timing of diagnosis, the severity of respiratory illness, or the likelihood of respiratory illnesses. Surgical removal of the lesions or lobe involved by open or thoracoscopic techniques is the general approach.[124–126] Controversy exists about the conservative management of asymptomatic postnatal diagnoses of c-CAM and extra lobar sequestration; however, congenital lobar emphysema may resolve spontaneously, so an observant approach is justified (evidence grade = very low).[119] Longitudinal research is required for these disorders.

REFERENCES

1. Landing BH, Dixon LG. Congenital malformations and genetic disorders of the respiratory tract (larynx, trachea, bronchi, and lungs). Am Rev Respir Dis 1979;120(1):151–85.
2. Chen JC, Holinger LD. Congenital tracheal anomalies: pathology study using serial macrosections and review of the literature. Pediatr Pathol 1994;14(3):513–37.
3. Chen JC, Holinger LD. Congenital laryngeal lesions: pathology study using serial macrosections and review of the literature. Pediatr Pathol 1994;14(2):301–25.
4. Mair EA, Parsons DS. Pediatric tracheobronchomalacia and major airway collapse. Ann Otol Rhinol Laryngol 1992;101(4):300–9.
5. Elluru RG, Whitsett JA. Potential role of Sox9 in patterning tracheal cartilage ring formation in an embryonic mouse model. Arch Otolaryngol Head Neck Surg 2004;130(6):732–6.
6. Altman KW, Wetmore RF, Marsh RR. Congenital airway abnormalities in patients requiring hospitalization. Arch Otolaryngol Head Neck Surg 1999;125(5):525–8.
7. Pillai JB, Smith J, Hasan A, et al. Review of pediatric airway malacia and its management, with emphasis on stenting. Eur J Cardiothorac Surg 2005;27(1):35–44.

8. Berrocal T, Madrid C, Novo S, et al. Congenital anomalies of the tracheobronchial tree, lung, and mediastinum: embryology, radiology, and pathology. Radiographics 2004;24(1):e17.

9. Liechty KW, Flake AW. Pulmonary vascular malformations. Semin Pediatr Surg 2008;17(1):9–16.

10. Barker PM, Esther CR Jr, Fordham LA, et al. Primary pulmonary lymphangiectasia in infancy and childhood. Eur Respir J 2004;24(3):413–9.

11. Esther CR Jr, Barker PM. Pulmonary lymphangiectasia: diagnosis and clinical course. Pediatr Pulmonol 2004;38(4):308–13.

12. Bellini C, Boccardo F, Campisi C, et al. Congenital pulmonary lymphangiectasia. Orphanet J Rare Dis 2006;1:43.

13. Smith GJ, Cooper DM. Laryngomalacia and inspiratory obstruction in later childhood. Arch Dis Child 1981;56(5):345–9.

14. Hoeve LJ, Rombout J. Pediatric laryngobronchoscopy. 1332 procedures stored in a data base. Int J Pediatr Otorhinolaryngol 1992;24(1):73–82.

15. Richter GT, Rutter MJ, deAlarcon A, et al. Late-onset laryngomalacia: a variant of disease. Arch Otolaryngol Head Neck Surg 2008;134(1):75–80.

16. Amin MR, Isaacson G. State-dependent laryngomalacia. Ann Otol Rhinol Laryngol 2007;106(11):887–90.

17. Bent J. Pediatric laryngotracheal obstruction: current perspectives on stridor. Laryngoscope 2006;116(7):1059–70.

18. Jacobs IN, Gray RF, Todd NW. Upper airway obstruction in children with Down syndrome. Arch Otolaryngol Head Neck Surg 1996;122(9):945–50.

19. Markert ML, Majure M, Harville TO, et al. Severe laryngomalacia and bronchomalacia in DiGeorge syndrome and CHARGE association. Pediatr Pulmonol 1997;24(5):364–9.

20. Masters IB, Chang AB, Patterson L, et al. Series of laryngomalacia, tracheomalacia, and bronchomalacia disorders and their associations with other conditions in children. Pediatr Pulmonol 2002;34(3):189–95.

21. Olney DR, Greinwald JH Jr, Smith RJ, et al. Laryngomalacia and its treatment. Laryngoscope 1999;109(11):1770–5.

22. Cicekcibasi AE, Keles B, Uyar M. The morphometric development of the fetal larynx during the fetal period. Int J Pediatr Otorhinolaryngol 2008;72(5):683–91.

23. Thompson DM. Abnormal sensorimotor integrative function of the larynx in congenital laryngomalacia: a new theory of etiology. Laryngoscope 2007;117(6 Pt 2 Suppl 114):1–33.

24. Shatz A, Goldberg S, Picard E, et al. Pharyngeal wall collapse and multiple synchronous airway lesions. Ann Otol Rhinol Laryngol 2004;113(6):483–7.

25. Shah UK, Wetmore RF. Laryngomalacia: a proposed classification form. Int J Pediatr Otorhinolaryngol 1998;46(1–2):21–6.

26. Giannoni C, Sulek M, Friedman EM, et al. Gastroesophageal reflux association with laryngomalacia: a prospective study. Int J Pediatr Otorhinolaryngol 1998; 43(1):11–20.

27. O'Donnell S, Murphy J, Bew S, et al. Aryepiglottoplasty for laryngomalacia: results and recommendations following a case series of 84. Int J Pediatr Otorhinolaryngol 2007;71(8):1271–5.

28. Rudman DT, Elmaraghy CA, Shiels WE, et al. The role of airway fluoroscopy in the evaluation of stridor in children. Arch Otolaryngol Head Neck Surg 2003; 129(3):305–9.

29. Carden KA, Boiselle PM, Waltz DA, et al. Tracheomalacia and tracheobronchomalacia in children and adults: an in-depth review. Chest 2005;127(3):984–1005.

30. Boogaard R, Huijsmans SH, Pijnenburg MW, et al. Tracheomalacia and bronchomalacia in children: incidence and patient characteristics. Chest 2005;128(5):3391-7.
31. Chen SJ, Lee WJ, Wang JK, et al. Usefulness of three-dimensional electron beam computed tomography for evaluating tracheobronchial anomalies in children with congenital heart disease. Am J Cardiol 2003;92(4):483-6.
32. Lee SL, Cheung YF, Leung MP, et al. Airway obstruction in children with congenital heart disease: assessment by flexible bronchoscopy. Pediatr Pulmonol 2002; 34(4):304-11.
33. Marchant JM, Masters IB, Taylor SM, et al. Evaluation and outcome of young children with chronic cough. Chest 2006;129(5):1132-41.
34. Chang AB, Gaffney JT, Eastburn MM, et al. Cough quality in children: a comparison of subjective vs. bronchoscopic findings. Respir Res 2005;6(1):3.
35. Wood RE. Localized tracheomalacia or bronchomalacia in children with intractable cough. J Pediatr 1990;116(3):404-6.
36. Thomson F, Masters IB, Chang AB. Persistent cough in children and the overuse of medications. J Paediatr Child Health 2002;38(6):578-81.
37. Murgu SD, Colt HG. Tracheobronchomalacia and excessive dynamic airway collapse. Respirology 2006;11(4):388-406.
38. Perl AK, Whitsett JA. Molecular mechanisms controlling lung morphogenesis. Clin Genet 1999;56(1):14-27.
39. Roth-Kleiner M, Post M. Genetic control of lung development. Biol Neonate 2003;84(1):83-8.
40. Miller LA, Wert SE, Clark JC, et al. Role of Sonic hedgehog in patterning of tracheal-bronchial cartilage and the peripheral lung. Dev Dyn 2004;231(1):57-71.
41. Shannon JM, Hyatt BA. Epithelial-mesenchymal interactions in the developing lung. Annu Rev Physiol 2004;66:625-45.
42. Warburton D, Bellusci S, De Langhe S, et al. Molecular mechanisms of early lung specification and branching morphogenesis. Pediatr Res 2005;57(5 Pt 2): 26R-37R.
43. Qi BQ, Merei J, Farmer P, et al. Tracheomalacia with esophageal atresia and tracheoesophageal fistula in fetal rats. J Pediatr Surg 1997;32(11):1575-9.
44. Merei J, Hasthorpe S, Farmer P, et al. Relationship between esophageal atresia with tracheoesophageal fistula and vertebral anomalies in mammalian embryos. J Pediatr Surg 1998;33(1):58-63.
45. Possoegel AK, Diez-Pardo JA, Morales C, et al. Notochord involvement in experimental esophageal atresia. Pediatr Surg Int 1999;15(3-4):201-5.
46. Xia H, Migliazza L, Diez-Pardo JA, et al. The tracheobronchial tree is abnormal in experimental congenital diaphragmatic hernia. Pediatr Surg Int 1999;15(3-4): 184-7.
47. Xia H, Otten C, Migliazza L, et al. Tracheobronchial malformations in experimental esophageal atresia. J Pediatr Surg 1999;34(4):536-9.
48. Beasley SW, Diez Pardo J, Qi BQ, et al. The contribution of the adriamycin-induced rat model of the VATER association to our understanding of congenital abnormalities and their embryogenesis. Pediatr Surg Int 2000;16(7):465-72.
49. Williams AK, Qi BQ, Beasley SW. Demonstration of abnormal notochord development by three-dimensional reconstructive imaging in the rat model of esophageal atresia. Pediatr Surg Int 2001;17(1):21-4.
50. Roberts CR, Rains JK, Pare PD, et al. Ultrastructure and tensile properties of human tracheal cartilage. J Biomech 1998;31(1):81-6.
51. Mankarious LA, Goetinck PF. Growth and development of the human cricoid cartilage: an immunohistochemical analysis of the maturation sequence of the

chondrocytes and surrounding cartilage matrix. Otolaryngol Head Neck Surg 2000;123(3):174–8.

52. Chen Q, Johnson DM, Haudenschild DR, et al. Progression and recapitulation of the chondrocyte differentiation program: cartilage matrix protein is a marker for cartilage maturation. Dev Biol 1995;172(1):293–306.

53. Mankarious LA, Adams AB, Pires VL. Patterns of cartilage structural protein loss in human tracheal stenosis. Laryngoscope 2002;112(6):1025–30.

54. Cherukupally SR, Adams AB, Mankarious LA. Age-related mechanisms of cricoid cartilage response to injury in the developing rabbit. Laryngoscope 2003;113(7):1145–8.

55. Kim JC, Mankarious LA. Novel cell proliferation marker for identification of a growth center in the developing human cricoid. Arch Otolaryngol Head Neck Surg 2000;126(2):197–202.

56. Roberts CR, Pare PD. Composition changes in human tracheal cartilage in growth and aging, including changes in proteoglycan structure. Am J Physiol 1991;261(2 Pt 1):L92–101.

57. Maki JM, Sormunen R, Lippo S, et al. Lysyl oxidase is essential for normal development and function of the respiratory system and for the integrity of elastic and collagen fibers in various tissues. Am J Pathol 2005;167(4):927–36.

58. Lu MM, Yang H, Zhang L, et al. The bone morphogenic protein antagonist gremlin regulates proximal-distal patterning of the lung. Dev Dyn 2001;222(4): 667–80.

59. Okamoto T, Yamamoto Y, Gotoh M, et al. Cartilage regeneration using slow release of bone morphogenetic protein-2 from a gelatin sponge to treat experimental canine tracheomalacia: a preliminary report. ASAIO J 2003;49(1):63–9.

60. Warburton D, Bellusci S, Del Moral PM, et al. Growth factor signaling in lung morphogenetic centers: automaticity, stereotypy and symmetry. Respir Res 2003;4:5.

61. Yamamoto Y, Okamoto T, Goto M, et al. Experimental study of bone morphogenetic proteins-2 slow release from an artificial trachea made of biodegradable materials: evaluation of stenting time. ASAIO J 2003;49(5):533–6.

62. Okamoto T, Yamamoto Y, Gotoh M, et al. Slow release of bone morphogenetic protein 2 from a gelatin sponge to promote regeneration of tracheal cartilage in a canine model. J Thorac Cardiovasc Surg 2004;127(2):329–34.

63. Crowley AR, Mehta SS, Hembree MJ, et al. Faulty bone morphogenetic protein signaling in esophageal atresia with tracheoesophageal fistula. J Pediatr Surg 2006;41(7):1208–13.

64. Cohen SR, Perelman N, Mahnovski V, et al. Whole organ evaluation of collagen in the developing human larynx and adjoining anatomic structures (hyoid and trachea). Ann Otol Rhinol Laryngol 1993;102(9):655–9.

65. Murgu S, Colt H. Tracheobronchomalacia untangling the Gordian knot. Journal of Bronchology 2005;12(4):239–44.

66. Couvreur J, Grimfeld A, Tournier G, et al [Tracheal dyskinesia (tracheomalacia) in children. Reflections apropos of 127 cases diagnosed by endoscopy]. Ann Pediatr (Paris) 1980;27(9):561–70 [in French].

67. Loundon N, Brugel L, Roger C, et al. Current approach of primary tracheal dyskinesia. Pediatr Pulmonol Suppl 1999;18:67–70.

68. Corre A, Chaudre F, Roger G, et al. Tracheal dyskinesia associated with midline abnormality: embryological hypotheses and therapeutic implications. Pediatr Pulmonol 2001;(Suppl 23):10–2.

69. Campbell AH. Definition and causes of the tracheobronchial collapse syndrome. Br J Dis Chest 1967;61(1):1–11.
70. Fletcher BD, Cohn RC. Tracheal compression and the innominate artery: MR evaluation in infants. Radiology 1989;170(1 Pt 1):103–7.
71. Mahboubi S, Harty MP, Hubbard AM, et al. Innominate artery compression of the trachea in infants. Int J Pediatr Otorhinolaryngol 1996;35(3):197–205.
72. Weber TR, Keller MS, Fiore A. Aortic suspension (aortopexy) for severe tracheomalacia in infants and children. Am J Surg 2002;184(6):573–7 [discussion 577].
73. Benjamin B. Tracheomalacia in infants and children. Ann Otol Rhinol Laryngol 1984;93(5 Pt 1):438–42.
74. Beasley SW, Qi BQ. Understanding tracheomalacia. J Paediatr Child Health 1998;34(3):209–10.
75. Shaffer TH, Wolfson MR, Panitch HB. Airway structure, function and development in health and disease. Paediatr Anaesth 2004;14(1):3–14.
76. Masters IB, Eastburn M, Francis PW, et al. Quantification of the magnification and distortion effects of a pediatric flexible video-bronchoscope. Respir Res 2005;6(1):16.
77. Masters IB, Eastburn MM, Wootton R, et al. A new method for objective identification and measurement of airway lumen in paediatric flexible videobronchoscopy. Thorax 2005;60(8):652–8.
78. Masters IB, Ware RS, Zimmerman PV, et al. Airway sizes and proportions in children quantified by a video-bronchoscopic technique. BMC Pulm Med 2006;6(1):5.
79. Masters IB, Zimmerman PV, Chang AB. Longitudinal quantification of growth and changes in primary tracheobronchomalacia sites in children. Pediatr Pulmonol 2007;42(10):906–13.
80. Aquino SL, Shepard JA, Ginns LC, et al. Acquired tracheomalacia: detection by expiratory CT scan. J Comput Assist Tomogr 2001;25(3):394–9.
81. Boiselle PM, Ernst A. Recent advances in central airway imaging. Chest 2002; 121(5):1651–60.
82. Boiselle PM. Multislice helical CT of the central airways. Radiol Clin North Am 2003;41(3):561–74.
83. Boiselle PM, Feller-Kopman D, Ashiku S, et al. Tracheobronchomalacia: evolving role of dynamic multislice helical CT. Radiol Clin North Am 2003;41(3):627–36.
84. Boiselle PM, Lee KS, Ernst A. Multidetector CT of the central airways. J Thorac Imaging 2005;20(3):186–95.
85. Boiselle PM, Ernst A. Tracheal morphology in patients with tracheomalacia: prevalence of inspiratory lunate and expiratory "frown" shapes. J Thorac Imaging 2006;21(3):190–6.
86. Boiselle PM, Lee KS, Lin S, et al. Cine CT during coughing for assessment of tracheomalacia: preliminary experience with 64-MDCT. AJR Am J Roentgenol 2006;187(2):W175–7.
87. Faust RA, Remley KB, Rimell FL. Real-time, cine magnetic resonance imaging for evaluation of the pediatric airway. Laryngoscope 2001;111(12):2187–90.
88. Long FR, Castile RG. Technique and clinical applications of full-inflation and end-exhalation controlled-ventilation chest CT in infants and young children. Pediatr Radiol 2001;31(6):413–22.
89. Faust RA, Rimell FL, Remley KB. Cine magnetic resonance imaging for evaluation of focal tracheomalacia: innominate artery compression syndrome. Int J Pediatr Otorhinolaryngol 2002;65(1):27–33.

90. Briganti V, Oriolo L, Buffa V, et al. Tracheomalacia in oesophageal atresia: morphological considerations by endoscopic and CT study. Eur J Cardiothorac Surg 2005;28(1):11–5.

91. Briganti V, Oriolo L, Mangia G, et al. Tracheomalacia in esophageal atresia. Usefulness of preoperative imaging evaluation for tailored surgical correction. J Pediatr Surg 2006;41(9):1624–8.

92. Murgu SD, Colt HG. Treatment of adult tracheobronchomalacia and excessive dynamic airway collapse: an update. Treat Respir Med 2006;5(2):103–15.

93. Masters IB, Zimmerman PV, Pandeya N, et al. Quantified tracheobronchomalacia disorders and their clinical profiles in children. Chest 2008;133(2): 461–7.

94. Chang AB, Landau LI, Van Asperen PP, et al. Cough in children: definitions and clinical evaluation. Med J Aust 2006;184(8):398–403.

95. Marchant JM, Masters IB, Chang AB. Defining paediatric chronic bronchitis. Respirology 2004;9(Suppl):A61.

96. Marchant JM, Masters IB, Chang AB. Chronic cough in children. Eur Respir J 2003;22(Suppl 45):176S.

97. Marchant JM, Masters IB, Taylor SM, et al. Utility of signs and symptoms of chronic cough in predicting specific cause in children. Thorax 2006;61(8): 694–8.

98. Masters IB, Chang AB. Interventions for primary (intrinsic) tracheomalacia in children. Cochrane Database Syst Rev 2005;(4):CD005304.

99. Newcombe PA, Sheffield JK, Juniper EF, et al. Development of a parent-proxy quality-of-life chronic cough-specific questionnaire: clinical impact vs psychometric evaluations. Chest 2008;133(2):386–95.

100. Hofhuis W, van der Wiel EC, Tiddens HA, et al. Bronchodilation in infants with malacia or recurrent wheeze. Arch Dis Child 2003;88(3):246–9.

101. Miller RW, Pollack MM, Murphy TM, et al. Effectiveness of continuous positive airway pressure in the treatment of bronchomalacia in infants: a bronchoscopic documentation. Crit Care Med 1986;14(2):125–7.

102. Ferguson GT, Benoist J. Nasal continuous positive airway pressure in the treatment of tracheobronchomalacia. Am Rev Respir Dis 1993;147(2):457–61.

103. Panitch HB, Allen JL, Alpert BE, et al. Effects of CPAP on lung mechanics in infants with acquired tracheobronchomalacia. Am J Respir Crit Care Med 1994; 150(5 Pt 1):1341–6.

104. Essouri S, Nicot F, Clement A, et al. Noninvasive positive pressure ventilation in infants with upper airway obstruction: comparison of continuous and bilevel positive pressure. Intensive Care Med 2005;31(4):574–80.

105. Dave S, Currie BG. The role of aortopexy in severe tracheomalacia. J Pediatr Surg 2006;41(3):533–7.

106. Ahel V, Banac S, Rozmanic V, et al. Aortopexy and bronchopexy for the management of severe tracheomalacia and bronchomalacia. Pediatr Int 2003;45(1): 104–6.

107. van der Zee DC, Bax NM. Thoracoscopic tracheoaortopexia for the treatment of life-threatening events in tracheomalacia. Surg Endosc 2007;21(11):2024–5.

108. Roberts CS, Othersen HB Jr, Sade RM, et al. Tracheoesophageal compression from aortic arch anomalies: analysis of 30 operatively treated children. J Pediatr Surg 1994;29(2):334–7 [discussion 337–8].

109. Kazim R, Berdon WE, Montoya CH, et al. Tracheobronchial anomalies in children with congenital cardiac disease. J Cardiothorac Vasc Anesth 1998; 12(5):553–5.

110. Fiore AC, Brown JW, Weber TR, et al. Surgical treatment of pulmonary artery sling and tracheal stenosis. Ann Thorac Surg 2005;79(1):38–46 [discussion 38].
111. Alsenaidi K, Gurofsky R, Karamlou T, et al. Management and outcomes of double aortic arch in 81 patients. Pediatrics 2006;118(5):e1336–41.
112. Brown JW, Ruzmetov M, Vijay P, et al. Surgical treatment of absent pulmonary valve syndrome associated with bronchial obstruction. Ann Thorac Surg 2006; 82(6):2221–6.
113. Burden RJ, Shann F, Butt W, et al. Tracheobronchial malacia and stenosis in children in intensive care: bronchograms help to predict outcome. Thorax 1999; 54(6):511–7.
114. Chang AB, Glomb WB. Guidelines for evaluating chronic cough in pediatrics: ACCP evidence-based clinical practice guidelines. Chest 2006;129(1 Suppl): 260S–83S.
115. Abdel-Rahman U, Ahrens P, Fieguth HG, et al. Surgical treatment of tracheomalacia by bronchoscopic monitored aortopexy in infants and children. Ann Thorac Surg 2002;74(2):315–9.
116. Imai Y, Mark EJ. Cystic adenomatoid change is common to various forms of cystic lung diseases of children: a clinicopathologic analysis of 10 cases with emphasis on tracing the bronchial tree. Arch Pathol Lab Med 2002;126(8):934–40.
117. Morikawa N, Kuroda T, Honna T, et al. Congenital bronchial atresia in infants and children. J Pediatr Surg 2005;40(12):1822–6.
118. Kim WS, Lee KS, Kim IO, et al. Congenital cystic adenomatoid malformation of the lung: CT-pathologic correlation. AJR Am J Roentgenol 1997;168(1):47–53.
119. Eber E. Antenatal diagnosis of congenital thoracic malformations: early surgery, late surgery, or no surgery? Semin Respir Crit Care Med 2007;28(3):355–66.
120. Azizkhan RG, Crombleholme TM. Congenital cystic lung disease: contemporary antenatal and postnatal management. Pediatr Surg Int 2008;24(6):643–57.
121. Volpe MV, Pham L, Lessin M, et al. Expression of Hoxb-5 during human lung development and in congenital lung malformations. Birth Defects Res A Clin Mol Teratol 2003;67(8):550–6.
122. Gonzaga S, Henriques-Coelho T, Davey M, et al. Cystic adenomatoid malformations are induced by localized FGF10 overexpression in fetal rat lung. Am J Respir Cell Mol Biol 2008;39:346–55.
123. Wagner AJ, Stumbaugh A, Tigue Z, et al. Genetic analysis of congenital cystic adenomatoid malformation reveals a novel pulmonary gene: fatty acid binding protein-7 (brain type). Pediatr Res 2008;64(1):11–6.
124. Tsai AY, Liechty KW, Hedrick HL, et al. Outcomes after postnatal resection of prenatally diagnosed asymptomatic cystic lung lesions. J Pediatr Surg 2008; 43(3):513–7.
125. Rothenberg SS. First decade's experience with thoracoscopic lobectomy in infants and children. J Pediatr Surg 2008;43(1):40–4 [discussion 45].
126. Vu LT, Farmer DL, Nobuhara KK, et al. Thoracoscopic versus open resection for congenital cystic adenomatoid malformations of the lung. J Pediatr Surg 2008; 43(1):35–9.

Obstructive Sleep Breathing Disorders

Chun Ting Au, MPhil, RPSGT, Albert Martin Li, MD*

KEYWORDS

- Sleep-disordered breathing • Obstructive sleep apnea • Child
- Snoring • Sleep disturbance

Sleep-disordered breathing (SDB) refers to a group of respiratory conditions that are exacerbated during sleep. SDB is increasingly being recognized as an important disease entity, and if the condition is left untreated, significant morbidity and even mortality can result.[1] The most prominent SDB condition in children is obstructive sleep apnea (OSA), which belongs to the severe end of a spectrum, ranging in severity from primary or simple snoring through upper airway resistance syndrome, obstructive hypopnea syndrome, to its most severe form, OSA (**Box 1**). The American Thoracic Society defines childhood OSA as a disorder that is characterized by repeated episodes of partial or complete upper airway obstruction during sleep that result in disruption of normal ventilation and sleep patterns.[2]

EPIDEMIOLOGY

The accurate identification of the prevalence of childhood OSA should allow better resource allocation and clinicians to perform more targeted screening. In relation to research, recognizing differences in the prevalence of the condition among races may allow a better understanding of its etiology. A recent review stressed that published literature on the prevalence of childhood OSA is fraught with difficulty because of a variety of methodologic issues.[3] Within these limitations, review of relevant literature suggests a prevalence of OSA from 0.1% to 13%, but most studies report a figure between 1% and 4%. There are accumulating data to suggest that OSA is more common among overweight or obese boys. This condition peaks between the ages of 2 and 8 years, coinciding with the peak age of lymphoid hyperplasia. Some data do suggest a higher prevalence among African Americans in the United States, but whether such a racial

Department of Pediatrics, Prince of Wales Hospital, The Chinese University of Hong Kong, Shatin, Hong Kong
* Corresponding author.
E-mail address: albertmli@cuhk.edu.hk (A. Li).

Pediatr Clin N Am 56 (2009) 243–259
doi:10.1016/j.pcl.2008.10.012
0031-3955/08/$ – see front matter © 2009 Elsevier Inc. All rights reserved.

Box 1
Continuum of obstructive sleep-disordered breathing
Primary snoring: increased airway resistance without other symptoms
Upper airway resistance syndrome: sleep disturbance with normal blood gas profile
Obstructive hypopnea syndrome: hypopnea, sleep disturbance without desaturation
OSA: apnea, hypopnea, sleep disturbance with desaturation

difference also holds true for other population remains to be examined. **Table 1** shows the prevalence of OSA reported after diagnostic testing in 13 studies.

ETIOLOGY

The most common cause for childhood OSA is adenotonsillar hypertrophy, but the large tonsils and adenoids alone cannot account for the entire pathophysiologic process. There is accumulating evidence to suggest that OSA is related to an interaction of structural and neuromuscular variables within the upper airway. Although several studies showed that children with OSA have larger tonsils and adenoids when compared with age-matched controls, a linear relation between the size of lymphoid tissues and severity of OSA has never been documented.[17–19] Some patients with no other known risk factors have persistent OSA despite having their tonsils and adenoids removed. A recent study revealed that childhood OSA was related to impaired response of the central nervous system to mechanical stimulation of the respiratory system.[20] Thus, structural factors alone cannot be fully responsible for this condition.

Upper airway resistance increases during sleep even in normal humans because of the reduction in muscle tone of the pharyngeal dilator muscles.[21,22] When the upper airway resistance is further increased because of other factors, such as adenotonsillar hypertrophy or neuromotor function abnormalities, however, the upper airway collapses at a lower threshold.[23,24] In more general terms, the mechanism underlying this condition is related to some combination of three processes: (1) decreased upper airway patency (adenotonsillar hypertrophy, allergies associated with chronic rhinitis or nasal obstruction), (2) reduced capacity to maintain airway patency related to neuromuscular tone (obesity, neuromuscular disorder), and (3) decreased drive to breathe (brain stem injury).

There are a variety of medical conditions that are associated with an increased risk for OSA (**Table 2**). Since its first description in 1976, childhood OSA has been recognized as a different disease entity from adult OSA with respect to etiology, clinical manifestations, and management (**Table 3**).

CLINICAL FEATURES

The most common presenting complaint of childhood OSA is snoring, and the condition is unlikely in the absence of habitual snoring (snoring for most nights of the week), although many children with snoring do not have OSA. Nocturnal and daytime symptoms associated with the condition are shown in **Table 4**.

No combination of symptoms and physical findings has been found to distinguish OSA reliably from primary snoring.[25] In most cases, children have enlarged tonsils or adenoids and do not demonstrate breathing difficulties during clinical examination. There is no reliable relation between the size of the tonsils on direct inspection and the presence of OSA.[26]

Table 1
Prevalence of childhood obstructive sleep apnea

Author	No. Subjects	Country	Age (Years)	Diagnostic Technique	Prevalence of Obstructive Sleep Apnea Symptoms
Ali et al, 1993[4]	782 screened 132 monitored	United Kingdom	4–5	Pulse oximetry, video	0.7%
Gislason et al, 1995[5]	454	Iceland	0.5–6	PSG (AHI >3)	2.9%
Redline et al, 1999[6]	126	United States	2–18	PSG	1.6% (AHI >10) 10.3% (AHI >5)
Brunetti et al, 2001[7]	895 screened 12 monitored	Italy	3–11	PSG (AHI >3)	1.0%–1.8%
Anuntaseree et al, 2001[8]	1008 screened 8 monitored	Thailand	6–13	PSG (AHI >1)	0.69%
Sánchez-Armengol et al, 2001[9]	100	Spain	12–16	PSG (RDI >10)	2.0%
Ng et al, 2002[10]	200	Hong Kong	6.4 ± 4	PSG (AHI >1)	0.1%
Castronovo et al, 2003[11]	595 screened 265 monitored	Italy	3–6	Pulse oximetry	13%
Rosen CL, 2003[12]	243	United States	8–11	PSG (OAI >1)	1.9%
O'Brien et al, 2003[13]	5728	United States	5–7	PSG (AHI >5)	5.7%
Kaditis et al, 2004[14]	3680	Greece	1–18	PSG (AHI >5)	4.3%
Sogut et al, 2005[15]	1198	Turkey	3–11	PSG (AHI >3)	0.9%
Anuntaseree et al, 2005[16]	755	Thailand	9–10	PSG (AHI >1)	1.3%

Abbreviations: AHI, apnea hypopnea index; PSG, polysomnography; RDI, respiratory disturbance index.

Table 2	
Medical conditions associated with childhood obstructive sleep apnea	
Craniofacial syndromes	Crouzon syndrome
	Apert syndrome
	Treacher-Collins syndrome
	Goldenhar syndrome
	Pierre Robin syndrome
Neurologic diseases	Arnold-Chiari malformation
	Meningomyelocele
	Cerebral palsy
	Duchenne muscular dystrophy
Conditions with abnormal muscle tone	Down syndrome
	Prader-Willi syndrome
	Hypothyroidism
Conditions with reduced upper airway patency	Adenotonsillar hypertrophy
	Obesity
	Allergic rhinitis
	Macroglossia
	Laryngomalacia
	Subglottic stenosis
	Mucopolysaccharidoses/metabolic storage diseases

COMPLICATIONS ASSOCIATED WITH OBSTRUCTIVE SLEEP APNEA
Neurocognitive Abnormalities

In contrast to adult patients, affected children tend to have preserved sleep architecture;[27] therefore, excessive daytime sleepiness (EDS) is not a predominant feature. Despite the relative absence of EDS, childhood OSA and even nonapneic snoring

Table 3		
Comparison of obstructive sleep apnea in children and adults		
	Children	**Adults**
Estimated prevalence	1%–4%	2%–4%
Peak age	2–8 years	30–60 years
Gender (male/female)	1:1	3:1
Weight	Normal, decreased, increased	Overweight
Major cause	Adenotonsillar hypertrophy	Obesity
Gas exchange abnormalities	Always	Always
Duration of obstructive apneas	Any	>10 seconds
Abnormal AI (per hour)	>1	>5
Abnormal AHI (per hour)	>1	>10
Sleep architecture	Preserved	Always altered
Arousals	Occasional	Always
Daytime sleepiness	30%	>90%
Neurocognitive problems	Common	Less common
Common treatment	Adenotonsillectomy	CPAP

Abbreviations: AHI, apnea-hypopnea index; AI, apnea index; CPAP, continuous positive airway pressure.

Table 4
Symptoms of childhood obstructive sleep apnea

Nocturnal symptoms	Loud habitual snoring
	Difficulty breathing when asleep
	Apneic pauses
	Restless sleep
	Sweating
	Dry mouth
	Abnormal sleeping position
	Enuresis
	Night terrors/sleep walking
	Bruxism/teeth grinding
Daytime symptoms	Mouth breathing
	Morning headache
	Difficulty in waking up
	Mood changes
	Poor attention span/academic problems
	Increased nap/daytime sleepiness
	Chronic nasal congestion/rhinorrhea
	Frequent upper respiratory tract infections
	Difficulty in swallowing/poor appetite
	Hearing problems

seem to be associated with significant neurocognitive sequelae, for example, behavioral and learning problems, poor attention span, hyperactivity, and even lower than average intelligent quotient.[28] Indeed, one clinical study showed an alarmingly high prevalence of snoring and gas exchange abnormalities in children who were academically poor achievers, and significant improvement in school performance was seen after adenotonsillectomy.[29] This finding has subsequently been substantiated in other clinical studies,[30–32] establishing a causal relation between OSA and neurocognitive deficit.

It has been estimated that up to 30% of children with habitual snoring or OSA have inattention and hyperactivity.[30] The attention deficit hyperactivity disorder (ADHD) symptoms that these children exhibit may not be true ADHD but rather a lack of behavioral inhibition secondary to repeated sleep arousals and intermittent hypoxic episodes that affects working memory, motor control, and self-regulation of motivation.[33] These attention and behavioral problems have also been shown to have an adverse effect on cognition and school performance.[34] There is, however, recent evidence to suggest reversibility of such neurocognitive dysfunction after treatment.[31] A more recent study indicated that the behavioral problems in children with SDB were not only attributable to SDB-related impairments but to being overweight, to insufficient sleep, and to comorbid sleep disorders, especially insomnia.[35] Therefore, clinicians should consider the relative contributions of all these factors when assessing behavior in children with SDB.

Cardiovascular Consequences

Hypertension has long been recognized as one of the complications in adult OSA. From the Wisconsin Sleep Cohort, it was found that adults with an apnea hypopnea index (AHI) of 15 or greater had a three times higher chance of developing hypertension.[36] Corresponding data are scarce for the pediatric population, however, and the few published studies have provided conflicting results.[37–42] Marcus and colleagues[37] suggested that children with OSA had higher diastolic blood pressure (BP) during wakefulness and sleep compared with primary snorers. Amin and colleagues,[38] conversely, found lower diastolic BP among children with OSA during wakefulness. Guilleminault and colleagues[39] demonstrated that a subgroup of children with OSA were hypotensive rather than hypertensive. The mechanism behind this low BP group is not known; it was suggested to be attributable to dominant vagal discharge as a result of increased work of breathing. Kohyama and colleagues[40] showed that children with OSA had higher diastolic BP; furthermore, the diastolic BP was significantly correlated with the AHI. The group also found that 29% of patients in the group with an AHI greater than 10 lacked a sleep-related decrease in BP versus 19% of patients in the lower AHI group (AHI <10). Similarly, Enright and colleagues[41] found that obesity, sleep efficiency, and respiratory disturbance index (RDI) were associated with an increase in BP in preadolescent children. A recent study by Leung and colleagues,[42] however, failed to confirm such a positive association between BP and severity of OSA. These inconsistent findings in BP measurements in children with OSA might have been related to the small sample sizes and the lack of normal healthy subjects for comparison. A meta-analysis concluded that there was inadequate evidence for an increased risk for elevated BP in children with SDB. Zintzaras and Kaditis[43] also found marked heterogeneity among published series and emphasized the need for further studies to clarify this important issue in childhood OSA. The authors' group has recently completed a large-scale community-based study further confirming the positive association between childhood OSA and elevated daytime and nighttime BP and has demonstrated that OSA is an independent predictor of nocturnal hypertension.[44] Another clinical study revealed that increases in ambulatory BP in children with OSA could predict changes in left ventricular relative wall thickness.[45] These findings consolidate the linkage between SDB and BP elevation in children, and future research should concentrate on BP changes after treatment for OSA.

Changes in ventricular geometry have also been reported in children with OSA. Amin and colleagues[46] investigated the heart size of 28 and 19 patients who had OSA and primary snoring, respectively, and found that the left ventricular mass index and wall thickness were greater in children with OSA. Those with an AHI of 10 or more had a right and left ventricular mass greater than the ninety-fifth percentile. The same group later showed that there was a dose-dependent decrease in left ventricular diastolic function with increased severity of OSA.[47] Sánchez-Armengol and colleagues[48] studied a group of adolescents (mean age: 13.7 ± 1.6 years) and found that the posterior ventricular wall thickness could be predicted from desaturation events and RDI. The intermittent hypoxia that occurs in children with OSA may induce elevations of pulmonary artery pressure, and such events may lead to right ventricular dysfunction,[49,50] but the exact pathophysiologic mechanism leading to ventricular dysfunction and morphologic changes and the effects of treatment need to be further examined.

Arterial distensibility assessed in vivo by measurement of pulse wave velocity (PWV) is an important predictor of cardiovascular risk in adults.[51] The PWV and BP were examined in a group of children with primary snoring, and these children were documented to have higher systolic, diastolic, and mean BP in comparison to the control group. Furthermore, the PWV was increased in children with primary snoring, which signified decreased arterial distensibility.[52] A recent study has also provided evidence of endothelial dysfunction in children with OSA. Postocclusive hyperemia, a marker of endothelial function, was blunted in 26 children with OSA, and such altered endothelial function was reversible at 4 to 6 months after treatment, particularly in those without a family history of cardiovascular disease.[53]

Insulin Resistance

There has been an alarming increase in the prevalence of type 2 diabetes mellitus (DM) in children, and in recent years, type 2 DM has become the most frequent endocrine disorder affecting glucose metabolism in children.[54] Insulin resistance is considered an important risk factor for the development of type 2 DM, and therefore provides an early intervention parameter for prevention of the disease and its significant long-term consequences.[55]

The term *metabolic syndrome*, a well-established risk factor for cardiovascular disease in adults, refers to clustering of insulin resistance, an abnormal lipid profile, hypertension, and obesity. Up to the time of writing, there is no clear-cut agreed-on definition of the metabolic syndrome for children.[56] Using adult criteria, the overall prevalence of metabolic syndrome among 12- to 19-year-old adolescents in the United States was found to be 4.2%.[57] Weiss and colleagues[58] found that the risk for metabolic syndrome was nearly 50% in severely obese adolescents and that the risk increased with every 0.5-unit increment in body mass index (BMI). Raised fasting insulin levels and increased BMI during childhood are strong predictors for the development of metabolic syndrome in adulthood.[59] Furthermore, insulin resistance in childhood is associated with an increased risk for later cardiovascular-related morbidity and mortality.[60]

Similar to obesity, there is accumulating evidence to suggest OSA as an important risk factor for insulin resistance in adults.[61,62] There are, however, limited data in the literature on the same subject in pediatrics. Previous pediatric studies that examined the relation between OSA, obesity, and insulin resistance[63–68] have reported conflicting results. In a large cohort of nonobese and obese snoring children, Tauman and colleagues[63] showed that insulin resistance (assessed by insulin/glucose ratio and homeostatic model assessment) and lipid dysregulation (evidence of increased plasma triglyceride and decreased plasma high-density lipoprotein concentration) were primarily determined by the degree of adiposity and that OSA played a minimal, if any, role in the occurrence of insulin resistance. These findings have been confirmed in a study involving Greek nonobese children.[64] In other studies conducted in obese children with OSA, however, insulin resistance was found to correlate with the severity of the respiratory disease independent of the degree of obesity.[65–67] More recently, Gozal and colleagues[68] further confirmed that OSA seemed to induce insulin resistance in obese but not nonobese children. Moreover, follow-up study demonstrated significant improvements in lipid profiles and apolipoprotein B levels after adenotonsillectomy. This finding suggested a causal role for OSA in lipid homeostasis independent of the degree of adiposity, but the complex interaction between insulin, obesity, OSA, and metabolic dysfunction needs further investigation.

Growth Failure

The pathogenesis associated with failure to thrive in children with OSA is likely to be an interplay among various mechanisms that include increased resting energy expenditure, difficulty with swallowing secondary to enlarged tonsils, and abnormal release of growth-related hormones.[69] Caloric intake and sleeping energy expenditure, in addition to anthropomorphic measurements, were taken before and after adenotonsillectomy in 14 children confirmed to have OSA. Average sleeping energy expenditure decreased and the mean weight z-score increased after surgery without any change in caloric intake.[70] The presence of poor appetite, difficulty in swallowing, and nausea with vomiting was reported more frequently in children with OSA compared with controls.[71] Statistically significant increases in weight and insulin-like growth factor-I levels were found in a group of children with OSA after adenotonsillectomy.[72] Fortunately, we are seeing less of this complication as parents are becoming more aware of this condition and seeking medical intervention early.

ROLE OF INFLAMMATION IN CHILDHOOD OBSTRUCTIVE SLEEP APNEA

Inflammation is a mechanism that may link OSA and cardiovascular disease.[73,74] Adults with OSA have higher levels of proinflammatory cytokines, tumor necrosis factor (TNF)-α, and interleukin-6,[75,76] which decrease after treatment for OSA.[77–79] C-reactive protein (CRP) is the most widely studied marker of systemic inflammation in children. Published studies have reported conflicting results, however.[80–83] In a study of 81 children with a mean age of 9.3 years, Tauman and colleagues[80] found raised levels of CRP, a strong marker of cardiovascular risk, in children with OSA compared with controls, with levels correlating with disease severity. A similar correlation between CRP and sleep apnea severity was also documented in a study involving older children with a mean age of 13.7 years.[81] These positive results were not confirmed by two other studies, however.[82,83] Adipose tissue is an important source of inflammatory cytokines, which are essential inducers for CRP production.[84] Obesity is therefore a confounding factor in the correlation between CRP and OSA, and that can partly explain discrepancies among results of published studies. Two recent studies have provided further support for the presence of systemic inflammation in children with OSA.[85,86] In both studies, these investigators (from the same research institute) demonstrated a significant reduction in CRP after treatment for OSA. The same research group also examined another marker of systemic inflammation, TNFα, and demonstrated that its serum levels were elevated in children with polysomnography (PSG) proved OSA and that the magnitude of the TNFα level was primarily correlated with the degree of respiratory event–induced sleep fragmentation.[87]

Children with OSA have also been documented to have elevated plasma levels of P-selectin, a marker of platelet activation, lending support to the premise that inflammatory processes are elicited by OSA in children and may contribute to an accelerated risk for cardiovascular morbidity.[88] Further large-scale controlled studies are needed to delineate the role of systemic inflammation in childhood OSA clearly; particularly important is the implication of such inflammation in future cardiovascular risk.

DIAGNOSIS OF OBSTRUCTIVE SLEEP APNEA

Many methods have been studied to diagnose OSA, starting with a history and physical examination; proceeding to audiotaping or videotaping; and ending with pulse oximetry, abbreviated PSG, and full PSG. Although PSG is the current gold standard for the diagnosis of OSA, many authorities have questioned its usefulness and feasibility in routine clinical practice. Arguments, such as cost and lack of consensus on the interpretation of PSG findings, are enough for many physicians to consider PSG not necessary for diagnosis. Conversely, a history and physical examination alone are poor at predicting OSA,[25] and abbreviated studies tend to be helpful if results are positive but have a poor predictive value if the results are negative.[1]

PSG is a cumbersome examination and may not accurately reflect the child's sleep in his or her habitual environment. The parameters originally used to evaluate childhood PSG were based on adult values. PSG has not been well standardized in its performance or interpretation, especially within the pediatric population. Normative standards for PSG determination have been chosen on the basis of statistical distribution of data, and it has not been established that those standards have any validity as predictors of long-term outcome. Most pediatric respiratory clinicians consider an obstructive apnea index greater than 1 to be abnormal.[89] This criterion does not take into account episodes of hypopnea, however, and, recently, an obstructive apnea-hypopnea index greater than 1 has been proposed as diagnostic for OSA.[90]

TREATMENT OF OBSTRUCTIVE SLEEP APNEA
Medical Treatment

Broad-spectrum antibiotics may offer temporary improvement, particularly if snoring and obstruction occur intermittently and are associated with recurrent tonsillitis or adenoiditis.[91] The use of antibiotics does not seem to obviate the need for surgery in most cases with adenotonsillar hypertrophy, however.[92] Nasal corticosteroids have been examined as an alternative to adenotonsillectomy in otherwise healthy children with OSA.[93,94] In a prospective, randomized, double-blind study, children with mild to moderate OSA were treated with a 6-week course of nasal corticosteroids or placebo. The researchers were able to demonstrate a moderate improvement in cases treated with nasal corticosteroids. This was associated with concomitant decreases of approximately 50% in the desaturation index and the movement arousal index. In contrast, the placebo group did not show any improvement.[93] Nasal corticosteroids work by exerting lympholytic action and effects on inflammation and upper airway edema.[95] In an open-labeled study, the leukotriene receptor antagonist montelukast was found to be clinically effective in reducing disease severity in children with mild OSA.[96] In a subsequent study, a combination of intranasal steroids and leukotriene modifier was found to be useful in children with residual OSA after adenotonsillectomy.[97]

Surgical Treatment

Treating children with OSA depends on the child's underlying abnormalities, the site of obstruction, and the presence or absence of contributing neurologic or functional abnormalities. Adenotonsillectomy is considered the cardinal treatment of childhood OSA, and the procedure is superior to adenoidectomy or tonsillectomy alone.[98] Nevertheless, a recent study reported that complete surgical cure of OSA occurred in only 25% of children, with another 50% showing significant improvements in their OSA parameters. The following groups of patients have been identified to be at a higher risk for persistent OSA despite surgery: initial severe OSA, obesity, and those with a positive family history of OSA.[99] Another recent study showed that initial BMI, gain velocity of BMI, and African-American race confer an independent increased risk for recurrence of SDB after adenotonsillectomy.[100] This implied that good weight control is important after surgical treatment. Other surgical procedures, such as nasal septoplasty, epiglottoplasty, uvulopharyngopalatoplasty, and maxillofacial surgery, are seldom performed in children but may be indicated in selected cases.[101]

Mechanical Treatment

Nasal continuous positive airway pressure (CPAP) provides positive pressure to the lumen of the airway and decreases airway collapsibility. It is of utmost importance that the initial approach to the family and child be performed correctly and successfully. CPAP therapy should be titrated during PSG to determine effective pressures, and children on CPAP therapy should be followed regularly to ensure compliance and proper fit of the mask interface. CPAP may be indicated in the following clinical situations:

- Adenotonsillectomy not indicated or contraindicated
- Adenotonsillectomy fails to resolve symptoms completely, usually in children with additional risk factors, such as obesity
- Before surgery in children with severe OAS[98]

Bilevel positive airway pressure (BiPAP) also allows setting of a backup rate and provides some ventilatory assistance. This is especially important for patients with sleep-related hypoventilation caused by muscle weakness, neurologic disease, or obesity.

CPAP and BiPAP are highly efficacious in pediatric obstructive apnea, but treatment is associated with a high dropout rate, and even in those adherent children, nighttime use is still suboptimal considering the long sleep hours in children.[102] One potential

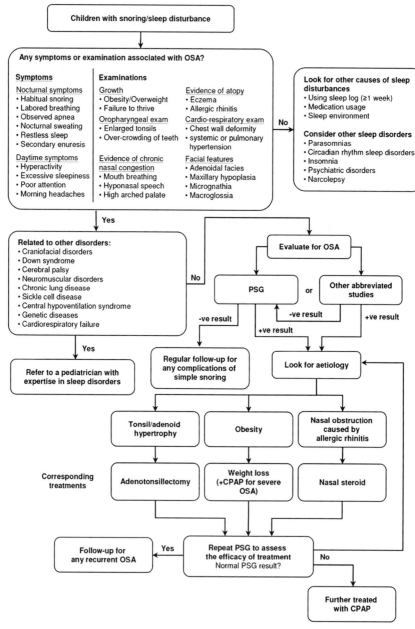

Fig. 1. Diagnosis and treatment of childhood OSA.

complication of long-term nasal mask CPAP or BiPAP is midface hypoplasia. In children on long-term nasal positive-pressure therapy, maxillomandibular growth should be monitored carefully and regularly.

Oral appliances, such as mandibular advancing devices and tongue retainers, are rarely used in children with OSA. Supplemental oxygen therapy abolishes desaturation episodes associated with OSA, but it does not treat the underlying obstruction and may worsen hypoventilation.

WHAT DO I DO WHEN A CHILD WITH SNORING OR SLEEP DISTURBANCE PRESENTS?

Fig. 1 is a proposed algorithm describing how children with snoring or sleep disturbance can be dealt with in clinical practice. The following is a summary of the algorithm:

1. Features suggestive of OSA should be sought during history taking.
2. Patients who have certain medical conditions (see diagram) are at higher risk for developing OSA, and their further management is best managed by a specialist.
3. Clinical symptoms alone are not able to discriminate between simple snoring and OSA. The gold standard for the diagnosis of childhood OSA is overnight PSG. Because of its high running cost, however, the service is not widely available. Other

Table 5
Recommendations of treatment for childhood obstructive sleep apnea

Medication or Intervention	Recommendation	Grading of Eecommendation (Based on Evidence of Benefit)	Quality of Supporting Evidence
Adenotonsillectomy	Recommended as first-line therapy for children with OSA secondary to adenotonsillar hypertrophy	Strong	High
Weight loss	Recommended as supplementary therapy for obese patients	Strong	High
Nasal steroids with or without leukotriene receptor antagonist	An option for children with mild OSA related to nasal obstruction caused by allergic rhinitis	Weak	Low
Noninvasive positive-pressure ventilation	Recommended for children who are not candidates for surgery or whose symptoms are not completely resolved after surgery	Strong	High
Oral appliances	Rarely used in childhood OSA	Weak	Low
Oxygen supplementation	Not suitable as monotherapy because it can aggravate carbon dioxide retention	Weak	Low

abbreviated studies, such as nocturnal pulse oximetry, daytime nap studies, and unattended home PSG, may also be considered. These studies have high rates of false-negative results, however.

4. Children with normal PSG should also be followed up to determine if symptoms of OSA appear and if any possible complications of snoring, such as hypertension and neurocognitive behavioral problems, emerge.

5. Children with positive overnight PSG or other abbreviated studies should be treated according to the underlying causes. One should take note that an individual patient can have multiple causes of OSA (**Table 5**).

6. Overnight PSG should be repeated after treatment to determine whether additional therapy is required.

Even though our understanding and knowledge of childhood OSA have expanded exponentially over the past few years, there are still many unanswered diagnostic and mechanistic questions on the condition. Recent evidence indicates that childhood OSA cannot be easily classified into simple clinical entities. The associated symptoms in children may vary and, many times, are difficult to detect. The diagnosis of the condition in children is far from being "straightforward," with the use of PSG in separating snoring children into categories being a gross simplification. Further advancement in this important field of pediatric medicine can only be made with international collaborative research using evidence-based definitions, standardized techniques, and diagnostic criteria. Further research work should give a better insight of the origins of adult morbidity resulting from childhood sleep-related breathing problems and how they can be prevented.

REFERENCES

1. American Academy of Pediatrics. Clinical practice guideline: diagnosis and management of childhood obstructive sleep apnea syndrome. Pediatrics 2002;109(4):704–12.
2. American Thoracic Society. Standards and indications for cardiopulmonary sleep studies in children. Am J Respir Crit Care Med 1996;153(2):866–78.
3. Lumeng JC, Chervin RD. Epidemiology of pediatric obstructive sleep apnea. Proc Am Thorac Soc 2008;5(2):242–52.
4. Ali NJ, Pitson DJ, Stradling JR. Snoring, sleep disturbance, and behaviour in 4–5 year olds. Arch Dis Child 1993;68(3):360–6.
5. Gislason T, Benediktsdóttir B. Snoring, apneic episodes, and nocturnal hypoxemia among children 6 months to 6 years old. An epidemiologic study of lower limit of prevalence. Chest 1995;107(4):963–6.
6. Redline S, Tishler PV, Schluchter M, et al. Risk factors for sleep-disordered breathing in children. Associations with obesity, race, and respiratory problems. Am J Respir Crit Care Med 1999;159(5 Pt 1):1527–32.
7. Brunetti L, Rana S, Lospalluti ML, et al. Prevalence of obstructive sleep apnea syndrome in a cohort of 1,207 children of southern Italy. Chest 2001;120(6):1930–5.
8. Anuntaseree W, Rookkapan K, Kuasirikul S, et al. Snoring and obstructive sleep apnea in Thai school-age children: prevalence and predisposing factors. Pediatr Pulmonol 2001;32(3):222–7.
9. Sánchez-Armengol A, Fuentes-Pradera MA, Capote-Gil F, et al. Sleep-related breathing disorders in adolescents aged 12 to 16 years: clinical and polygraphic findings. Chest 2001;119(5):1393–400.

10. Ng DK, Kwok KL, Poon G, et al. Habitual snoring and sleep bruxism in a paediatric outpatient population in Hong Kong. Singapore Med J 2002; 43(11):554–6.
11. Castronovo V, Zucconi M, Nosetti L, et al. Prevalence of habitual snoring and sleep-disordered breathing in preschool-aged children in an Italian community. J Pediatr 2003;142(4):377–82.
12. Rosen CL, Larkin EK, Kirchner HL, et al. Prevalence and risk factors for sleep-disordered breathing in 8- to 11-year-old children: association with race and prematurity. J Pediatr 2003;142(4):383–9.
13. O'Brien LM, Holbrook CR, Mervis CB, et al. Sleep and neurobehavioral characteristics of 5- to 7-year-old children with parentally reported symptoms of attention-deficit/hyperactivity disorder. Pediatrics 2003;111(3):554–63.
14. Kaditis AG, Finder J, Alexopoulos EI, et al. Sleep-disordered breathing in 3,680 Greek children. Pediatr Pulmonol 2004;37(6):499–509.
15. Sogut A, Altin R, Uzun L, et al. Prevalence of obstructive sleep apnea syndrome and associated symptoms in 3–11-year-old Turkish children. Pediatr Pulmonol 2005;39(3):251–6.
16. Anuntaseree W, Kuasirikul S, Suntornlohanakul S. Natural history of snoring and obstructive sleep apnea in Thai school-age children. Pediatr Pulmonol 2005; 39(5):415–20.
17. Brooks LJ, Stephens BM, Bacevice AM. Adenoid size is related to severity but not the number of episodes of obstructive apnea in children. J Pediatr 1998; 132(4):682–6.
18. Fernbach SK, Brouillette RT, Riggs TW, et al. Radiologic evaluation of adenoids and tonsils in children with obstructive sleep apnea: plain films and fluoroscopy. Pediatr Radiol 1983;13(5):258–65.
19. Laurikainen E, Erkinjuntti M, Alihanka J, et al. Radiological parameters of the bony nasopharynx and the adenotonsillar size compared with sleep apnea episodes in children. Int J Pediatr Otorhinolaryngol 1987;12(3):303–10.
20. Huang J, Colrain IM, Melendres MC, et al. Cortical processing of respiratory afferent stimuli during sleep in children with the obstructive sleep apnea syndrome. Sleep 2008;31(3):403–10.
21. Tangel DJ, Mezzanotte WS, White DP. Influence of sleep on tensor palatini EMG and upper airway resistance in normal men. J Appl Phys 1991;70(6):2574–81.
22. Wiegand DA, Latz B, Zwillich CW, et al. Upper airway resistance and geniohyoid muscle activity in normal men during wakefulness and sleep. J Appl Phys 1990; 69(4):1252–61.
23. Marcus CL, McColley SA, Carroll JL, et al. Upper airway collapsibility in children with obstructive sleep apnea syndrome. J Appl Phys 1994;77(2): 918–24.
24. Marcus CL. Pathophysiology of childhood obstructive sleep apnea: current concepts. Respir Physiol 2000;119(2–3):143–54.
25. Carroll JL, McColley SA, Marcus CL, et al. Inability of clinical history to distinguish primary snoring from obstructive sleep apnea syndrome in children. Chest 1995;108(3):610–8.
26. Li AM, Hui S, Wong E, et al. Obstructive sleep apnoea in children with adenotonsillar hypertrophy: prospective study. Hong Kong Med J 2001;7(3): 236–40.
27. Goh DY, Galster P, Marcus CL. Sleep architecture and respiratory disturbances in children with obstructive sleep apnea. Am J Respir Crit Care Med 2000; 162(2 Pt 1):682–6.

28. Beebe DW. Neurobehavioral morbidity associated with disordered breathing during sleep in children: a comprehensive review. Sleep 2006;29(9):1115–34.

29. Gozal D. Sleep-disordered breathing and school performance in children. Pediatrics 1998;102(3 Pt 1):616–20.

30. Chervin RD, Archbold KH, Dillon JE, et al. Inattention, hyperactivity, and symptoms of sleep-disordered breathing. Pediatrics 2002;109(3):449–56.

31. Chervin RD, Ruzicka DL, Giordani BJ, et al. Sleep-disordered breathing, behavior, and cognition in children before and after adenotonsillectomy. Pediatrics 2006;117(4):e769–78.

32. Gozal D, Pope DW Jr. Snoring during early childhood and academic performance at ages thirteen to fourteen years. Pediatrics 2001;107(6): 1394–9.

33. Chervin RD, Dillon JE, Bassetti C, et al. Symptoms of sleep disorders, inattention, and hyperactivity in children. Sleep 1997;20(12):1185–92.

34. Hiscock H, Canterford L, Ukoumunne OC, et al. Adverse associations of sleep problems in Australian preschoolers: national population study. Pediatrics 2007;119(1):86–93.

35. Owens JA, Mehlenbeck R, Lee J, et al. Effect of weight, sleep duration, and comorbid sleep disorders on behavioral outcomes in children with sleep-disordered breathing. Arch Pediatr Adolesc Med 2008;162(4):313–21.

36. Peppard PE, Young T, Palta M, et al. Prospective study of the association between sleep-disordered breathing and hypertension. N Engl J Med 2000; 342(19):1378–84.

37. Marcus CL, Greene MG, Carroll JL. Blood pressure in children with obstructive sleep apnea. Am J Respir Crit Care Med 1998;157(4 Pt 1):1098–103.

38. Amin RS, Carroll JL, Jeffries JL, et al. Twenty-four-hour ambulatory blood pressure in children with sleep-disordered breathing. Am J Respir Crit Care Med 2004;169(8):950–6.

39. Guilleminault C, Khramsov A, Stoohs RA, et al. Abnormal blood pressure in prepubertal children with sleep-disordered breathing. Pediatr Res 2004;55(1): 76–84.

40. Kohyama J, Ohinata JS, Hasegawa T. Blood pressure in sleep disordered breathing. Arch Dis Child 2003;88(2):139–42.

41. Enright PL, Goodwin JL, Sherrill DL, et al. Tucson children's assessment of sleep apnea study. Blood pressure elevation associated with sleep-related breathing disorder in a community sample of white and Hispanic children: the Tucson children's assessment of sleep apnea study. Arch Pediatr Adolesc Med 2003; 157(9):901–4.

42. Leung LC, Ng DK, Lau MW, et al. Twenty-four-hour ambulatory BP in snoring children with obstructive sleep apnea syndrome. Chest 2006;130(4): 1009–17.

43. Zintzaras E, Kaditis AG. Sleep-disordered breathing and blood pressure in children: a meta-analysis. Arch Pediatr Adolesc Med 2007;161(2):172–8.

44. Li AM, Au CT, Sung RY, et al. Ambulatory blood pressure in children with obstructive sleep apnoea—a community based study. Thorax 2008;63(9):803–9.

45. Amin R, Somers VK, McConnell K, et al. Activity-adjusted 24-hour ambulatory blood pressure and cardiac remodeling in children with sleep disordered breathing. Hypertension 2008;51(1):84–91.

46. Amin RS, Kimball TR, Bean JA, et al. Left ventricular hypertrophy and abnormal ventricular geometry in children and adolescents with obstructive sleep apnea. Am J Respir Crit Care Med 2002;165(10):1395–9.

47. Amin RS, Kimball TR, Kalra M, et al. Left ventricular function in children with sleep-disordered breathing. Am J Cardiol 2005;95(6):801–4.
48. Sánchez-Armengol A, Rodríguez-Puras MJ, Fuentes-Pradera MA, et al. Echocardiographic parameters in adolescents with sleep-related breathing disorders. Pediatr Pulmonol 2003;36(1):27–33.
49. Tal A, Leiberman A, Margulis G, et al. Ventricular dysfunction in children with obstructive sleep apnea: radionuclide assessment. Pediatr Pulmonol 1988; 4(3):139–43.
50. Shiomi T, Guilleminault C, Stoohs R, et al. Obstructed breathing in children during sleep monitored by echocardiography. Acta Paediatr 1993;82(10): 863–71.
51. Blacher J, Asmar R, Djane S, et al. Aortic pulse wave velocity as a marker of cardiovascular risk in hypertensive patients. Hypertension 1999;33(5):1111–7.
52. Kwok KL, Ng DK, Cheung YF. BP and arterial distensibility in children with primary snoring. Chest 2003;123(5):1561–6.
53. Gozal D, Kheirandish-Gozal L, Serpero LD, et al. Obstructive sleep apnea and endothelial function in school-aged nonobese children: effect of adenotonsillectomy. Circulation 2007;116(20):2307–14.
54. Vivian EM. Type 2 diabetes in children and adolescents—the next epidemic? Curr Med Res Opin 2006;22(2):297–306.
55. Gahagan S, Silverstein J. American Academy of Pediatrics Committee on Native American Child Health; American Academy of Pediatrics Section on Endocrinology. Prevention and treatment of type 2 diabetes mellitus in children, with special emphasis on American Indian and Alaska Native children. American Academy of Pediatrics Committee on Native American Child Health. Pediatrics 2003;112(4):e328–47.
56. Tresaco B, Bueno G, Pineda I, et al. Homeostatic model assessment (HOMA) index cut-off values to identify the metabolic syndrome in children. J Physiol Biochem 2005;61(2):381–8.
57. Cook S, Weitzman M, Auinger P, et al. Prevalence of a metabolic syndrome phenotype in adolescents: findings from the Third National Health and Nutrition Examination Survey, 1988–1994. Arch Pediatr Adolesc Med 2003;157(8): 821–7.
58. Weiss R, Dziura J, Burgert TS, et al. Obesity and the metabolic syndrome in children and adolescents. N Engl J Med 2004;350(23):2362–74.
59. Srinivasan SR, Myers L, Berenson GS. Predictability of childhood adiposity and insulin for developing insulin resistance syndrome (syndrome X) in young adulthood: the Bogalusa Heart Study. Diabetes 2002;51(1):204–9.
60. Cruz ML, Huang TT, Johnson MS, et al. Insulin sensitivity and blood pressure in black and white children. Hypertension 2002;40(1):18–22.
61. Punjabi NM, Sorkin JD, Katzel LI, et al. Sleep-disordered breathing and insulin resistance in middle-aged and overweight men. Am J Respir Crit Care Med 2002;165(5):677–82.
62. Ip MS, Lam B, Ng MM, et al. Obstructive sleep apnea is independently associated with insulin resistance. Am J Respir Crit Care Med 2002;165(5):670–6.
63. Tauman R, O'Brien LM, Ivanenko A, et al. Obesity rather than severity of sleep-disordered breathing as the major determinant of insulin resistance and altered lipidemia in snoring children. Pediatrics 2005;116(1):e66–73.
64. Kaditis AG, Alexopoulos EI, Damani E, et al. Obstructive sleep-disordered breathing and fasting insulin levels in nonobese children. Pediatr Pulmonol 2005;40(6):515–23.

65. de la Eva RC, Baur LA, Donaghue KC, et al. Metabolic correlates with obstructive sleep apnea in obese subjects. J Pediatr 2002;140(6):654–9.
66. Li AM, Chan MH, Chan DF, et al. Insulin and obstructive sleep apnea in obese Chinese children. Pediatr Pulmonol 2006;41(12):1175–81.
67. Verhulst SL, Schrauwen N, Haentjens D, et al. Sleep-disordered breathing and the metabolic syndrome in overweight and obese children and adolescents. J Pediatr 2007;150(6):608–12.
68. Gozal D, Sans Capdevila O, Kheirandish-Gozal L. Metabolic alterations in obstructive sleep apnea among non-obese and obese prepubertal children. Am J Respir Crit Care Med 2008;117(10):1142–9.
69. Li AM, Yin J, Chan D, et al. Sleeping energy expenditure in paediatric patients with obstructive sleep apnoea syndrome. Hong Kong Med J 2003; 9(5):353–6.
70. Marcus CL, Carroll JL, Koerner CB, et al. Determinants of growth in children with the obstructive sleep apnea syndrome. J Pediatr 1994;125(4):556–62.
71. Bland RM, Bulgarelli S, Ventham JC, et al. Total energy expenditure in children with obstructive sleep apnoea syndrome. Eur Respir J 2001;18(1):164–9.
72. Bar A, Tarasiuk A, Segev Y, et al. The effect of adenotonsillectomy on serum insulin-like growth factor-I and growth in children with obstructive sleep apnea syndrome. J Pediatr 1999;135(1):76–80.
73. Parish JM, Somers VK. Obstructive sleep apnea and cardiovascular disease. Mayo Clin Proc 2004;79(8):1036–46.
74. Ryan S, Taylor CT, McNicholas WT. Selective activation of inflammatory pathways by intermittent hypoxia in obstructive sleep apnea syndrome. Circulation 2005;112(17):2660–7.
75. Alberti A, Sarchielli P, Gallinella E, et al. Plasma cytokine levels in patients with obstructive sleep apnea syndrome: a preliminary study. J Sleep Res 2003; 12(4):305–11.
76. Vgontzas AN, Papanicolaou DA, Bixler EO, et al. Elevation of plasma cytokines in disorders of excessive daytime sleepiness: role of sleep disturbance and obesity. J Clin Endocrinol Metab 1997;82(5):1313–6.
77. Kataoka T, Enomoto F, Kim R, et al. The effect of surgical treatment of obstructive sleep apnea syndrome on the plasma TNF-alpha levels. Tohoku J Exp Med 2004;204(4):267–72.
78. Ohga E, Tomita T, Wada H, et al. Effects of obstructive sleep apnea on circulating ICAM-1, IL-8, and MCP-1. J Appl Phys 2003;94(1):179–84.
79. Yokoe T, Minoguchi K, Matsuo H, et al. Elevated levels of C-reactive protein and interleukin-6 in patients with obstructive sleep apnea syndrome are decreased by nasal continuous positive airway pressure. Circulation 2003; 107(8):1129–34.
80. Tauman R, Ivanenko A, O'Brien LM, et al. Plasma C-reactive protein levels among children with sleep-disordered breathing. Pediatrics 2004;113(6): e564–9.
81. Larkin EK, Rosen CL, Kirchner HL, et al. Variation of C-reactive protein levels in adolescents: association with sleep-disordered breathing and sleep duration. Circulation 2005;111(15):1978–84.
82. Tam CS, Wong M, McBain R, et al. Inflammatory measures in children with obstructive sleep apnoea. J Paediatr Child Health 2006;42(5):277–82.
83. Kaditis AG, Alexopoulos EI, Kalampouka E, et al. Morning levels of C-reactive protein in children with obstructive sleep-disordered breathing. Am J Respir Crit Care Med 2005;171(3):282–6.

84. Juge-Aubry CE, Henrichot E, Meier CA. Adipose tissue: a regulator of inflammation. Best Pract Res Clin Endocrinol Metab 2005;19(4):547–66.
85. Kheirandish-Gozal L, Capdevila OS, Tauman R, et al. Plasma C-reactive protein in nonobese children with obstructive sleep apnea before and after adenotonsillectomy. J Clin Sleep Med 2006;2(3):301–4.
86. Gozal D, Serpero LD, Sans Capdevila O, et al. Systemic inflammation in nonobese children with obstructive sleep apnea. Sleep Med 2008;9(3):254–9.
87. Tauman R, Serpero LD, Capdevila OS, et al. Adipokines in children with sleep disordered breathing. Sleep 2007;30(4):443–9.
88. O'Brien LM, Serpero LD, Tauman R, et al. Plasma adhesion molecules in children with sleep-disordered breathing. Chest 2006;129(4):947–53.
89. Marcus CL, Omlin KJ, Basinki DJ, et al. Normal polysomnographic values for children and adolescents. Am Rev Respir Dis 1992;146(5 Pt 1):1235–9.
90. American Academy of Sleep Medicine. The international classification of sleep disorders, diagnostic and coding manual. 2nd edition. Westchester (IL): American Academy of Sleep Medicine; 2005. p. 58.
91. Sclafani AP, Ginsburg J, Shah MK, et al. Treatment of symptomatic chronic adenotonsillar hypertrophy with amoxicillin/clavulanate potassium: short- and long-term results. Pediatrics 1998;101(4 Pt 1):675–81.
92. Don DM, Goldstein NA, Crockett DM, et al. Antimicrobial therapy for children with adenotonsillar hypertrophy and obstructive sleep apnea: a prospective randomized trial comparing azithromycin vs placebo. Otolaryngol Head Neck Surg 2005;133(4):562–8.
93. Brouillette RT, Manoukian JJ, Ducharme FM, et al. Efficacy of fluticasone nasal spray for pediatric obstructive sleep apnea. J Pediatr 2001;138(6):838–44.
94. Demain JG, Goetz DW. Pediatric adenoidal hypertrophy and nasal airway obstruction: reduction with aqueous nasal beclomethasone. Pediatrics 1995; 95(3):355–64.
95. Kiely JL, Nolan P, McNicholas WT. Intranasal corticosteroid therapy for obstructive sleep apnoea in patients with co-existing rhinitis. Thorax 2004;59(1):50–5.
96. Goldbart AD, Goldman JL, Veling MC, et al. Leukotriene modifier therapy for mild sleep-disordered breathing in children. Am J Respir Crit Care Med 2005; 172(3):364–70.
97. Kheirandish L, Goldbart AD, Gozal D. Intranasal steroids and oral leukotriene modifier therapy in residual sleep-disordered breathing after tonsillectomy and adenoidectomy in children. Pediatrics 2006;117(1):e61–6.
98. Kirk V, Kahn A, Brouillette RT. Diagnostic approach to obstructive sleep apnea in children. Sleep Med Rev 1998;2(4):255–69.
99. Tauman R, Gulliver TE, Krishna J, et al. Persistence of obstructive sleep apnea syndrome in children after adenotonsillectomy. J Pediatr 2006;149(6):803–8.
100. Amin R, Anthony L, Somers V, et al. Growth velocity predicts recurrence of sleep-disordered breathing 1 year after adenotonsillectomy. Am J Respir Crit Care Med 2008;177(6):654–9.
101. Shine NP, Coates HL, Lannigan FJ. Obstructive sleep apnea, morbid obesity, and adenotonsillar surgery: a review of the literature. Int J Pediatr Otorhinolaryngol 2005;69(11):1475–82.
102. Marcus CL, Rosen G, Ward SL, et al. Adherence to and effectiveness of positive airway pressure therapy in children with obstructive sleep apnea. Pediatrics 2006;117(3):e442–51.

Chronic Respiratory Failure and Neuromuscular Disease

J. Declan Kennedy, MD, FRCP, FRACP[a,b,*],
A. James Martin, MRCP, FRACP[b]

KEYWORDS

- Noninvasive ventilation • Neuromuscular disease
- Respiratory failure • Child health • Pathophysiology

Over the past 2 decades, there have been significant developments in the understanding of the pathophysiology and management of respiratory complications of neuromuscular disorders (NMDs) in children, resulting in an increase in life expectancy, reduction in hospital admissions, and increase in the quality of life for the patient and his or her caregivers. A major driver of these changes has been the availability of sophisticated technology to investigate and treat affected children. Other important factors include recognition that affected children require close monitoring by a well-coordinated multidisciplinary team, timely use of airway clearance techniques, improved recognition of those at risk for respiratory failure, and the provision of noninvasive ventilation (NIV) for those in respiratory failure. Expert assessment and management of orthopedic, nutritional, and cardiac complications of NMDs have also added to improved prognosis (**Table 1**).

Despite advances in clinical practice and undoubtedly improved prognosis, the evidence on which some management principles are based is relatively sparse, with the number of consensus statements on the use of NIV in children exceeding that of randomized trials of its use. There is, however, no doubt that the outlook for a child with significant respiratory muscle weakness in this decade is markedly improved, with the mean age of survival in Duchenne muscular dystrophy (DMD) increasing by 30% from 19 to 25 years.[1] Even for those with the most severe disorder, type 1 spinal muscular atrophy (SMA-1), the prognosis for those treated in some specialized

[a] Discipline of Paediatrics, Faculty of Health Sciences, Medical School, University of Adelaide, South Australia 5005, Australia
[b] Department of Pulmonary Medicine, University of Adelaide, Women's and Children's Hospital, 72 King William Road, North Adelaide, South Australia 5006, Australia
* Corresponding author. Department of Pulmonary Medicine, University of Adelaide, Women's and Children's Hospital, 72 King William Road, North Adelaide, South Australia, 5006, Australia.
E-mail address: declan.kennedy@adelaide.edu.au (J.D. Kennedy).

Pediatr Clin N Am 56 (2009) 261–273
doi:10.1016/j.pcl.2008.10.011
0031-3955/08/$ – see front matter. Crown Copyright © 2009 Published by Elsevier Inc. All rights reserved.

Table 1
Grading of evidence of interventions in respiratory care of children who have neuromuscular disorders

Assessment/Intervention	Recommendation	Grading of Recommendation	Quality of Supporting Evidence
Symptoms or signs of respiratory failure	Close clinical monitoring of patient	Strong	Strong
FVC <1 L	Urgent respiratory review because survival risk is poor, NIV if not previously started	Strong	Moderate
FVC <40% indicative of nocturnal hypoventilation	Refer for sleep study or polysomnogram	Strong	Weak
Maximal inspiratory pressure <40 cm H_2O	Polysomnogram with evaluation of day/night CO_2 levels	Moderate	Weak
Peak cough flows (PCFs) <270 L/min in older children	Monitor patient closely because there is a risk for respiratory failure with LRTI	Strong	Strong
When wheelchair bound	Overnight sleep monitoring	Moderate	Weak
Intervention: supplemental oxygen	Not recommended	Strong	Moderate
If upper airway obstruction but not significant respiratory muscle weakness	Adenotonsillectomy (or CPAP if no adenotonsillar hypertrophy)	Moderate	Weak
If acute respiratory failure or chronic or nocturnal and diurnal hypercarbia	NIV	Strong	Moderate

Abbreviations: CO_2, carbon dioxide; CPAP, continuous positive airway pressure; FVC, forced vital capacity; LRTI, lower respiratory tract infection; PCF, peak cough flow.

centers has improved from 9.6 ± 4.0 months of age to 65.2 ± 45.8 months of age (range: 11–153 months).[2] The increase in longevity has and is bringing its own challenges to patients, caregivers, and the health system.[3] The picture is further complicated by variation in service provision between and within countries based on available resources and different ethical views.

The primary purpose of this article is to review the principles of pathophysiology, investigation, and management of the respiratory complications of children with NMDs. The management of orthopedic, nutritional, and cardiac complications is not within the remit of this review. NMDs of childhood can be broadly classified into muscular dystrophies, metabolic and congenital myopathies, anterior horn cell disorders, peripheral neuropathies, and diseases affecting the neuromuscular junction. The two disorders that are the most common and exemplify the important principles of assessment, investigation, and management that apply to all these disorders are DMD and SMA. This review concentrates on these two conditions.

PHYSIOLOGIC EFFECTS OF RESPIRATORY MUSCLE WEAKNESS

Understanding the physiologic sequelae of evolving respiratory muscle weakness is important because it facilitates the prediction and early recognition of symptoms and physical signs, which are often subtle in slowly evolving neuromuscular conditions.[4] The normal infant and young child are at a physiologic disadvantage compared with older children and adults, and this is further compounded when respiratory muscle weakness is superimposed. The lung is relatively stiff compared with the highly compliant chest wall in infants and young children,[5] impeding the generation of adequate tidal volumes.[6] In those with significant muscular weakness, however, functional residual capacity (FRC) is not maintained because of an even more compliant chest wall and failure to maintain inspiratory muscle tone, predisposing to airway closure and microatelectasis. Upper and lower airways are of smaller caliber in younger children, with a greater amount of intrathoracic airway resistance occurring in the smaller airways.[7] In addition, the large central airways are more collapsible because of increased compliance.[7] The respiratory pump power is further challenged by the younger child's horizontal ribs and reduced zone of apposition of the diaphragm.[8] Thus, any disease of the lower airways in a young child quickly brings added stress to an already stressed system. If challenged, therefore, the infant with severe neuromuscular weakness cannot easily increase minute ventilation and respiratory failure quickly follows. The infant also has poorer collateral ventilation. The pores of Kohn and the other interalveolar pathways are not well developed; therefore any lower respiratory disease adds further to compromise because the collateral channels are less available for compensation.[9] Add to this the fact that infants have fewer alveoli in total and reduced elastic recoil; thus, it is surprising that the infant with significant neuromuscular disease can breathe at all.

With the ongoing development of neuromuscular weakness, chest wall compliance decreases because of the gradual stiffening of costosternal and costovertebral articulations, which become ankylosed with lack of use.[10] In SMA-1, pectus excavatum develops with concomitant paradoxical respiration because as the diaphragm contracts, the abdomen expands and the anterior chest wall sinks in.[11] As patients who have SMA-1 slowly get older, although still in infancy, respiratory muscles that are not functioning at their optimal length tension relations because of weakness undergo significant changes, with resultant loss of normal elasticity and plasticity.[11] When scoliosis develops, lung volumes are further reduced, whereas the intercostal muscles are placed at further mechanical disadvantage. The consensus view is that control of breathing is normal in NMD, but in chronic respiratory failure a "blunting" of central chemoreceptors is thought to occur as a result of chronic carbon dioxide (CO_2) retention.[12]

AIRWAY-PROTECTIVE MECHANISMS IN NEUROMUSCULAR WEAKNESS

With loss of expiratory muscle strength, cough power is reduced and is further compromised by inspiratory muscle weakness, because a precough inspiration in excess of 60% of total lung capacity is optimally required.[13] Transmural airway pressures decrease, thereby reducing the cough flow transients that aid mucus clearance from the airway, and bulbar weakness impairs glottis closure, thereby further impairing cough strength.[13]

If a lower respiratory tract infection is "imposed" on the vulnerable respiratory physiology of a child with NMD, a marked increase in respiratory work occurs at a time when the pump muscles are further weakened by the viral infection itself.[14,15] Airway resistance increases as a result of increased airway secretions that cannot be effectively cleared by an impaired cough. Lung compliance decreases as a result of increasing mucus plugging and atelectasis. Acute respiratory failure ensues, and the child may succumb if not mechanically ventilated by NIV or an endotracheal tube. A presentation that is an all too common scenario in childhood NMD is rushing the child in acute respiratory failure attributable to a lower respiratory tract infection or pneumonia to the emergency department. Incidences of 0.8 to 1 per year have been reported in NMDs.[16] A similar presentation can also be the result of aspiration secondary to swallowing dysfunction.[17]

SLEEP AND RESPIRATORY FAILURE

It is during sleep that physiologic changes are magnified, thereby increasing the likelihood of respiratory compromise. In normal children, while sleeping, the respiratory pattern of wakefulness changes in a characteristic way—ventilatory control inputs from higher centers are lost; chemoreceptor, medullary, and cortical arousal center sensitivity decreases; respiratory muscle power diminishes; and upper airway muscle tone decreases. As a result, tidal volume decreases and there is a mild decrease in oxygen saturation and increase in CO_2.[18] During rapid eye movement (REM) sleep, respiratory control is at its nadir, skeletal muscle atonia is maximal with loss of accessory muscle power, and diaphragmatic function is maintained. Depending on the severity and distribution of respiratory muscle weakness in a child with NMD, the "sleep-induced" effects on muscle power are heightened as NMD-induced diaphragmatic weakness accentuates the normal muscle atonia of REM. Thus, in a child with NMD, sleep does not "knit up the ravell'd sleeve of care" but may, in a true sense, be the "death of each day's life".[19]

The net result of the physiologic changes outlined previously is the development in NMD of hypoventilation, first during rapid eye movement sleep, then during no rapid eye movement, and, subsequently, during wakefulness. Depending on the distribution of respiratory muscle weakness, however, the pattern may vary. For example, if diaphragmatic function is not significantly impaired while upper airway musculature is weak and tonsils and adenoids are enlarged, upper airway obstruction may predominate during sleep.[18]

SYMPTOMS AND SIGNS OF RESPIRATORY COMPROMISE IN NEUROMUSCULAR DISORDERS

In severe early-onset respiratory muscle weakness, as encountered in SMA-1, physical examination may reveal a bell-shaped chest with tachypnea, paradoxical breathing, and head bobbing in the context of severe generalized hypotonia. In more slowly evolving respiratory failure, such as that of DMD, the development of symptoms may be insidious and often missed. Those symptoms that should be specifically sought relate to the effects of nocturnal hypoventilation with resultant hypoxia and sleep fragmentation, including daytime behavioral and neurocognitive problems, hyperactivity or tiredness, morning headaches, nocturnal arousals and frequent repositioning, and daytime sleepiness.[6,20] Anorexia at breakfast and cyanosis during meals and on transfer from a wheelchair may also occur.[21] Symptoms may be poorly predictive of sleep breathing difficulties, however.[22,23] Mellies and colleagues[4] recently reported that a structured symptom questionnaire was poorly predictive of sleep-disordered breathing (SDB) or nocturnal hypercapnic ventilation in a group of 49 children with NMDs of varying etiologies. The deficit in general intellectual functioning in boys with DMD further complicates ascertainment of significant symptoms, and in the clinical setting of a pediatric outpatient visit, these boys often sit quietly with their parents saying little about their concerns. Thus, in summary, symptoms of respiratory failure are often not reported or are subtle and overlooked.

RESPIRATORY MONITORING IN CHILDHOOD NEUROMUSCULAR DISORDERS
Role of Lung Function Testing in Predicting Respiratory Failure

Serial monitoring of lung function is mandated for all children with NMD when it is able to be performed—usually after the age of 5 years.[24,25] The rate of decline in forced vital capacity (FVC) in DMD is variable (2%–39% per year), with a median of 8%, whereas a FVC of less than 1 L in DMD is associated with a median survival of 3.1 years and a 5-year survival rate of only 8%.[26] Bourke and Gibson[27] suggest that FVC may be a better measure of overall survival in DMD than nocturnal hypoxia. A recent report suggested that a FVC of greater than 60% represented a low risk for nocturnal hypoventilation, whereas a FVC less than 40% was a good predictor of nocturnal hypoventilation in children with NMDs of varying etiologies.[25] Daytime $Paco_2$ levels greater than 45 mm Hg, in combination with spirometry, have also been used to predict SDB,[28] whereas Mellies and colleagues[4] asserted that SDB with nocturnal hypercapnic hypoventilation could be predicted by a $Paco_2$ greater than 40 mm Hg (92% sensitivity, 72% specificity) and inspiratory vital capacity less than 40% (96% sensitivity, 88% specificity) in a group of 49 children and adolescents who had NMD of mixed etiology (aged 11.3 ± 4.4 years). These researchers also reported that a maximum peak inspiratory pressure less than 4 kPa and less than 2.5 kPa predicted SDB onset and nocturnal hypercapnia, respectively.[4] Similarly maximum expiratory mouth pressure (MEP) has been used to measure effective cough capacity (MEP >60 cm H_2O is adequate, and MEP <45 cm H_2O is insufficient),[29] whereas a maximum inspiratory mouth pressure (MIP) less than 60 cm has been suggested as indicative of the need to consider NIV.[30] Peak cough flows (PCFs) are now recognized as important measures of the capacity for mucociliary clearance. Consensus documents have accepted 270 L/min as the acceptable level of flow;[24,25] at greater than that level, there is a reduced risk for developing respiratory failure during upper respiratory tract infections, whereas a level lower than that target value identifies patients who would benefit from manually assisted cough techniques.[31] In adult patients who have NMD, however, with PCF values of 270 L/min while well, these values often decrease to less than 160 L/min during acute viral infections,[31] a level insufficient to clear airway secretions. The target PCF value of 270 L/min may not be appropriate for children because those younger than 13 years of age are often not able to generate values of 270 L/min.[13] PCFs less than 270 L/min are more likely when FVC is <2.1 L in children who have DMD.[32] It is worth noting that PCF can be increased by breath stacking.

In those with the most severe form of NMD, SMA-1, infant lung function testing is technically demanding and untested in this clinical setting, but monitoring with polysomnography (PSG), or with oximetry if the former is not available, particularly during sleep, is extremely helpful in assessing evolving respiratory muscle weakness and resultant hypoventilation.[17] There is a clear consensus in the literature[24,25,30] that serial monitoring of lung function is mandated for all children who are old enough to perform it. For spirometric evaluation, MIP, MEP, and PCF, this is usually after the age of 5 years.

When to Refer for Specialized Respiratory Review

Although a recent American Thoracic Society consensus statement[24] recommended that those who have DMD be reviewed by a pediatric respiratory physician twice yearly after FVC has decreased to less than 80% of that predicted, or if aged 12 years or when confined to a wheel chair, many respiratory pediatricians believe that they should review all children with NMD after the diagnosis has been confirmed. This allows the pediatric respiratory physician and respiratory team to meet with the family before respiratory complications have developed to discuss their potential evolution and the methods of assessing and treating them. This is important to facilitate before the family undertakes "Internet surfing," wherein management techniques with varying levels of scientific support may be promulgated. The frequency of specialized respiratory assessment depends on clinical progress.[25] In children whose respiratory muscle weakness is evolving more slowly, annual monitoring with spirometry and overnight PSG is reasonable initially. The timing of further overnight studies may be varied depending on the PSG results. The more difficult question to answer is when to begin overnight monitoring, although guidelines are outlined elsewhere in this article.

Timing of Polysomnography

In children who have DMD, consensus guidelines[24] suggest that overnight monitoring should be considered from the time the child becomes a wheelchair user or when clinically indicated. As outlined previously, symptoms of nocturnal hypoxemia and sleep fragmentation may often be subtle. PSG should be considered annually when FVC is less than 60% and more often if it is less than 40%. A MIP less than 60%[30] and daytime $Paco_2$ greater than 40 mm Hg[4] are also helpful in prompting a referral for PSG evaluation. These target values are general guidelines only, because not infrequently in clinical practice, one sees children whose FVC is greater than 70% of that predicted but whose PSGs demonstrate significant alveolar hypoventilation.

TREATMENT OF RESPIRATORY FAILURE IN NEUROMUSCULAR DISORDERS

Although one of the major changes in the treatment of respiratory failure in NMDs has been the introduction of NIV, the literature evidence on which its effectiveness is based is not clear-cut. In a recent Cochrane review, the conclusions of Annane and colleagues[33] were that "current evidence about the therapeutic benefit of mechanical ventilation (in NMD) is weak, but directionally consistent suggesting alleviation of the symptoms of chronic hypoventilation in the short term." They suggested that large randomized trials were needed to confirm long-term beneficial effects of NIV on symptoms, quality of life, unplanned hospital admissions, and mortality and, finally, to evaluate its cost-effectiveness. For this review, only eight trials in the literature were deemed eligible for evaluation because entry criteria dictated that they had to be quasirandomized or randomized controlled studies and most patients studied were adults. It is against this backdrop that one needs to consider the pros and cons of NIV treatment in pediatric patients who have NMD.

Although noninvasive positive-pressure ventilation was first used in the 1960s,[34,35] it was not until the 1980s, after the development of the continuous positive airway pressure mask,[36] that Rideau and colleagues[37] in Europe and Bach and colleagues[35] in the United States suggested that noninvasive positive-pressure ventilation (NIV) be used to treat respiratory failure in NMD. With the subsequent development of suitable children's masks, NIV gained acceptance in pediatric practice during the 1990s. In a recent review of NIV in children, Norregaard[6] noted that knowledge of NIV application in children depended in the main on reports of case series, with little firm evidence of when to initiate NIV in this age group. It is also salutary to note how far pediatric clinical practice has come since the findings of a consensus conference,[38] which reported that "nasal mask ventilation in young children must be considered an investigational technique for research and/or use only by experienced centers." Notwithstanding the conclusions of the Cochrane report outlined previously, NIV is now accepted as one of the major strategies in the treatment of respiratory failure in children who have NMD and is strongly supported by several consensus statements.[17,24,25] There is not a clear consensus in the literature as to when one should initiate NIV, however.

EVIDENCE THAT NONINVASIVE VENTILATION IS EFFECTIVE IN RESPIRATORY FAILURE IN NEUROMUSCULAR DISORDERS

The evidence for NIV's effectiveness in NMD is based mainly on case series, nonrandomized trials, and comparisons with historical controls. Despite this, the weight of evidence is persuasive. Eagle and colleagues[1] reported that the mean age of death in patients who had DMD and were treated with NIV had increased from 19 to 25 years when compared with historical controls who did not receive this treatment, whereas Simonds and colleagues[39] found a one year and five year survival rate of 85% and 73%, respectively, in DMD patients treated with NIV. There are now a series of studies that report improvements not only in survival but in symptoms of nocturnal hypoventilation, gas exchange during the day and night, preservation of lung function, quality of life, and frequency of hospital admissions.[21,31,39–46] John Bach has been a tireless advocate over many years of NIV in the treatment of respiratory failure in NMD, and his results even in severe muscle weakness, such as SMA-1,[2,47] are impressive. He reported that as a result of noninvasive management in his clinic (which included monitoring of oximetry, mechanical-assisted coughing techniques, and short-term intubations for acute respiratory infections), 80 of 115 patients who had SMA-1 were still alive without tracheostomy at 4 years, with 8 children older than 8 years of age and 2 older than 10 years of age.[48] The management of children who have SMA-1 is a highly controversial area, however, and as outlined by Bush and colleagues,[49] individual physicians may discourage long-term daytime NIV but "many will disagree with this approach in good faith." What Bach's approach may be demonstrating is that with aggressive management of respiratory failure with NIV, close monitoring of ventilation with oximetry, and the early introduction of mechanical-assisted coughing in acute respiratory infections, the long-term outlook for many children with neuromuscular weakness of varying etiologies may be enhanced.

WHEN TO START NONINVASIVE VENTILATION

There is little consensus in the literature regarding when to start NIV, with some advocating its introduction if the patient is hypercapnic or hypoxic during sleep or wakefulness (in DMD).[50] Others (in congenital muscular dystrophies, SMA-2, and congenital myopathies) advocate its initiation in those with acute respiratory failure, symptomatic diurnal hypercapnia or symptomatic nocturnal hypoventilation in the absence of daytime hypercapnia, failure to thrive, or more than three chest infections per year, with its use in nonsymptomatic nocturnal hypercapnia or hypopnea being considered on an individual basis.[25] As outlined previously, symptoms are often subtle.

Mallory[51] suggests that its use should commence early, that is, before the onset of respiratory failure. The American Thoracic Society consensus statement[24] suggests that NIV be used to treat "sleep-related upper airway obstruction and chronic respiratory insufficiency" in DMD, although no definitive guidelines are given as to levels of severity that would mandate NIV. A second consensus statement[30] suggests NIV use in NMD if the patient has symptoms, such as fatigue, morning headache, and one of the following: (1) $Paco_2$ of 45 mm Hg or greater, (2) nocturnal oxygen saturation of 88% or less for 5 consecutive minutes, or (3) maximal inspiratory pressures less than 60 cm H_2O or FVC less than 50% of that predicted. Ward and colleagues[44] make the point that these recommendations are not based on controlled studies and that the oxygen saturation guidelines were not based on evidence but partly on

Medicare guidelines for oxygen therapy in chronic obstructive pulmonary disease.[52] These researchers performed one of the few randomized controlled trials of NIV in a group of patients who had NMD (of mixed etiology).[44] They randomized 26 subjects, aged 7 to 51 years, with an FVC less than 50% of that predicted with nocturnal hypercapnia (peak $Tcco_2$ >6.5 kPa) but normal daytime CO_2 levels to nocturnal NIV or to a control group without NIV. Nocturnal ventilation improved in the treated group, but 9 of 10 controls needed NIV after a mean of 8.3 months (SD = 7.3). These findings support the conclusion that once nocturnal hypoventilation is present, NIV treatment should be considered.[40] A recent index, the "Breathing Intolerance Index," was developed by Koga and colleagues[53] calculated from the formula of inspiratory time (T_i) divided by total respiratory time (T_{tot}), multiplied by the result of tidal volume (V_t) divided by vital capacity (VC) [ie, (T_i/T_{tot}) × (V_t/VC)]. These investigators found that a value greater than 0.15 was noted for all subjects on NIV.

One of the studies often quoted in the literature as demonstrating the possible hazard of initiating NIV early is that of Raphael and colleagues.[54] Its importance lies in its being one of the few randomized trials of NIV use in children. These researchers' aim was to evaluate the use of "prophylactic" NIV in a group of 70 teenaged patients who had DMD with a FVC from 20% to 50% of that predicted and who had not developed diurnal hypercapnia by randomizing them to NIV or standard treatment. The worrying result was a fourfold increase in mortality in the NIV group, with most resulting from respiratory infections. These investigators thought that the putative reason for the increase in mortality was the false sense of security in patients using NIV, thereby resulting in a delay in seeking medical help during a significant respiratory infection. The study has subsequently been criticized by many investigators for limitations in design and analysis, including failure to document patient compliance with NIV or to use assisted cough techniques, a higher proportion of patients with cardiac dysfunction in the NIV group,[52] and the absence of PSG data before and after NIV initiation.[55]

The initiation of NIV should optimally be electively planned after discussions with family and patients. Unfortunately, in practice, this is not always what happens. Sritippayawan and colleagues[56] reported that of 73 children who had NMD of mixed etiologies, only 21% had NIV commenced electively. Some authorities have suggested that the reticence to discuss long-term ventilatory support with patients might be because of health providers' assessments of the patients' poor quality of life.[57,58] As outlined by Kohler and colleagues,[59] however, even patients who have DMD with advanced muscle weakness report a high quality of life despite their illness, which was not correlated with physical limitation or need for NIV.

The long-term positive effects of NIV in children who have NMD have been demonstrated in two recent studies. Mellies and colleagues[43] reported that in 30 patients who had NMD of varying etiologies, NIV normalized nocturnal and daytime gas exchange and sleep and that the effects persisted over 25.3 ± 12.7 months. In 15 children who had varying types of NMD, Katz and colleagues[45] found that over at least a 1-year period, NIV resulted in an 85% reduction in days in the hospital and a 68% reduction in days in intensive care. The physiologic reasons for this improvement in respiratory failure parameters have been recently explored by Nickol and colleagues,[60] who found that increased ventilatory response to CO_2 was the main contributor. An intriguing aspect of NIV use is its possible positive effects on lung and chest wall growth. Bach and Bianchi[11] have advocated its use for this purpose, suggesting "high span positive inspiratory pressure plus positive end-expiratory pressure" to improve lung compliance and prevent pectus excavatum in SMA-1. The effectiveness of NIV in promoting lung and chest wall growth awaits further elucidation. The long-term potential effect of NIV on facial development also needs to be remembered because a recent study of

40 children using NIV (cystic fibrosis [n = 10], obstructive sleep apnea [n = 16], and NMD [n = 14]) found a prevalence of global facial flattening in 68%. No correlation was found with age or daily or cumulative use of NIV.[61]

The increasing use of NIV in neuromuscular disease in children must be seen against the background of other developments that have, in concert, improved the quality and quantity of life for affected children. The importance of airway clearance methods using manual-assisted techniques (manual-assisted coughing with increased inspiratory capacity facilitated by glossopharyngeal breathing, breath stacking, or self-inflating bag and mask) has been highlighted in recent studies and consensus statements.[24,25,31] In addition, mechanical insufflator-exsufflators play an important role in mobilizing airway secretions, especially in those whose PCFs are ineffective, and their efficacy in NMD has been highlighted in several recent studies.[31,62–64] Chatwin and colleagues[65] demonstrated in 22 patients with NMD, 8 of whom were children, that the insufflator-exsufflator produced a greater increase in PCFs than voluntary unassisted cough or cough assisted by physiotherapy or noninvasive positive-pressure ventilation. Two newer mucus clearance devices whose benefit awaits clarification include high-frequency chest wall oscillation and intrapulmonary percussive ventilation.[66,67]

The continued improvement in outlook from a respiratory point of view for children who have NMD has also been aided by the early use of antibiotics in acute respiratory infections, influenza, and pneumococcal vaccinations; improved intensive care techniques; and specialized regional care centers. Nonrespiratory interventions, such as the use of oral steroids in DMD to improve muscle strength and respiratory function[68] (although not uniformly accepted),[24] surgical correction of scoliosis,[69] early intervention and treatment of cardiac dysfunction,[70,71] recognition and treatment of gastroesophageal reflux and aspiration,[17] close monitoring of nutritional status, and intervention with gastrostomy in those failing to thrive[24] are all integral to optimal management of these complex patients.

In summary, the management of respiratory complications of children who have neuromuscular disease has markedly improved in the past 15 years. The reasons for this are many and include a better appreciation of the symptoms of hypoventilation during sleep, which are often subtle; a greater understanding of the importance of close monitoring by a respiratory pediatrician with serial lung function testing and overnight monitoring; the acceptance of the importance of NIV in treating acute and chronic hypoventilation; and improved airway clearance techniques, including assisted coughing and insufflator-exsufflators. The role of the respiratory pediatrician is vital in coordinating all these aspects of care.

Further improvements in the quality and quantity of life for children who have NMD are likely in the years ahead with gene- and cell-based treatments. This should also have a significant impact on patients' families and health systems. Governments need to be made aware of the demands that are likely to be made on the health systems as a result. There is an urgent need for improvement in the home care and respite opportunities provided in addition to education and skills training for young adults. We have come some way, but there is much to be done.

ACKNOWLEDGMENTS

The authors gratefully acknowledge the assistance of Dr. Cameron van den Heuvel at the University of Adelaide in formatting and proofreading this manuscript.

REFERENCES

1. Eagle M, Baudouin SV, Chandler C, et al. Survival in Duchenne muscular dystrophy: improvements in life expectancy since 1967 and the impact of home nocturnal ventilation. Neuromuscul Disord 2002;12(10):926–9.
2. Bach JR, Saltstein K, Sinquee D, et al. Long-term survival in Werdnig-Hoffmann disease. Am J Phys Med Rehabil 2007;86(5):339–45.
3. Birnkrant D. New challenges in the management of prolonged survivors of pediatric neuromuscular diseases: a pulmonologist's perspective. Pediatr Pulmonol 2006;41:1113–7.
4. Mellies U, Ragette R, Schwake C, et al. Daytime predictors of sleep disordered breathing in children and adolescents with neuromuscular disorders. Neuromuscul Disord 2003;13(2):123–8.
5. Papastamelos C, Panitch HB, Allen JL. Chest wall compliance in infants and children with neuromuscular disease. Am J Respir Crit Care Med 1996;154(4 Pt 1):1045–8.
6. Norregaard O. Noninvasive ventilation in children. Eur Respir J 2002;20(5):1332–42.
7. Gaultier C. Developmental anatomy and physiology of the respiratory system. In: Taussig LM, Landau L, Le Souef PN, et al, editors. Pediatric respiratory medicine. St. Louis (MO): Mosby; 1999. p. 18–37.
8. Devlieger H, Daniels H, Marchal G, et al. The diaphragm of the newborn infant: anatomical and ultrasonographic studies. J Dev Physiol 1991;16(6):321–9.
9. Rosenberg DE, Lyons HA. Collateral ventilation in excised human lungs. Respiration 1979;37(3):125–34.
10. Estenne M, Heilporn A, Delhez L, et al. Chest wall stiffness in patients with chronic respiratory muscle weakness. Am Rev Respir Dis 1983;128(6):1002–7.
11. Bach JR, Bianchi C. Prevention of pectus excavatum for children with spinal muscular atrophy type 1. Am J Phys Med Rehabil 2003;82(10):815–9.
12. Perrin C, Unterborn JN, D' Ambrosio CD, et al. Pulmonary complications of chronic neuromuscular diseases and their management. Muscle Nerve 2004;29(1):5–27.
13. Panitch HB. Respiratory issues in the management of children with neuromuscular disease. Respir Care 2006;51(8):885–93.
14. Mier-Jedrzejowicz A, Brophy C, Green M. Respiratory muscle weakness during upper respiratory tract infections. Am Rev Respir Dis 1988;138(1):5–7.
15. Poponick JM, Jacobs I, Supinski G, et al. Effect of upper respiratory tract infection in patients with neuromuscular disease. Am J Respir Crit Care Med 1997;156(2 Pt 1):659–64.
16. Bach JR, Rajaraman R, Ballanger F, et al. Neuromuscular ventilatory insufficiency: effect of home mechanical ventilator use v oxygen therapy on pneumonia and hospitalization rates. Am J Phys Med Rehabil 1998;77(1):8–19.
17. Wang CH, Finkel RS, Bertini ES, et al. Consensus statement for standard of care in spinal muscular atrophy. J Child Neurol 2007;22(8):1027–49.
18. Givan D. Sleep and breathing in children with neuromuscular disease. In: Loughlin GM, Carroll JL, Marcus CL, editors. Sleep and breathing in children—a developmental approach, vol. 147. New York: Marcel Dekker AG; 2000. p. 691–735.
19. Macbeth, II, ii. Jaggard and Blount, First Folio. 1623.
20. Mellies U, Dohna-Schwake C, Ragette R, et al. [Nocturnal noninvasive ventilation of children and adolescents with neuromuscular diseases: effect on sleep and symptoms]. Wien Klin Wochenschr 2003;115(24):855–9 [in German].

21. Simonds AK, Ward S, Heather S, et al. Outcome of paediatric domiciliary mask ventilation in neuromuscular and skeletal disease. Eur Respir J 2000;16(3): 476–81.
22. Young HK, Lowe A, Fitzgerald DA, et al. Outcome of noninvasive ventilation in children with neuromuscular disease. Neurology 2007;68(3):198–201.
23. Suresh S, Wales P, Dakin C, et al. Sleep related breathing disorder in Duchenne muscular dystrophy: disease spectrum in the pediatric population. J Paediatr Child Health 2005;41:500–3.
24. Finder JD, Birnkrant D, Carl J, et al. Respiratory care of the patient with Duchenne muscular dystrophy: ATS consensus statement. Am J Respir Crit Care Med 2004; 170(4):456–65.
25. Wallgren-Pettersson C, Bushby K, Mellies U, et al. 117th ENMC workshop: ventilatory support in congenital neuromuscular disorders—congenital myopathies, congenital muscular dystrophies, congenital myotonic dystrophy and SMA (II). 4–6 April 2003, Naarden, The Netherlands. Neuromuscul Disord 2004;14(1): 56–69.
26. Phillips MF, Quinlivan RC, Edwards RH, et al. Changes in spirometry over time as a prognostic marker in patients with Duchenne muscular dystrophy. Am J Respir Crit Care Med 2001;164(12):2191–4.
27. Bourke SC, Gibson GJ. Sleep and breathing in neuromuscular disease. Eur Respir J 2002;19(6):1194–201.
28. Hukins CA, Hillman DR. Daytime predictors of sleep hypoventilation in Duchenne muscular dystrophy. Am J Respir Crit Care Med 2000;161(1):166–70.
29. Szeinberg A, Tabachnik E, Rashed N, et al. Cough capacity in patients with muscular dystrophy. Chest 1988;94(6):1232–5.
30. Consensus Conference. Clinical indications for noninvasive positive pressure ventilation in chronic respiratory failurre due to restrictive lung disease, COPD, and nocturnal hypoventilation. A consensus conference report. Chest 1999; 116:521–34.
31. Tzeng AC, Bach JR. Prevention of pulmonary morbidity for patients with neuromuscular disease. Chest 2000;118(5):1390–6.
32. Gauld LM, Boynton A. Relationship between peak cough flow and spirometry in Duchenne muscular dystrophy. Pediatr Pulmonol 2005;39(5):457–60.
33. Annane D, Orlikowski D, Chevret S. Nocturnal mechanical ventilation for chronic hypoventilation in patients with neuromuscular and chest wall disorders. Cochrane Database Syst Rev 2007;(4):1–28.
34. Alba A, Khan A, Lee M. Mouth IPPV for sleep. Rehabilitation Gazette 1981;24: 47–9.
35. Bach JR, Alba A, Mosher R, et al. Intermittent positive pressure ventilation via nasal access in the management of respiratory insufficiency. Chest 1987;92(1): 168–70.
36. Sullivan CE, Issa FG, Berthon-Jones M, et al. Reversal of obstructive sleep apnoea by continuous positive airway pressure applied through the nares. Lancet 1981;1(8225):862–5.
37. Rideau Y, Gatin G, Bach J, et al. Prolongation of life in Duchenne's muscular dystrophy. Acta Neurol (Napoli) 1983;5(2):118–24.
38. Make BJ, Hill NS, Goldberg AI, et al. Mechanical ventilation beyond the intensive care unit. Report of a consensus conference of the American College of Chest Physicians. Chest 1998;113(Suppl 5):289S–344S.
39. Simonds AK, Muntoni F, Heather S, et al. Impact of nasal ventilation on survival in hypercapnic Duchenne muscular dystrophy. Thorax 1998;53(11):949–52.

40. Simonds AK. Recent advances in respiratory care for neuromuscular disease. Chest 2006;130(6):1879–86.
41. Vianello A, Bevilacqua M, Salvador V, et al. Long-term nasal intermittent positive pressure ventilation in advanced Duchenne's muscular dystrophy. Chest 1994; 105(2):445–8.
42. Bach JR, Ishikawa Y, Kim H. Prevention of pulmonary morbidity for patients with Duchenne muscular dystrophy. Chest 1997;112(4):1024–8.
43. Mellies U, Ragette R, Dohna Schwake C, et al. Long-term noninvasive ventilation in children and adolescents with neuromuscular disorders. Eur Respir J 2003; 22(4):631–6.
44. Ward S, Chatwin M, Heather S, et al. Randomised controlled trial of non-invasive ventilation (NIV) for nocturnal hypoventilation in neuromuscular and chest wall disease patients with daytime normocapnia. Thorax 2005;60(12):1019–24.
45. Katz S, Selvadurai H, Keilty K, et al. Outcome of non-invasive positive pressure ventilation in paediatric neuromuscular disease. Arch Dis Child 2004;89(2):121–4.
46. Dohna-Schwake C, Podlewski P, Voit T, et al. Non-invasive ventilation reduces respiratory tract infections in children with neuromuscular disorders. Pediatr Pulmonol 2008;43(1):67–71.
47. Bach JR, Baird JS, Plosky D, et al. Spinal muscular atrophy type 1: management and outcomes. Pediatr Pulmonol 2002;34(1):16–22.
48. Bach JR. There are other ways to manage spinal muscular atrophy type 1. Chest 2005;127(4):1463.
49. Bush A, Fraser J, Jardine E, et al. Respiratory management of the infant with type 1 spinal muscular atrophy. Arch Dis Child 2005;90(7):709–11.
50. Wagner KR, Lechtzin N, Judge DP. Current treatment of adult Duchenne muscular dystrophy. Biochim Biophys Acta 2007;1772(2):229–37.
51. Mallory GB. Pulmonary complications of neuromuscular disease. Pediatr Pulmonol Suppl 2004;26:138–40.
52. Mehta S, Hill NS. Noninvasive ventilation. Am J Respir Crit Care Med 2001;163(2): 540–77.
53. Koga T, Watanabe K, Sano M, et al. Breathing intolerance index. Am J Phys Med Rehabil 2005;85:24–30.
54. Raphael JC, Chevret S, Chastang C, et al. Randomised trial of preventive nasal ventilation in Duchenne muscular dystrophy. French Multicentre Cooperative Group on Home Mechanical Ventilation Assistance in Duchenne de Boulogne Muscular Dystrophy. Lancet 1994;343(8913):1600–4.
55. Fauroux B, Lofaso F. Non-invasive mechanical ventilation: when to start for what benefit? Thorax 2005;60(12):979–80.
56. Sritippayawan S, Kun SS, Keens TG, et al. Initiation of home mechanical ventilation in children with neuromuscular diseases. J Pediatr 2003;142(5):481–5.
57. Bach JR, Campagnolo DI, Hoeman S. Life satisfaction of individuals with Duchenne muscular dystrophy using long-term mechanical ventilatory support. Am J Phys Med Rehabil 1991;70(3):129–35.
58. Gibson B. Long-term ventilation for patients with Duchenne muscular dystrophy: physicians' beliefs and practices. Chest 2001;119(3):940–6.
59. Kohler M, Clarenbach CF, Boni L, et al. Quality of life, physical disability, and respiratory impairment in Duchenne muscular dystrophy. Am J Respir Crit Care Med 2005;172(8):1032–6.
60. Nickol AH, Hart N, Hopkinson NS, et al. Mechanisms of improvement of respiratory failure in patients with restrictive thoracic disease treated with non-invasive ventilation. Thorax 2005;60(9):754–60.

61. Fauroux B, Lavis JF, Nicot F, et al. Facial side effects during noninvasive positive pressure ventilation in children. Intensive Care Med 2005;31(7):965–9.
62. Winck JC, Goncalves MR, Lourenco C, et al. Effects of mechanical insufflation-exsufflation on respiratory parameters for patients with chronic airway secretion encumbrance. Chest 2004;126(3):774–80.
63. Bach JR, Niranjan V, Weaver B. Spinal muscular atrophy type 1: a noninvasive respiratory management approach. Chest 2000;117(4):1100–5.
64. Miske LJ, Hickey EM, Kolb SM, et al. Use of the mechanical in-exsufflator in pediatric patients with neuromuscular disease and impaired cough. Chest 2004;125(4):1406–12.
65. Chatwin M, Ross E, Hart N, et al. Cough augmentation with mechanical insufflation/exsufflation in patients with neuromuscular weakness. Eur Respir J 2003; 21(3):502–8.
66. Plioplys AV, Lewis S, Kasnicka I. Pulmonary vest therapy in pediatric long-term care. J Am Med Dir Assoc 2002;3(5):318–21.
67. Toussaint M, De Win H, Steens M, et al. Effect of intrapulmonary percussive ventilation on mucus clearance in Duchenne muscular dystrophy patients: a preliminary report. Respir Care 2003;48(10):940–7.
68. Biggar WD, Harris VA, Eliasoph L, et al. Long-term benefits of deflazacort treatment for boys with Duchenne muscular dystrophy in their second decade. Neuromuscul Disord 2006;16(4):249–55.
69. Eagle M, Bourke J, Bullock R, et al. Managing Duchenne muscular dystrophy—the additive effect of spinal surgery and home nocturnal ventilation in improving survival. Neuromuscul Disord 2007;17(6):470–5.
70. Bushby K, Muntoni F, Bourke JP. 107th ENMC international workshop: the management of cardiac involvement in muscular dystrophy and myotonic dystrophy. 7th-9th June 2002, Naarden, The Netherlands. Neuromuscul Disord 2003;13(2): 166–72.
71. Cardiovascular health supervision for individuals affected by Duchenne or Becker muscular dystrophy. Pediatrics 2005;116(6):1569–73.

Domiciliary Oxygen for Children

Ian M. Balfour-Lynn, MBBS, MD, FRCP, FRCPCH, FRCS(Ed), DHMSA

KEYWORDS

• Oxygen • Domiciliary • Home • Neonatal lung disease

The pediatric use of domiciliary oxygen (supplemental oxygen delivered in the home) has been steadily increasing since its first reported use in children in the 1970s.[1] Like much pediatric practice, because of a scarcity of good evidence to inform clinicians, there is a lack of consensus over many issues. Most available evidence relates to infants discharged home with chronic neonatal lung disease (CNLD), which is easily the largest patient group receiving domiciliary oxygen. Because this article is part of a series on "evidence-based management," much of it relates to CNLD; however, other conditions are also covered, remembering the adage "lack of evidence of benefit is not the same as evidence for lack of benefit" (**Box 1**). Nevertheless, whenever possible, recommendations are accompanied by a grade indicating quality of evidence and strength of the recommendation using the GRADE system.[2]

DEFINITIONS

Although domiciliary refers to the home, in the context of oxygen therapy, it refers to delivery of supplemental oxygen outside the hospital because it may also be used outside the home, especially by children. Modes of delivery fall into three categories. Long-term oxygen therapy (LTOT) is defined as the provision of oxygen for continuous use at home for patients who have chronic hypoxemia (attributable to any cause) to maintain oxygen saturation (SaO_2) at or greater than 92% (depending on the type of oximeter) or PaO_2 greater than 8 kPa.[3] It may be required 24 hours per day or during periods of sleep only; thus, the adult definition that includes a requirement for more than 15 hours per day is not relevant. Ambulatory oxygen therapy (AOT) refers to the provision of portable oxygen that can be used outside the home. In adult patients, this is not always necessary because many are house-bound (although they may still need to attend hospital appointments). All children on LTOT require facilities for portable AOT unless they only use nighttime oxygen. This particularly applies to the infant age group (who spend periods during the day sleeping) because parents need to be able to take the baby outside the home to lead as normal a life as possible. Short burst oxygen therapy (SBOT)

Department of Paediatric Respiratory Medicine, Royal Brompton Hospital, Sydney Street, London SW3 6NP, UK
E-mail address: i.balfourlynn@ic.ac.uk

Pediatr Clin N Am 56 (2009) 275–296
doi:10.1016/j.pcl.2008.10.010
0031-3955/08/$ – see front matter © 2009 Elsevier Inc. All rights reserved.

> **Box 1**
> **Principal pediatric conditions that may require long-term oxygen therapy**
>
> CNLD (bronchopulmonary dysplasia)
>
> Other neonatal lung conditions (eg, pulmonary hypoplasia)
>
> Congenital heart disease with pulmonary hypertension
>
> Pulmonary hypertension secondary to pulmonary disease
>
> Interstitial lung disease
>
> Obliterative bronchiolitis
>
> Cystic fibrosis and non-cystic fibrosis bronchiectasis
>
> Obstructive sleep apnea syndrome and other sleep-related disorders
>
> Neuromuscular conditions requiring noninvasive ventilation
>
> Disorders of the chest wall (eg, thoracic dystrophy, severe kyphoscoliosis)
>
> Sickle cell disease
>
> End-of-life palliative care

refers to acute use of short-term oxygen, and there are few indications specific to children, although it is undoubtedly used that way in many families (eg, during seizures).

NORMAL OXYGEN LEVELS

Painful arterial stabs result in a crying (and sometimes hypoxic) child, which gives unreliable results; thus, studies of oxygen levels in children are invariably performed using pulse oximetry. The issue here, however, is that pulse oximeters do not all give equivalent readings of SaO_2; thus, it is necessary to know which oximeter was used when comparing studies. A group of investigators have studied children at varying ages using the same equipment (**Table 1**). Their study of healthy term infants in the first month of life measured by pulse oximetry found in the first week of life that the baseline SaO_2 ranged from 92% to 100% (median of 97.6%), whereas in weeks 2 through 4, it ranged from 87% to 100% (median of 98.0%).[4] Episodes of desaturation ($SaO_2 \leq 80\%$ for ≥ 4 seconds) occurred in 35% of recordings in week 1 and in 60% in weeks 2 through 4. These investigators also studied 67 older healthy full-term infants aged 4 to 8 weeks and found that their baseline SaO_2, measured by pulse oximetry, ranged from 97% to 100% (median of 99.8%).[5] Short

Table 1
Normal oxygen saturation levels in healthy children, measured by the same group of investigators using pulse oximetry

Age	n	Median	Range	Reference
Ex-preterm babies at term	66	99.4	89–100	6
1 week	50	97.6	92–100	4
2–4 weeks	50	98.0	87–100	4
4–8 weeks	67	99.8	97–100	5
2–16 (mean 8) years	70	99.5	96–100	8

episodes of desaturation to 80% or less were found in 81% of infants, occurring at a median of 0.9 per hour, with a median duration of 1.2 seconds (97% were for less than 4 seconds). They studied 66 preterm infants born at a gestational age of 25 to 36 weeks (median of 34 weeks) when they had reached term.[6] Their baseline SaO_2 ranged from 89% to 100% (median of 99.4%). Desaturations were more frequent (median of 5.4 per hour) and longer (median of 1.5 seconds) than in the term infants, however.[5] High altitude affects SaO_2 and may need to be taken into account when interpreting normal values (and publications).[7] Finally, they studied 70 healthy older children with a mean age of 8 years (range: 2–16 years) using a pulse oximeter.[8] Baseline SaO_2 was a median of 99.5% (range: 95.8%–100%, fifth centile = 96.6%). The number of desaturations of 90% or less decreased with age, with episodic decreases seen in 47% of 2- to 6-year-olds and in 13% of 13- to 16-year-olds. A more recent study in 100 third-grade primary school children (mean age = 9.3 years) recorded overnight SaO_2 measured by pulse oximetry.[9] The median SaO_2 was 97% (range: 94%–100%), and a baseline SaO_2 less than 97% was uncommon. Furthermore, although intermittent desaturations by 4% or more were frequent, the SaO_2 rarely decreased to 90% or less.

WHAT ARE THE ADVERSE EFFECTS OF CHRONIC LOW OXYGEN SATURATION?

This, of course, depends on the degree and duration of the low SaO_2 levels, and it is likely that mild hypoxemia has no adverse effects. Newborns and infants younger than 1 year of age, however, have an increased tendency to ventilation-perfusion mismatch, making them particularly susceptible to hypoxemic episodes, especially if they are ill or in the presence of airway hypoxia.[7] There are several factors that contribute to this greater risk for developing hypoxemia: the presence of fetal hemoglobin (with the oxygen dissociation curve shifted to the left), tendency to pulmonary vasoconstriction in the presence of airway hypoxia, tendency to bronchoconstriction in the presence of airway hypoxia, relatively fewer alveoli, compliant rib cage, and smaller airway diameter.[7] In addition, in the first 2 months of life, infants may show a paradoxical inhibition of the respiratory drive causing apnea or hypoventilation in response to hypoxia or infection.[7] Some of the more recognized adverse effects are outlined in this article.

Pulmonary Arterial Hypertension

Chronic alveolar hypoxia leads to an increase in systolic pulmonary artery pressure resulting from pulmonary vasoconstriction and increased pulmonary vascular resistance. There is adaptation of the pulmonary endothelium with pulmonary artery remodeling.[10] This can lead to right ventricular hypertrophy and dysfunction, and eventually to right heart failure.

Acute Life-Threatening Events and Sudden Infant Death

It is known that hypoxia can cause apnea and hypoventilation; thus, the greatest concern is that a period of hypoxia may lead to an acute life-threatening event or actual sudden infant death (SID).

Neurodevelopmental Problems

Intermittent oxygen desaturations are associated with significant learning difficulties in animal studies.[11] Chronic or intermittent hypoxia has been shown to affect cognitive and behavioral outcomes adversely, particularly in some children with congenital cyanotic heart disease and sleep-disordered breathing.[12]

- **Suboptimal growth**
  In infants with chronic hypoxemia, this is best demonstrated by the fact that growth velocities improve when the babies are given supplemental oxygen. This may relate to the effects of hypoxemia on nutrient absorption from the gastrointestinal tract[13] or may be attributable to changes in growth hormone secretion.[14]
- **Increased airway resistance**
  This may result from hypoxia in infants with CNLD, a finding that was not seen in healthy infants.[15]
- **Increased airway inflammation**
  This can result from hypoxia attributable to up-regulated cytokine expression and neutrophil inflammation in CF.[16]

WHAT ARE THE ADVERSE EFFECTS OF CHRONIC HIGH OXYGEN SATURATION?

The effect of too much oxygen on the developing retina is well established, although less relevant at the stage at which the baby is being considered for hospital discharge. Oxygen toxicity, particularly in premature infants, can inhibit lung healing and contribute to ongoing lung injury through the formation of reactive oxygen intermediates and peroxidation of membrane lipids.[17] The Benefits of Oxygen Saturation Targeting (BOOST) study showed a nonsignificant excess) of deaths from pulmonary causes in the babies kept at a higher SaO_2.[18] The Supplemental Therapeutic Oxygen for Prethreshold Retinopathy of Prematurity (STOP-ROP) study found an increased rate of adverse pulmonary sequelae (pneumonia and exacerbations of CNLD), although not deaths, in the high-saturation group; this group also had more infants still requiring supplemental oxygen at 3 months.[19] Oxidative stress from a high oxygen concentration may also be a contributing factor to the development of bronchopulmonary dysplasia (BPD),[20] and it is suggested that a fraction of inspired oxygen (FiO_2) of 0.8 to 1.0 for 24 hours is associated (but not necessarily causative) with the occurrence of BPD.[1] In addition, animal work has shown a possible permanent blunting of the ventilatory response to hypoxia after exposure to high oxygen concentrations during a critical developmental period.[11] This could lead to an increase in sleep-disordered breathing and even sudden death.

WHAT IS THE EVIDENCE THAT SUPPLEMENTAL OXYGEN IS BENEFICIAL TO PATIENTS AND THAT DOMICILIARY OXYGEN IS PREFERABLE TO HOSPITAL BASED OXYGEN?

These questions are answered for a variety of conditions outlined in this article, accepting that evidence is often lacking. Benefit is considered in terms of symptoms (eg, breathlessness, respiratory distress, exercise tolerance), growth and neurodevelopment, school attendance and hospitalization rates, quality of life, psychologic impact, and survival. Obviously, these parameters are not applicable to all patient groups.

This section deals with the issues of LTOT and AOT because almost all children receiving LTOT should not be confined to their home; thus, equipment for AOT must be provided (unless LTOT is used at nighttime only). The indications for LTOT are therefore identical to those for AOT.

Chronic Neonatal Lung Disease

The definitions of CNLD and BPD keep evolving. CNLD is said to be present in babies born before term who require continuous oxygen at 36 weeks of gestational age, or if they are born at greater than 32 weeks of gestational age, they still require supplemental oxygen at 28 days of age. BPD is defined as the need for supplemental oxygen for at least 28 days after birth, and it is graded according to the oxygen flow rate required near to term.[21] CNLD is the main indication for LTOT in children; data from the Children's Home Oxygen Record database for England and Wales indicate that CNLD is the underlying cause in 57% of cases. Data from surviving babies (born between 1997 and 2002) weighing less than 1500 g showed that 22% developed BPD.[22] They often require a prolonged period of mechanical ventilation and continued to need supplemental oxygen once extubated. With increased survival of extremely low birth weight premature infants, the incidence of CNLD is also likely to increase,[23] as is the need for LTOT.

There have been no controlled studies on the effects of mild hypoxemia on mortality in infants who have CNLD. It has been suggested that the use of supplementary oxygen may reduce mortality from SID, however.[24] This may be because oxygen therapy reduces the number of apneic and cyanotic episodes, in addition to the frequency of intermittent desaturations.[24] Certainly, supplemental oxygen significantly reduces pulmonary arterial hypertension in infants who have CNLD, and this effect is achieved at an oxygen concentration that is deliverable at home (2–3 L/min by nasal cannulae).[25] Measurement of infant lung function has shown that supplemental oxygen reduced total pulmonary resistance and increased compliance in babies who had severe BPD and reversible obstructive lung disease.[26] The effect of oxygen on sleep quality is difficult to interpret, but it seems that although desaturations are reduced, this is at the cost of sleep disruption.[27–29]

Home oxygen has been shown to improve growth to the level of healthy term infants, and premature discontinuation of the supplementation (against medical advice) caused a significant deceleration in weight gain.[30–32] The effect of supplemental oxygen on neurodevelopment is difficult to assess, but it is likely to be beneficial.[33] Further, it reduces the risk for nosocomial infection and it is believed to be good for parent-child bonding.[33] Although there have been no randomized trials of babies on LTOT, it is suggested that caring for babies on supplementary oxygen at home is preferable to a prolonged hospital stay.[34] Finally, it is beneficial in terms of freed resources for neonatal units and reduces the total cost of care for an infant.[34–37]

Recommendation: Domiciliary LTOT should be considered for infants who have CNLD and are otherwise ready for hospital discharge. Recommendation B, quality of evidence: moderate.

Other (Oxygen-Dependent) Neonatal Lung Conditions

Other relevant neonatal lung conditions include pulmonary hypoplasia, congenital pneumonia, and meconium aspiration syndrome; however, compared with CNLD, these cases are rare. Survivors of congenital diaphragmatic hernia repair not uncommonly develop chronic lung disease, mainly attributable to pulmonary hypoplasia or lung damage resulting from mechanical ventilation. Some require domiciliary oxygen, but this is unusual beyond 2 years of age.[38] Randomized controlled trials have not been (nor could they be) conducted; hence, the low-level recommendation, Nevertheless, it is likely that outcomes from receiving LTOT at home would be no different from those in babies with CNLD.

Recommendation: Domiciliary LTOT should be considered for infants with other oxygen-dependent neonatal lung conditions who are otherwise ready for hospital discharge. Recommendation I, quality of evidence: poor.

Congenital Heart Disease: Acyanotic and Cyanotic

It is likely that only those with pulmonary hypertension (without Eisenmenger syndrome) need to be at home on long-term oxygen. In cyanotic congenital heart disease, oxygen has little effect in raising SaO_2 and is not indicated, although the degree of polycythemia may be reduced.[39] In some cases with chronic left-to-right shunting, however, irreversible pulmonary vascular disease can develop and cause right-to-left shunting (Eisenmenger syndrome). The resulting pulmonary hypertension is not responsive to oxygen. However, in a small but important controlled study, 100% oxygen given for a minimum of 12 hours per day for up to 5 years significantly improved survival in children with pulmonary vascular disease too severe to have corrective surgery.[40] This was not the case in a recent 2-year study of adults with advanced Eisenmenger syndrome, however, in which nocturnal oxygen had no impact on survival, exercise capacity, or quality of life.[41] Some children with congenital heart disease who are awaiting corrective surgery (without Eisenmenger syndrome), and who have raised pulmonary artery pressure that is oxygen responsive, may benefit from LTOT, as can some children after surgery.[42] In addition, children with severe right ventricular failure and resting hypoxemia need long-term oxygen, but are unlikely to be at home.[39] Decisions in these cases should be made by a specialist pediatric cardiologist.

Recommendation: Domiciliary LTOT should be considered for children with pulmonary hypertension accompanying Eisenmenger syndrome (if they have symptomatic relief) and in children who have pulmonary vascular disease too severe for corrective surgery, who are otherwise ready for hospital discharge. Recommendation B, quality of evidence: low.

Pulmonary Hypertension (Secondary and Primary)

Pulmonary hypertension resulting from pulmonary disease (secondary) is caused by chronic hypoxia and considerably worsens the overall prognosis of the underlying disease.[10] There are several associated pulmonary disorders (reviewed by Roy and Couriel).[43] Acute hypoxia causes smooth muscle contraction in pulmonary arteries, and chronic hypoxia leads to pulmonary vasoconstriction and endothelial dysfunction. Children have a more reactive pulmonary circulation in response to hypoxemia than adults, and oxygen is the most important vasodilator for maintenance of pulmonary vascular tone.[43] LTOT reverses or at least slows the progress of the hypoxic-induced changes to the pulmonary vascular bed and can contribute to improved survival.[10]

Primary pulmonary hypertension has a poor prognosis in children (median survival <1 year). Some of the children desaturate during sleep (especially during the early morning hours) because of mild hypoventilation, which may lead to severe dyspnea, and the resulting hypoxemia can be eliminated by supplemental oxygen.[39] These children also need oxygen available at home for emergency use (eg, when they have viral upper respiratory tract infections) because some tend to desaturate.

Recommendation: Domiciliary LTOT should be considered for children with pulmonary hypertension who are otherwise ready for hospital discharge. Recommendation B, quality of evidence: low.

Interstitial Lung Disease

Interstitial lung disease represents a spectrum of rare conditions with a variable but often poor outlook (eg, chronic pneumonitis of infancy, nonspecific interstitial pneumonitis, desquamative interstitial pneumonitis, immunodeficiency) in which oxygen exchange is impaired. Drug therapy (usually systemic corticosteroids or hydroxychloroquine) is sometimes beneficial. Many of the children are hypoxic and require LTOT. The European Respiratory Society Task Force on Chronic Interstitial Lung Disease reported that 26% of all children with interstitial lung disease were on long-term oxygen, including 55% of those younger than 2 years of age.[44] There has been a single unpublished adult study (reported in a Cochrane review) with the finding that domiciliary oxygen had no effect on mortality after 3 years.[45] A randomized controlled trial of domiciliary oxygen can never be conducted; hence, the low level of the evidence-based recommendation. Nevertheless, in reality, the recommendation is to offer it.

Recommendation: Domiciliary LTOT should be considered for hypoxic children who have interstitial lung disease and are otherwise ready for hospital discharge. Recommendation I, quality of evidence: poor.

Obliterative Bronchiolitis

Obliterative bronchiolitis leads to severe obstructive lung disease, and although it may occur after a viral infection (eg, adenovirus), the cause is often unknown. There is no specific therapy, and, again, the outlook is variable. Many of the children are hypoxic and require LTOT, although, again, there is no evidence base to back this up. In a recent large review, there is no mention of oxygen in the section on treatment.[46] In one study of 18 children in Chile who had postadenoviral bronchiolitis obliterans, 28% children required home oxygen but it could be discontinued after 1 year in all the children.[47] A smaller study from Malaysia of children on home oxygen found that those with bronchiolitis obliterans required a longer duration, with a median of 28 months (interquartile range: 14–66 months).[48]

Recommendation: Domiciliary LTOT should be considered for hypoxic children who have obliterative bronchiolitis and are otherwise ready for hospital discharge. Recommendation I, quality of evidence: poor.

Cystic Fibrosis and Non-Cystic Fibrosis Bronchiectasis

As therapy improves, there are fewer children with cystic fibrosis (CF) who are hypoxic and require supplemental oxygen, and pulmonary hypertension is uncommon in children who have CF. Hypoxemia may be associated with infective chest exacerbations when ventilation-perfusion mismatch is worsened. It is estimated that 1% to 2% of children who have CF receive LTOT.[3] There is, however, no clear-cut definition of hypoxia in CF, and little evidence to guide when supplemental oxygen is indicated.[16] Oxygenation problems are not limited to those who have severe disease; a study of 24 children (median age of 9.5 years) showed that 96% of children with normal lung function or mild to moderate lung disease (defined as forced expiratory volume in 1 second, percentage predicted of 40%–60% and 60%–80%, respectively) had desaturation events during sleep, although they would not be classified as having nocturnal hypoxia (SaO_2 <90% for >5% of the time).[49] There was a degree of correlation of nocturnal oxygenation with clinical, radiographic, and growth parameters. Although the proportion of children who had CF and had desaturations was similar to that in a study of normal children,[9] the children who had CF had a lower mean and minimum SaO_2 and more desaturation events.

There is surprisingly little evidence for the benefit of LTOT in CF, and although it led to an improvement in school or work attendance, there was no effect on mortality, frequency of hospitalization, or disease progression in a small study (n = 28).[50] A problem with that study was that nocturnal oxygen was titrated to normalize daytime SaO_2, which is not necessarily predictive of nocturnal hypoxemia; thus, some of the patients may have been undertreated. It is not clear how many of the subjects were children, although all were older than 12 years of age; two of four of the recruiting hospitals were children's CF units. It is recommended that LTOT be reserved for those patients who have CF who obtain symptomatic relief,[51] particularly because adherence to treatment is usually poor if the child feels no benefit. The potential adverse psychologic effect of starting oxygen at home must be also considered. It is often taken as an indicator of a serious deterioration in the child's condition and has rightly been described as an "emotional life event" for a patient who has CF.[52] It is yet another burden of treatment; thus, the patient and family must be motivated and convinced of the need.

In two small adult studies comparing noninvasive ventilation (NIV) with supplemental oxygen, it was noted that in those receiving supplemental oxygen alone, the improvement in oxygenation was accompanied by an increase in transcutaneous carbon dioxide (CO_2), which caused morning headaches in a few patients.[53,54] Studies have not been performed in children, but there is no reason to suggest that this would be different in adolescents having severe lung disease, who are the ones likely to be receiving home oxygen. It is therefore recommended that monitoring of transcutaneous CO_2 levels be performed when oxygen therapy is initiated.

A Cochrane systematic review has summarized the effects of supplemental oxygen on exercise from three studies (which included a few children only); there was an improvement in exercise duration and peak performance.[55] In reality, use of supplemental oxygen for exercise would not be an indication for domiciliary oxygen in children. There are other causes of bronchiectasis in children (although in approximately 50% cases, no underlying cause is found), and LTOT is occasionally necessary for those with severe disease.

Recommendation: Domiciliary LTOT should be considered for hypoxic children who have CF as a means to improve school attendance and for those who obtain symptomatic relief. Monitoring of transcutaneous CO_2 levels should be performed when oxygen therapy is initiated. Recommendation B, quality of evidence: low.

Obstructive Sleep Apnea Syndrome

In cases in which the obstruction can be relieved, any pulmonary hypertension that may have developed is usually reversible and resolves rapidly.[43] Obstructive sleep apnea syndrome may require NIV if the obstruction cannot be relieved. Occasionally, supplemental oxygen alone is used if the child does not tolerate face mask ventilation (eg, some children with Down's syndrome). As a temporary treatment, it seems to be safe and has a beneficial effect on oxygenation and sleep quality.[56] Oxygen does not suppress the ventilatory drive in most children who have obstructive sleep apnea syndrome, but $PaCO_2$ levels should still be monitored.[57]

Recommendation: Domiciliary LTOT can be considered for children who have obstructive sleep apnea syndrome and do not tolerate NIV as long as $PaCO_2$ levels are monitored. Recommendation B, quality of evidence: low.

Chronic Hypoventilation: Central, Neuromuscular Weakness, Chest Wall Disorders

There are some patients who require long-term NIV because of chronic hypoventilation (to control hypercapnia and hypoxemia). Oxygen alone is inadequate for most children with chronic hypoventilation. A UK survey in 1997 estimated the number of children receiving NIV to be 141, of whom 93 (65%) were at home.[58] The incidence was shown to have increased over the previous decade, and this figure is likely to continue to increase in the future. The children had a variety of conditions, principally neuromuscular disorders (46%), congenital central hypoventilation syndrome (13%), spinal injury (12%), craniofacial syndromes (7%), and BPD (4%). There was a variety of other less frequent causes (18%). In 35% of cases, they had access to supplemental oxygen at home as well (E. Jardine, personal communication, 2004). It is likely that these children have other problems affecting the lungs (eg, recurrent infection attributable to aspiration from swallowing difficulties and gastroesophageal reflux) that lead to the oxygen requirement. In one UK series of children with neuromuscular and skeletal disease requiring NIV, 5 of 40 children required supplemental oxygen at night (to maintain SaO_2 >90%), and 2 of the children stopped the oxygen after 6 months of NIV.[59] Core guidelines have suggested that children on home ventilation should have a stable oxygen requirement with an FiO_2 requirement of less than 40%.[60]

Recommendation: Domiciliary LTOT can be considered for children with chronic hypoventilation who remain hypoxic despite NIV with optimal CO_2 control. Recommendation I, quality of evidence: low.

Sickle Cell Disease

It is important that children who have sickle cell disease and upper airway obstruction do not become hypoxemic during sleep because it can lead to debilitating episodes of sickling.[61] Low overnight SaO_2 has been linked to cerebrovascular disease and frequent episodes of acute pain.[62] In addition, in a recent study of 75 children aged older than 6 years, the prevalence of elevated pulmonary artery pressure was 30%, which was similar to that in adults.[63] This was significantly associated with a low SaO_2 documented in the clinic. Because pulmonary hypertension confers a high risk for death in sickle cell disease (at least in adults),[64] it is obvious that chronic hypoxemia must be prevented. For this reason, domiciliary oxygen should be provided for children with persistent nocturnal hypoxia after other causes (eg, adenotonsillar hypertrophy) have been treated. It is recommended in the UK guideline for sickle cell disease in childhood that overnight SaO_2 should be measured if there is a history of snoring, or nocturnal enuresis after the age of 6 years.[62] The UK guideline also recommends an annual measurement of SaO_2 when the child is well and is in outpatient treatment; if it is less than 95%, overnight monitoring should be undertaken.[62] Furthermore, home oxygen is suggested as one of the therapies for chronic sickle lung, although the UK guideline gives no evidence to back up this recommendation.

Recommendation: Domiciliary LTOT should be considered for children who have sickle cell disease and nocturnal hypoxia. Recommendation I, quality of evidence: low.

Palliative Care and End-of-Life Care

There are no data on the management of terminal dyspnea in patients who have neuromuscular disorders and CF.[65] Most published data are on adult patients who have terminal cancer; a double-blind crossover trial in 14 adults showed that oxygen at a rate of 5 L/min delivered by mask improved the subjective sensation of dyspnea.[66] A recent meta-analysis, however, found that oxygen did not provide symptomatic benefit for patients who had cancer with refractory dyspnea and were mildly or nonhypoxemic.[67] It has been suggested that supplemental oxygen may be effective in relieving dyspnea in children who cannot tolerate NIV (especially when they are not hypercapnic).[68] With chronic hypercapnia, the hypercarbic drive to breathe may be blunted, and in these circumstances, when the primary drive to breathe is hypoxemia, this may be removed by supplemental oxygen. Although this may lead to hypopnea or even apnea, this is less of a concern in an end-of-life situation.[68] It may also be important for the family to have a full view of their child's face; thus, nasal cannulae may be preferable to a NIV face mask.[68] Clinical experience shows that some children do get a degree of symptomatic relief from supplemental oxygen, although, of course, it does not affect the final outcome. In addition, reversing hypoxemia can cause pulmonary vasodilation and prevent the intracranial vasodilation that can be a cause of headaches.[68] For these reasons, oxygen can be offered, but children are likely to continue with it only if they find it helpful.

Recommendation: Domiciliary LTOT can be considered for children undergoing palliative care who obtain symptomatic relief from supplemental oxygen. Recommendation I, quality of evidence: low.

INDICATIONS FOR ACUTE USE OF DOMICILIARY OXYGEN
Neurodisability: Recurrent Seizures

It is apparent that some children with seizures are receiving home oxygen, which is administered at the time of the seizure. There has been a study of respiratory function observed during 101 seizures in 37 children.[69] An increase in respiratory rate was noted in 66% of the 21 generalized seizures, but this was not associated with apnea or hypoxemia (measured by pulse oximetry). No respiratory abnormalities were seen during the 40 absence seizures. Nevertheless, the 40 focal seizures were often associated with respiratory abnormalities, 70% by frequent respiratory pauses and 30% by apnea, and significant hypoxemia (defined as SaO_2 <85%) was observed in 40% of seizures. Supplemental oxygen is unlikely to be beneficial because the brief period of hypoxia does not respond to oxygen while the child is not breathing, and the hypoxia is self-limited and brief anyway. The UK guideline referred to on the National Institute for Clinical Excellence Web site does, however, suggest that oxygen be administered to patients in the hospital having generalized tonic-clonic status epilepticus.[70]

Recommendation: domiciliary acute oxygen therapy is not recommended for children with neurodisability who have recurrent seizures. Recommendation I, quality of evidence: low.

Acute Asthma

Any child with an acute asthma episode severe enough to require oxygen should be in the hospital and not at home. There are, however, a few children who have such severe asthma that they need supplemental oxygen while waiting for an ambulance to take them to the hospital; thus, it must be available at home. In addition, these severely asthmatic children may need an oxygen supply to drive their nebulizer while waiting for the ambulance. Generally, spacer devices are preferred for administering bronchodilators,[71] but there are occasions when the child is only able to use a nebulizer. Home nebulizers are usually driven by room air, but nebulized salbutamol can cause an initial decrease in SaO_2 in asthmatic children and wheezy infants, more commonly with air-than with oxygen-driven nebulization.[72,73] This may be clinically significant if the child is already hypoxemic and on the steep part of the oxygen dissociation curve from the acute bronchoconstriction. For those children with recurrent severe life-threatening episodes, it is better to have oxygen available in the home for use with their nebulizer before transfer to the hospital.

Recommendation: domiciliary acute oxygen therapy is recommended for children with recurrent episodes of severe acute asthma as a temporary therapy before ambulance transfer to the hospital. Recommendation B, quality of evidence: moderate.

Acute Bronchiolitis

The need for supplemental oxygen in an infant with acute bronchiolitis has generally been regarded as an indication for hospital admission. The recommendation in the Scottish Intercollegiate Guideline Network (SIGN) guideline is that infants with an SaO_2 of 92% or less require inpatient care, and they can be considered for discharge when their SaO_2 is greater than 94%.[74] Nevertheless, there has since been a randomized trial of 92 infants aged 2 to 24 months presenting with acute bronchiolitis and hypoxia, defined as an SaO_2 of 87% or less.[75] After an 8-hour observation period, 70% of those randomized for discharge with home oxygen could be discharged (some no longer required oxygen, and some failed to meet the discharge criteria). Of those sent home, 97% were treated successfully with oxygen at a rate of 1 L/min by means of nasal cannulae as outpatients; 1 infant, however, had to be admitted after a cyanotic spell that occurred after 24 hours at home. This certainly opens up a potential alternative to hospital admission, but if financial considerations were excluded, the author's suspicion is that most parents would opt for a short hospital stay. It must also be remembered that these patients presumably had the US definition of bronchiolitis (it is not defined in the paper) and that some of them would have been diagnosed outside the United States as having acute viral wheeze or infantile asthma.

Recommendation: domiciliary acute oxygen therapy can be considered for children who have acute bronchiolitis after a period of hospital observation. Recommendation B, quality of evidence: moderate.

ASSESSMENT OF INITIATION OF LONG-TERM OXYGEN THERAPY (WHEN TO START)

The following sections on assessment and follow-up are mainly concerned with infants who have CNLD. This is the largest patient group and is distinguished by having a good prognosis; there are few other patients who can be weaned off the oxygen over time.

Assessment in Infancy

Suitability for domiciliary oxygen therapy should be assessed by a specialist with appropriate experience in the care of the relevant condition; this is usually a respiratory pediatrician or neonatologist (but may be a pediatric cardiologist, general pediatrician, or palliative care specialist). The family must also be assessed as competent to manage home oxygen therapy and be able to cope with all aspects of the baby's care. In adults, measurement of arterial PaO_2 is considered critical, but this is neither possible nor practical in infants. In pediatric practice, SaO_2 measured by pulse oximetry remains the main form of assessment, because an arterial stab in a crying (hypoxic) child is unreliable, whereas capillary PaO_2 does not correlate well with arterial PaO_2.[76] Single measurements are insufficient, and before discharge, SaO_2 must be measured continuously for at least 6 to 12 hours, including periods of sleep, wakefulness, and activity or feeding (watching for the effects of movement artifact). It is important to include all levels of activity because infants have an increased oxygen requirement when active and infants who have CNLD may develop feeding-related hypoxemia.[77] In addition, some children may only be hypoxemic at night, without daytime hypoxemia. An instrument should be used that has been validated in infants, and although it has been suggested that pulse oximeter readings should be verified by an arterial gas measurement at the start of the study, this is impractical and is not essential. It is important to remember that correlation between SaO_2 and arterial PaO_2 is such that at 94% saturation, the PaO_2 may vary from 9 to 17 kPa.[78] Although correlation is particularly poor in the saturation range of 85% to 90%,[79] this should not matter because all infants with SaO_2 less than 90% should receive LTOT anyway.

Most of the work in infancy relates to CNLD, and there is only limited evidence to recommend a minimally acceptable level of oxygenation; hence, the lack of consensus on who requires home oxygen.[80] Normal SaO_2 is around 96%, and supplemental oxygen is usually considered for infants who cannot maintain SaO_2 at 93% or greater when asleep or quietly awake; oxygen therapy is then given to achieve SaO_2 greater than 92%.[3] Previously, some researchers have recommended keeping SaO_2 at 95% or greater,[24] but there is a trend toward lower levels now. This resulted from concerns over oxygen lung toxicity after two important trials. The first was the BOOST trial of 358 premature infants who still required oxygen at 32 weeks of postmenstrual age.[18] This showed that maintaining SaO_2 at 95% to 98% had no advantage over 91% to 94% in terms of growth and neurodevelopment at 1 year of age (using oximeters). The study also found that the group with the higher target oxygen level had an excess of deaths from pulmonary causes, albeit not statistically significant. This was in keeping with the second study, the STOP-ROP trial on retinopathy of prematurity.[19] Here, 649 preterm infants were randomly assigned to different target oxygen levels (89%–94% vs. 96%–99%) for at least 2 weeks, using oximeters that are calibrated to display SaO_2 that is 1.6% saturation points lower than other commercial oximeters. The study found an increased rate of adverse pulmonary sequelae (pneumonia and exacerbations of CNLD), although not deaths, in the high-saturation group when assessed at 3 months after the due date of the infant (13.2% versus 8.5%). The high-saturation group also had more infants still requiring supplemental oxygen at 3 months (47% versus 37%). Further studies are underway using lower target saturations (85%–89%), and results of these trials are to be combined in a meta-analysis.[81] It must be remembered that the correct target saturation for a preterm baby who has not yet reached term is likely to differ from that of an infant who is old enough to be at home, albeit with supplemental oxygen.

Recommendation: Oxygen therapy should aim to keep SaO_2 at 92% to 94% in infants, particularly during the preterm period, with no more than 5% of time spent at lower than 90% saturation. Assessment of SaO_2 must be for at least 6 to 12 hours and include periods of sleep, wakefulness, and activity or feeding. Recommendation B, quality of evidence: moderate.

Assessment in Older Children

For older children, adult criteria for oxygen prescription may be acceptable, although specific studies on upper and lower limits of PaO_2 for LTOT are lacking. It is important to include an entire night (with at least 4 hours of uninterrupted sleep) in case the child only develops nocturnal hypoxemia, such as in CF, in which nocturnal hypoxemia usually precedes daytime desaturation. In children with hypoventilation, such as in neuromuscular disease, it is important to check the CO_2 status because in the presence of hypercapnia, NIV is necessary rather than LTOT alone. Measurement of overnight transcutaneous or end-tidal CO_2 is ideal, although capillary CO_2 taken just as the child wakes up may be useful if either of the former is not available. Full polysomnography is not usually required.

DISCHARGE CRITERIA

A multidisciplinary meeting should ensure that discharge planning is achieved properly because extensive collaboration is required between the parents and multidisciplinary team. The goal is to select the infants and families most likely to cope at home and to get the timing of discharge right.[82] Each neonatal unit has its own criteria, but some general principles follow:[3]

- The oxygen requirement must be stable with mean SaO_2 of 93% or greater, without frequent episodes of desaturation. SaO_2 should not drop lower than 90% for more than 5% of the artifact-free recording period.
- No other clinical conditions should preclude discharge, and the child must be medically stable with satisfactory growth. There should be no apneic episodes for at least 2 weeks.
- Immunizations should be up to date. Palivizumab may be considered at the appropriate time of year for infants who have CNLD requiring home oxygen.
- Parents are willing and believed to be capable of taking the baby home while still on oxygen.

- Home conditions must be satisfactory, and, preferably, a landline telephone is installed (in addition to a mobile phone). A visit from a member of the home care team is required before discharge.
- Parents are trained and have written information on the use of home oxygen and also cardiopulmonary resuscitation in the case of infants. Vigilance for an empty oxygen supply, dislodged cannulae, or blocked valve is critical. A structured education program can be useful.[83]
- Advice is given about no smoking in the home. It needs to be strongly discouraged, but help to do so must be offered. In a study of burns affecting 27 adults on home oxygen, 89% were smoking at the time; thus, parents must be aware of the danger.[84] Advice must also be given about open flames (eg, birthday cake candles).[85] Notification to local fire services is recommended.
- Older children also need to have training on how to use their oxygen equipment.
- Parents must be advised about travel with cylinders and inform their home and car insurers.
- Appropriate support must be in place (eg, community nursing, nurse specialists, health visitor, social worker).
- Communication with a general practitioner has taken place, and roles are clarified for delivering clinical care.
- Parents must have a list of telephone numbers for advice and emergency help, including a telephone number for repair of equipment breakdown.
- Arrangements are in place for open access to the local pediatric unit.

Recommendation: Children can be discharged from the neonatal unit when their oxygen requirement is stable with a mean SaO_2 of 93% or greater and without frequent episodes of desaturation. The SaO_2 should not drop to lower than 90% for more than 5% of the artifact-free recording period. There should be no other clinical conditions precluding discharge, and the child must be medically stable with satisfactory growth. Recommendation B, quality of evidence: low.

FOLLOW-UP OF INFANTS ON DOMICILIARY OXYGEN

Arrangements for follow-up after discharge should be coordinated by the hospital specialist who has initiated domiciliary oxygen. Liaison must take place between the specialist, local or community pediatrician, general practitioner, nurse specialists, community pediatric nursing service, occupational therapist, and health visitor. The oxygen requirement is likely to change over time; it should be reduced in infants with CNLD but is likely to increase in most other conditions. Regular home monitoring with pulse oximetry is necessary and should be set up by community or specialist nurses. A visit within the first 24 hours is important to reassure parents. The first formal SaO_2 monitoring should take place within a week; subsequent recordings should occur as clinically indicated but rarely less often than every 3 to 4 weeks.[86] Recorded data can then be discussed with the supervising consultant, although protocols can be in place for experienced nursing teams to initiate changes.

These infants require a lot of input from health care professionals. Emotional support is necessary because parents display marked pre- and postdischarge anxiety, which decreases as they see their baby's oxygen dependency resolving.[87] Mothers have also been reported to show low self-esteem, self-blame, and elements of grief and isolation[88] in addition to less vitality and more mental health problems.[89] A study in Oxford, United Kingdom, on 55 babies with CNLD at home with LTOT looked at health care use in 31 of the babies.[34] It was found that these families received a median of 43 visits per baby (range: 8–173 visits) from a pediatric community nurse and that these lasted a median of 45 minutes; 83% of families saw a health visitor, with a median of 12 visits (range: 2–82 visits), and the visits were for a median of 30 minutes; 83% of families saw a general practitioner, with a median of 6 visits (range: 1–140 visits), and the visits were for a median of 10 minutes. A lesser proportion of families also saw a hospital consultant (they almost all had hospital clinic visits, however, on a median of four occasions), social worker, physiotherapist, and speech therapist. In addition, infants with CNLD who require home oxygen have more frequent and longer hospital admissions, and more clinic attendances, than those sent home without oxygen; this means that their total cost of care was 40% greater.[90] This is particularly the case if they had been hospitalized in the first 2 years of life with respiratory syncytial virus infection, which had a significant impact on the cost of care.[91] In the Oxford study, 41% of the babies required readmission, on a median of 1 occasion (range: 0–10 occasions), staying for a median 9 days (range: 1–64 days).[34]

The children should be seen regularly by the hospital specialist in the clinic to monitor the underlying condition in addition to growth and neurodevelopment. There must be direct access for the child to be admitted to the hospital in the case of any emergency or acute deterioration in his or her condition, and the parents must have the telephone numbers of the team. Even a simple viral upper respiratory tract infection in a young infant on LTOT may necessitate admission, and winter (particularly the first) can be an anxious time for parents. If the caregivers believe the child requires an increase in oxygen, they can turn up the flow rate but must then seek advice from the home care team. Even when the child comes off oxygen, support must continue because the children may sometimes relapse and require further periods of oxygen therapy after an apparently complete recovery. This is usually related to intercurrent infection.

Recommendation: Regular home monitoring with pulse oximetry is necessary. After an initial visit within the first 24 hours, the first formal SaO_2 monitoring should take place within 1 week; subsequent recordings are done as clinically indicated but usually not less often than every 3 to 4 weeks. Recommendation B, quality of evidence: low.

WEANING INFANTS OFF LONG-TERM OXYGEN THERAPY (WHEN TO STOP)

The issue of weaning off oxygen principally applies to infants with CNLD and some other neonatal lung conditions. In children with congenital heart disease, only those having successful corrective surgery or transplantation no longer require LTOT. Some young children with interstitial lung disease or obliterative bronchiolitis may improve sufficiently to lose their oxygen dependency. The older children with progressive lung disease, such as CF or neuromuscular conditions, usually continue to require oxygen for the remainder of their lives. It is not easy to counsel the parents of children who have CNLD as to how long LTOT is needed. Although group data showed that capillary blood $PaCO_2$ measured near term correlates with length of oxygen dependency in CNLD, oxygen dependency is impossible to predict for an individual.[92] In general, however, those with a higher $PaCO_2$ are more likely to require oxygen for longer. The length of time that infants with CNLD remain on LTOT varies, but it is usually less than 12 months, although some require it for several years.[35,93,94] Persisting symptoms or failure to progress warrants review to rule out such conditions as tracheobronchomalacia, large airway stenosis or granuloma formation, gastroesophageal reflux, recurrent aspiration, or unsuspected congenital cardiac disease.

There is enormous variety of practice with regard to criteria used by pediatricians about when to discontinue LTOT in children with CNLD, which reflects a lack of evidence on which to base guidelines.[95] During periods of weaning or withdrawal of oxygen, more frequent monitoring is needed. It is not normally necessary for the child to have a SaO_2 monitor kept in the home because one can be provided for intermittent monitoring. Recording should include monitoring during daytime activity, feeding, and sleep. Short-term awake SaO_2 measurements do not predict prolonged sleeping SaO_2.[32] The same target saturations used to decide on initiation of supplementation are used for weaning purposes (92%–94%). Saturation targets in the physiologic range (95%–98%) may be thought to be desirable in infants with pulmonary hypertension. In a study using 2-hour room air challenges, most infants reached their lowest saturations within 40 minutes of discontinuing oxygen and a level of 92% or greater best predicted readiness for weaning judged by 6 months of follow-up.[96] Furthermore, infants requiring an oxygen flow rate of 0.02 L/min per kilogram of body weight were most likely to be successfully weaned.[96]

Some units wean infants from continuous low-flow oxygen to nighttime and naps only, whereas others maintain continuous oxygen until the child has no requirement at all; there is no evidence to recommend which approach is best. When the oxygen requirement is minimal, the children should have supervised weaning into air with continuous monitoring (including active periods and sleep). The babies tend to be weaned down to an oxygen flow rate of 0.1 L/min using a low-flow meter, and from that level, they can usually be weaned straight to air. Although extremely low (or ultralow) flow meters exist (range: 0.025–0.2 L/min), allowing the flow to be reduced even further before weaning to air, this is usually unnecessary. There is also concern that some caregivers may become confused by the decimal points. Weaning is preferably done at home because this minimizes the chances of nosocomial infection, although a child may sometimes need a brief hospital admission. It is usually prudent to ensure that the child has coped with at least one viral upper respiratory tract infection without problems before the equipment is removed from the home, and it should be left there for a few months, especially in the winter.

Recommendation: The same target saturations used to decide on initiation of supplementation should be used for weaning purposes (92%–94%). Higher saturation targets (95%–98%) may be used in infants with pulmonary hypertension. Recommendation B, quality of evidence: low.

Infants can be weaned from continuous low-flow oxygen to provision of oxygen during nighttime and naps only or remain in continuous oxygen on a 24-hour basis until the child has no requirement at all. Recommendation I, quality of evidence: poor.

EQUIPMENT

Provision of equipment depends on local arrangements and availability, but there are some general principles.[3]

- Oxygen concentrators are usually the preferred devices with large back-up cylinders for breakdown (which must be secured to a wall). They work by filtering room air and removing the nitrogen to increase the oxygen concentration.
- Oxygen concentrators need two outlets, one in the child's bedroom and one in the main living room area.
- Portable cylinders are required for ambulatory use. Although many find lightweight cylinders easier to handle, the standard-weight cylinders last longer outside the home.

- Oxygen cylinders may be more appropriate if initial flow rates are lower than 0.3 L/min and the anticipated duration of oxygen therapy is less than 3 months. A back-up cylinder must be available for those on continuous oxygen. Particular attention must be paid to safety and securing of cylinders in the presence of young children.
- Low-flow meter (0.1–1 L/min) must be available for infants and extremely young children.
- A humidification system is often required for those on flow rates greater than 1 L/min for nasal comfort. Cold bubble humidifiers may be used for this purpose, but they only achieve 40% relative humidity and are inadequate for direct airway humidification (eg, by means of a tracheostomy). Heated humidification is less convenient for domestic use and is only effective at flow rates of 4 L/min or higher delivered by a concentrator because water can block the tubing at lower flow rates.
- Appropriately sized soft twin-prong nasal cannulae (small children rarely tolerate >2 L/min by nasal cannulae), a face mask, and nonkinking extension tubing must be provided. Stomahesive (or equivalent) should also be provided to protect the skin in those using nasal cannulae.
- An oxygen conserver is a device to ensure that oxygen is delivered from the cylinder only during inspiration, which prolongs the cylinder life up to threefold. They are said to be usable in older children (>8 years of age) but are generally not used in pediatric practice because of the often irregular and shallow breathing patterns of children.
- Ambulatory equipment must be available as part of the oxygen delivery systems unless oxygen is only required at night. This must be lightweight so that older children can handle it themselves, and for infants, it must fit on to a pram or push chair. Parents need advice on the type of pram to buy (ie, one with a metal basket underneath that is safe and strong enough to hold the cylinder).
- Children in wheelchairs need to have cylinder fitting provided by their wheelchair service to maintain safety.

Oxygen Saturation Monitor (Pulse Oximeter)

The issue of whether parents should be provided with their own saturation monitor has been an area of debate in the United Kingdom. If a child requires continuous monitoring, it is unlikely that he or she is ready for hospital discharge. There is no evidence that provision of oximeters improves the outcome of babies on home oxygen (or that it does not); however, in practice, they may lead to excessive adjustments of the flow rate by the caregivers.[86] They may also give false reassurance, and SaO_2 is only one aspect of the baby's respiratory status. Some parents, however, request one for spot measurements as a guide to when oxygen needs increasing, during, for example, a viral cold. In fact, the baby should be seen in these circumstances, usually by the home care nurse, who can then make a proper assessment. In addition, the use as an overnight "alarm" is often unsatisfactory because of the number of false alarms, mostly from movement artifact. Nevertheless, the American Thoracic Society has supported the provision of oximeters to parents, but their rationale seems to be mostly cost based in terms of reducing hospital and office visits.[97]

OXYGEN OUTSIDE THE HOME
School

There is a small but important demand for oxygen therapy to be available in schools. Liaison is required between the specialist pediatric respiratory team and education health services, and this is usually coordinated by community pediatric services. The following need particular consideration:

- Oxygen delivery equipment must be lightweight and easy for the child to handle and adjust.
- Safety devices must be in place for stabilizing oxygen cylinders or other equipment.
- Insurance coverage must be obtained by the school for the staff and premises.
- Adequate technical back-up must be available.
- School staff must be trained in the use of oxygen therapy.
- School staff must have easily identified health care contacts.
- Provision must be made for ambulatory oxygen for the journey to and from school.

Holidays and Airplanes

Arrangements can and should be made for oxygen concentrators and cylinders to be in place so that families can go away on holiday. Oxygen-dependent children need an increased flow rate during air flight because of the drop in air pressure, and hence equivalent FIO_2 to 0.15 at cruising altitude; the issue of preflight testing has been reviewed recently.[98]

SUMMARY

The use of domiciliary oxygen is significant, with approximately 3500 children receiving it in England and Wales. The evidence base behind this is poor, although evidence for its use in CNLD (the most common indication) is reasonable. Lack of evidence should not mean, however, that it is wrong to prescribe domiciliary oxygen, and common sense and clinical experience must prevail. Studies are urgently needed because, currently, we are not even sure of the ideal target SaO_2.

REFERENCES

1. MacLean JE, Fitzgerald DA. A rational approach to home oxygen use in infants and children. Paediatr Respir Rev 2006;7:215–22.
2. Atkins D, Best D, Briss PA, et al. GRADE Working Group. Grading quality of evidence and strength of recommendations. BMJ 2004;328:1490.
3. Balfour-Lynn IM, Primhak RA, Shaw BN. Home oxygen for children: who, how and when? Thorax 2005;60:76–81.
4. Poets CF, Stebbens VA, Lang JA, et al. Arterial oxygen saturation in healthy term neonates. Eur J Pediatr 1996;155:219–23.
5. Stebbens VA, Poets CF, Alexander JR, et al. Oxygen saturation and breathing patterns in infancy. 1: full term infants in the second month of life. Arch Dis Child 1991;66:569–73.
6. Poets CF, Stebbens VA, Alexander JR, et al. Oxygen saturation and breathing patterns in infancy. 2: preterm infants at discharge from special care. Arch Dis Child 1991;66:574–8.
7. Samuels MP. The effects of flight and altitude. Arch Dis Child 2004;89:448–55.
8. Poets CF, Stebbens VA, Samuels MP, et al. Oxygen saturation and breathing patterns in children. Pediatrics 1993;92:686–90.
9. Urschitz MS, Wolff J, Von Einem V, et al. Reference values for nocturnal home pulse oximetry during sleep in primary school children. Chest 2003;123:96–101.

10. Higenbottam T, Cremona G. Acute and chronic hypoxic pulmonary hypertension. Eur Respir J 1993;6:1207–12.
11. Halbower AC, McGrath SA. Home oxygen therapy: the jury is still in session. J Perinatol 2004;24:59–61.
12. Bass JL, Corwin M, Gozal D, et al. The effect of chronic or intermittent hypoxia on cognition in childhood: a review of the evidence. Pediatr 2004;114:805–16.
13. Bernstein D, Bell JG, Kwong L, et al. Alterations in postnatal intestinal function during chronic hypoxemia. Pediatr Res 1992;31:234–8.
14. Fitzgerald D, Van Asperen P, O'Leary P, et al. Sleep, respiratory rate, and growth hormone in chronic neonatal lung disease. Pediatr Pulmonol 1998;26:241–9.
15. Teague WG, Pian MS, Heldt GP, et al. An acute reduction in the fraction of inspired oxygen increases airway constriction in infants with chronic lung disease. Am Rev Respir Dis 1988;137:861–5.
16. Urquhart DS, Montgomery H, Jaffé A. Assessment of hypoxia in children with cystic fibrosis. Arch Dis Child 2005;90:1138–43.
17. Weinberger B, Laskin DL, Heck DE, et al. Oxygen toxicity in premature infants. Toxicol Appl Pharmacol 2002;181:60–7.
18. Askie LM, Henderson-Smart DJ, Irwig L, et al. Oxygen-saturation targets and outcomes in extremely preterm infants. N Engl J Med 2003;349:959–67.
19. Supplemental Therapeutic Oxygen for Prethreshold Retinopathy of Prematurity (STOP-ROP), a randomized, controlled trial. I: primary outcomes. Pediatrics 2000;105:295–310.
20. Saugstad OD. Chronic lung disease: oxygen dogma revisited. Acta Paediatr 2001;90:113–5.
21. Baraldi E, Filippone M. Chronic lung disease after premature birth. N Engl J Med 2007;357:1946–55.
22. Fanaroff AA, Stoll BJ, Wright LL, et al. NICHD Neonatal Research Network. Trends in neonatal morbidity and mortality for very low birthweight infants. Am J Obstet Gynecol 2007;196:147e1–8.
23. Hack M, Fanaroff AA. Outcomes of children of extremely low birthweight and gestational age in the 1990s. Semin Neonatol 2000;5:89–106.
24. Poets CF. When do infants need additional inspired oxygen? A review of the current literature. Pediatr Pulmonol 1998;26:424–8.
25. Abman SH, Wolfe RR, Accurso FJ, et al. Pulmonary vascular response to oxygen in infants with severe bronchopulmonary dysplasia. Pediatrics 1985;75:80–4.
26. Tay-Uyboco JS, Kwiatkowski K, Cates DB, et al. Hypoxic airway constriction in infants of very low birth weight recovering from moderate to severe bronchopulmonary dysplasia. J Pediatr 1989;115:456–9.
27. Harris MA, Sullivan CE. Sleep pattern and supplementary oxygen requirements in infants with chronic neonatal lung disease. Lancet 1995;345:831–2.
28. Fitzgerald D, Van Asperen P, Leslie G, et al. Higher SaO$_2$ in chronic neonatal lung disease: does it improve sleep? Pediatr Pulmonol 1998;26:235–40.
29. Simakajornboon N, Beckerman RC, Mack C, et al. Effect of supplemental oxygen on sleep architecture and cardiorespiratory events in preterm infants. Pediatrics 2002;110:884–8.
30. Groothuis JR, Rosenberg AA. Home oxygen promotes weight gain in infants with bronchopulmonary dysplasia. Am J Dis Child 1987;141:992–5.
31. Hudak BB, Allen MC, Hudak ML, et al. Home oxygen therapy for chronic lung disease in extremely low-birth-weight infants. Am J Dis Child 1989;143:357–60.

32. Moyer-Mileur LJ, Nielson DW, Pfeffer KD, et al. Eliminating sleep-associated hypoxemia improves growth in infants with bronchopulmonary dysplasia. Pediatrics 1996;98:779–83.
33. Kotecha S, Allen J. Oxygen therapy for infants with chronic lung disease. Arch Dis Child Fetal Neonatal Ed 2002;87:F11–4.
34. Hallam L, Rudbeck B, Bradley M. Resource use and costs of caring for oxygen-dependent children: a comparison of hospital and home-based care. J Neonatal Nursing 1996;2:25–30.
35. Baraldi E, Carra S, Vencato F, et al. Home oxygen therapy in infants with bronchopulmonary dysplasia: a prospective study. Eur J Pediatr 1997;156:878–82.
36. Spinner SS, Girifalco RB, Gibson E, et al. Earlier discharge of infants from neonatal intensive care units: a pilot program of specialized case management and home care. Delaware Valley Child Health Alliance. Clin Pediatr (Phila) 1998;37: 353–7.
37. Greenough A, Alexander J, Burgess S, et al. High versus restricted use of home oxygen therapy, health care utilisation and the cost of care in chronic lung disease. Eur J Ped 2004;163:292–6.
38. Jaillard SM, Pierrat V, Dubois A, et al. Outcome at 2 years of infants with congenital diaphragmatic hernia: a population-based study. Ann Thorac Surg 2003;75: 250–6.
39. Widlitz A, Barst RJ. Pulmonary arterial hypertension in children. Eur Respir J 2003;21:155–76.
40. Bowyer JJ, Busst CM, Denison DM, et al. Effect of long term oxygen treatment at home in children with pulmonary vascular disease. Br Heart J 1986;55: 385–90.
41. Sandoval J, Aguirre JS, Pulido T, et al. Nocturnal oxygen therapy in patients with Eisenmenger syndrome. Am J Crit Care Med 2001;164:1682–7.
42. Ohashi N, Matsushima M, Maeda M, et al. Advantages of oxygen inhalation therapy for postoperative pulmonary hypertension. Pediatr Cardiol 2005;26:90–2.
43. Roy R, Couriel JM. Secondary pulmonary hypertension. Paediatr Respir Rev 2006;7:36–44.
44. Clement A, Ers Task Force. Task force on chronic interstitial lung disease in immunocompetent children. Eur Respir J 2004;24:686–97.
45. Crockett AJ, Cranston JM, Antic N, Domiciliary oxygen for interstitial lung disease. Cochrane Database Syst Rev 2001;(3):CD002883.
46. Kurland G, Michelson P. Bronchiolitis obliterans in children. Pediatr Pulmonol 2005;39:193–208.
47. Castro-Rodriguez JA, Daszenies C, Garcia M, et al. Adenovirus pneumonia in infants and factors for developing bronchiolitis obliterans: a 5-year follow-up. Pediatr Pulmonol 2006;41:947–53.
48. Norzila MZ, Azizi BH, Norrashidah AW, et al. Home oxygen therapy for children with chronic lung diseases. Med J Malaysia 2001;56:151–7.
49. Uyan ZS, Ozdemir N, Ersu R, et al. Factors that correlate with sleep oxygenation in children with cystic fibrosis. Pediatr Pulmonol 2007;42:716–22.
50. Zinman R, Corey M, Coates AL, et al. Nocturnal home oxygen in the treatment of hypoxemic cystic fibrosis patients. J Pediatr 1989;114:368–77.
51. Schidlow DV, Taussig LM, Knowles MR. Cystic Fibrosis Foundation consensus conference report on pulmonary complications of cystic fibrosis. Pediatr Pulmonol 1993;15:187–98.

52. Tiddens HAWM, Devadason SG, et al. Delivery of therapy to the cystic fibrosis lung. In: Hodson ME, Geddes D, Bush A, et al, editors. Cystic fibrosis. 3rd edition. London: Hodder Arnold; 2007. p. 184–98.

53. Gozal D. Nocturnal ventilatory support in patients with cystic fibrosis: comparison with supplemental oxygen. Eur Respir J 1997;10:1999–2003.

54. Young AC, Wilson JW, Kotsimbos TC, et al. Randomised placebo controlled trial of non-invasive ventilation for hypercapnia in cystic fibrosis. Thorax 2008;63: 72–7.

55. Mallory GB, Fullmer JJ, Vaughan DJ, Oxygen therapy for cystic fibrosis. Cochrane Database Syst Rev 2005;(4):CD003884.

56. Aljadeff G, Gozal D, Bailey-Wahl SL, et al. Effects of overnight supplemental oxygen in obstructive sleep apnea in children. Am J Respir Crit Care Med 1996;153: 51–5.

57. Marcus CL, Carroll JL, Bamford O, et al. Supplemental oxygen during sleep in children with sleep-disordered breathing. Am J Respir Crit Care Med 1995;152: 1297–301.

58. Jardine E, O'Toole M, Paton JY, et al. Current status of long term ventilation in children in the United Kingdom: questionnaire survey. BMJ 1999;318:295–9.

59. Simonds AK, Ward S, Heather S, et al. Outcome of paediatric domiciliary mask ventilation in neuromuscular and skeletal disease. Eur Respir J 2000;16:476–81.

60. Jardine E, Wallis C. Core guidelines for the discharge home of the child on long term assisted ventilation in children in the United Kingdom. Thorax 1998;53: 762–7.

61. Blaisdell CJ. Sickle cell disease and breathing during sleep. Lung Biol Health Dis 2000;147:755–63.

62. NHS Sickle Cell and Thalassaemia Screening Programme in partnership with the Sickle Cell Society. Sickle cell disease in childhood. Detailed guidance standards and guidelines for clinical care. Available at: http://www.sickleandthal.org.uk/Documents/DETAILED_CLIN_Oct19.pdf. Accessed 2008.

63. Pashankar FD, Carbonella J, Bazzy-Asaad A, et al. Prevalence and risk factors of elevated pulmonary artery pressures in children with sickle cell disease. Pediatrics 2008;121:777–82.

64. Gladwin MT, Sachdev V, Jison ML, et al. Pulmonary hypertension as a risk factor for death in patients with sickle cell disease. N Engl J Med 2004;350:886–95.

65. Collins JJ, Fitzgerald DA. Palliative care and paediatric respiratory medicine. Paediatr Respir Rev 2006;7:281–7.

66. Bruera E, de Stoutz N, Velasco-Leiva A, et al. Effects of oxygen on dyspnoea in hypoxaemic terminal-cancer patients. Lancet 1993;342:13–4.

67. Uronis HE, Currow DC, McCrory DC, et al. Oxygen for relief of dyspnoea in mildly- or non-hypoxaemic patients with cancer: a systematic review and meta-analysis. Br J Cancer 2008;98:294–9.

68. Ullrich CK, Mayer OH. Assessment and management of fatigue and dyspnea in pediatric palliative care. Pediatr Clin North Am 2007;54:735–56.

69. O'Regan ME, Brown JK. Abnormalities in cardiac and respiratory function observed during seizures in childhood. Dev Med Child Neurol 2005;47:4–9.

70. Stokes T, Shaw EJ, Juarez-Garcia A, et al. Clinical guidelines and evidence review for the epilepsies: diagnosis and management in adults and children in primary and secondary care. 2004 London: Royal College of General Practitioners. Available at: http://www.nice.org.uk/nicemedia/pdf/CG020fullguideline.pdf. Accessed 2008.

71. Cates CJ, Crilly JA, Rowe BH. Holding chambers (spacers) versus nebulisers for beta-agonist treatment of acute asthma. Cochrane Database Syst Rev 2006;(2): CD000052.
72. Gleeson JG, Green S, Price JF. Air or oxygen as driving gas for nebulised salbutamol. Arch Dis Child 1988;63:900–4.
73. Prendiville A, Rose A, Maxwell DL, et al. Hypoxaemia in wheezy infants after bronchodilator treatment. Arch Dis Child 1987;62:997–1000.
74. Scottish Intercollegiate Guidelines Network. Bronchiolitis in children. A national clinical guideline. 2006. Available at: http://www.sign.ac.uk/pdf/sign91.pdf. Accessed 2008.
75. Bajaj L, Turner CG, Bothner J. A randomized trial of home oxygen therapy from the emergency department for acute bronchiolitis. Pediatrics 2006;117:633–40.
76. Yildizdaş D, Yapicioğlu H, Yilmaz HL, et al. Correlation of simultaneously obtained capillary, venous, and arterial blood gases of patients in a paediatric intensive care unit. Arch Dis Child 2004;89:176–80.
77. Singer L, Martin RJ, Hawkins SW, et al. Oxygen desaturation complicates feeding in infants with bronchopulmonary dysplasia after discharge. Pediatrics 1992;90: 380–4.
78. Wasunna A, Whitelaw AG. Pulse oximetry in preterm infants. Arch Dis Child 1987; 62:957–8.
79. Roberts CM, Bugler JR, Melchor R, et al. Value of pulse oximetry in screening for long-term oxygen therapy requirement. Eur Respir J 1993;6:559–62.
80. Ellsbury DL, Acarregui MJ, McGuinness GA, et al. Controversy surrounding the use of home oxygen for premature infants with bronchopulmonary dysplasia. J Perinatol 2004;24:36–40.
81. Higgins RD, Bancalari E, Willinger M, et al. Executive summary of the workshop on oxygen in neonatal therapies: controversies and opportunities for research. Pediatrics 2007;119:790–6.
82. Gracey K, Talbot D, Lankford R, et al. The changing face of bronchopulmonary dysplasia: part 2. Discharging an infant home on oxygen. Adv Neonatal Care 2003;3:88–98.
83. Laubscher B. Home oxygen therapy: beware of birthday cakes. Arch Dis Child 2003;88:1125.
84. Robb BW, Hungness ES, Hershko DD, et al. Home oxygen therapy: adjunct or risk factor? J Burn Care Rehabil 2003;24:403–6.
85. Brown KA, Sauve RS. Evaluation of a caregiver education program: home oxygen therapy for infants. J Obstet Gynecol Neonatal Nurs 1994;23:429–35.
86. Primhak RA. Discharge and aftercare in chronic lung disease of the newborn. Semin Neonatol 2003;8:117–26.
87. Zanardo V, Freato F. Home oxygen therapy in infants with bronchopulmonary dysplasia: assessment of parental anxiety. Early Hum Dev 2001;65:39–46.
88. Manns SV. Life after the NNU: the long term effects on mothers' lives, managing a child at home with broncho-pulmonary dysplasia and on home oxygen. Neuro Endocrinol Lett 2004;25(Suppl 1):127–32.
89. McLean A, Townsend A, Clark J, et al. Quality of life of mothers and families caring for preterm infants requiring home oxygen therapy: a brief report. J Paediatr Child Health 2000;36:440–4.
90. Greenough A, Alexander J, Burgess S, et al. Home oxygen status and rehospitalisation and primary care requirements of infants with chronic lung disease. Arch Dis Child 2002;86:40–3.

91. Greenough A, Alexander J, Burgess S, et al. Health care utilisation of prematurely born, preschool children related to hospitalisation for RSV infection. Arch Dis Child 2004;89:673–8.
92. Victor S, Shaw B. Carbon dioxide levels do not predict duration of home oxygen requirement: a retrospective study. J Perinat Med 2002;30:333–5.
93. Sauve RS, McMillan DD, Mitchell I, et al. Home oxygen therapy. Outcome of infants discharged from NICU on continuous treatment. Clin Pediatr 1989;28:113–8.
94. Abman SH, Davis JM, et al. Bronchopulmonary dysplasia. In: Chernick V, Boat TF, Wilmott RW, et al, editors. Kendig's disorders of the respiratory tract in children. 7th edition. Philadelphia: WB Saunders; 2006. p. 342–58.
95. Solis A, Harrison G, Shaw BN. Assessing oxygen requirement after discharge in chronic lung disease: a survey of current practice. Eur J Pediatr 2002;161:428–30.
96. Simoes EA, Rosenberg AA, King SJ, et al. Room air challenge: prediction for successful weaning of oxygen-dependent infants. J Perinatol 1997;17:125–9.
97. American Thoracic Society. Statement on the care of the child with chronic lung disease of infancy and childhood. Am J Respir Crit Care Med 2003;168:356–96.
98. Bossley C, Balfour-Lynn IM. Taking young children on aeroplanes: what are the risks? Arch Dis Child 2008;93:528–33.

Index

Note: Page numbers of article titles are in **boldface** type.

A

Abscess, lung, 149
N-Acetylcysteine, for bronchiectasis, 164
Acoustic analysis, of noisy breathing, 12–14
Adenoid(s), hypertrophy of, obstructive sleep apnea in, 244, 251
Adenoidectomy or adenotonsillectomy
    for obstructive sleep apnea, 251, 253
    for otitis media, 106, 112–113
Airways
    congenital lesions of, **227–242**
    excessive secretions in, rattle in, 5
    hydration of, for bronchiectasis, 163–164
    obstruction of
        recurrent, 71–73
        recurrent shadowing in, 82
        sleep apnea in, 244
        stridor in, 5–6
        wheeze in, 3–4
Albuterol, for dyspnea, 45
Allergy, recurrent shadowing in, 83
Amebiasis, pulmonary, 147–148
American Thoracic Society, grading recommendations of, 192–193
Aminophylline, for asthma, 196, 199, 201
Amoxicillin
    for bronchiectasis, 163
    for pneumonia, 141, 143–144
Analgesics
    for otitis media, 106, 111
    for pharyngitis, 105, 109
Antacids, for aspiration lung disease, 184
Antibiotics
    for asthma, 196, 205
    for bronchiectasis, 162–163
    for cough, 22
    for lung abscess, 149
    for obstructive sleep apnea, 251
    for otitis media, 106, 111–113
    for pharyngitis, 105, 109
    for pneumonia, 141–144
    for rhinosinusitis, 104
    for sinusitis, 108

Pediatr Clin N Am 56 (2009) 297–315
doi:10.1016/S0031-3955(08)00231-9
0031-3955/08/$ – see front matter © 2009 Elsevier Inc. All rights reserved.

Moving?

Make sure your subscription moves with you!

To notify us of your new address, find your **Clinics Account Number** (located on your mailing label above your name), and contact customer service at:

E-mail: elspcs@elsevier.com

800-654-2452 (subscribers in the U.S. & Canada)
314-453-7041 (subscribers outside of the U.S. & Canada)

Fax number: 314-523-5170

Elsevier Periodicals Customer Service
11830 Westline Industrial Drive
St. Louis, MO 63146

*To ensure uninterrupted delivery of your subscription, please notify us at least 4 weeks in advance of move.